Acneiform Eruptions in Dermatology

Joshua A. Zeichner
Editor

Acneiform Eruptions in Dermatology

A Differential Diagnosis

Springer

Editor
Joshua A. Zeichner, M.D.
Assistant Professor
Director of Cosmetic and Clinical Research
Dermatology Department
Mount Sinai Medical Center
New York, NY, USA

ISBN 978-1-4614-8343-4 ISBN 978-1-4614-8344-1 (eBook)
DOI 10.1007/978-1-4614-8344-1
Springer New York Heidelberg Dordrecht London

Library of Congress Control Number: 2013951661

Printed on acid-free paper

Springer is part of Springer Science+Business Media (www.springer.com)

To Cori, Jake, and Chloe, whose bright smiles and unconditional love inspire me every day. To my parents, without whose support I would not be where I am today.

Joshua A. Zeichner, M.D.

Preface

An estimated 40–50 million people in the United States suffer from acne, and up to 85 % of people experience acne at some point in their lives. Dermatologists, primary care doctors, and pediatricians see these patients every day in practice. It is important to treat the skin effectively not only to reduce the risk of physical scarring but also to address the negative psychosocial impact this disease carries. Improving the skin can improve self-confidence, interpersonal relationships, and performance in school or at work.

While the majority of acne patients seen in practice truly have run-of-the-mill acne, not all "acne" is really acne vulgaris. It may be exception rather than the rule for a patient to have a condition that mimics acne, but it is our responsibility as health care providers to be up to date and educated on acne's broad differential diagnosis. If patients do not have any comedonal lesions, if they have an atypical medical history, or if they are not responding to traditional therapies, then alternative diagnoses should be considered. Proper diagnosis will allow us to prescribe proper treatments and ultimately improve clinical outcomes and patient satisfaction.

This book will help to provide a broad overview of acne vulgaris itself as well as conditions that manifest with acneiform eruptions in the skin.

New York, NY, USA — Joshua A. Zeichner, M.D.

Acknowledgment

We are all influenced by the people with whom we surround ourselves. I have had the privilege of learning from the greatest minds in Dermatology, who have shaped the person I am today. While I have had countless mentors touch my career, I must take this opportunity to acknowledge one person in particular. Dr. Mark Lebwohl is truly a mentor of mentors. He has taught me not only how to be a good dermatologist, but also, more importantly, how to be a great doctor, colleague, and teacher. This book would not have been possible without his support, advice, and encouragement.

Contents

Contributors

Yasser Albahrani, M.D. Department of Dermatology, Mt. Sinai School of Medicine, New York, NY, USA

Andrew F. Alexis, M.D., M.P.H. Department of Dermatology, St. Luke's-Roosevelt Hospital Center, New York, NY, USA

Hilary Baldwin, M.D. Department of Dermatology, SUNY Downstate School of Medicine, Brooklyn, NY, USA

Annelyse Ballin, M.D. Private Practice, Dr. Brandt Dermatology Associates, Coral Gables, FL, USA

Sebastian Bernardo, M.D. Department of Dermatology, Mt. Sinai School of Medicine, New York, NY, USA

Diane Berson, M.D. Department of Dermatology, Weill Cornell Medical College, New York, NY, USA

Neal Bhatia, M.D. Division of Dermatology, Harbor-UCLA Medical Center, Torrance, CA, USA

Joseph Bikowski, M.D. Director, Bikowski Skin Care Center, Sewickley, PA, USA

Whitney P. Bowe, M.D. Department of Dermatology, SUNY Downstate Medical Center, Brooklyn, NY, USA

Valerie D. Callender, M.D. Callender Dermatology & Cosmetic Center, Glenn Dale, MD, USA

Cristina Caridi, B.A. Department of Dermatology, Mt. Sinai School of Medicine, New York, NY, USA

Yvonne Clark, MPAS-C Department of Dermatology, Sharp Rees-Stealy, La Mesa, CA, USA

Shinjita Das, M.D. Department of Dermatology, Harvard Combined Dermatology Residency Program, Boston, MA, USA

Consuelo Vera David, M.D. Division of Dermatology, Harbor-UCLA Medical Center, Torrance, CA, USA

James Del Rosso, D.O. Touro University College of Osteopathic Medicine, Henderson, NV, USA

Ha K. Do, M.D. Department of Dermatology, Indiana University School of Medicine, New York, NY, USA

Zoe Diana Draelos, M.D. Department of Dermatology, Duke University School of Medicine, Durham, NC, USA

Lynn A. Drake, M.D. Department of Dermatology, Massachusetts General Hospital, Boston, MA, USA

Lawrence F. Eichenfield, M.D. Division of Pediatric and Adolescent Dermatology, Rady Children's Hospital, San Diego, San Diego, CA, USA

Boni Elewski, M.D. Department of Dermatology, University of Alabama, Birmingham, Birmingham, AL, USA

Jason Emer, M.D. Department of Dermatology, Mount Sinai School of Medicine, New York, NY, USA

Joseph C. English III, M.D. Department of Dermatology, University of Pittsburgh, Pittsburgh, PA, USA

Rachel Epstein, D.O. Department of Dermatology, Loma Linda University, Loma Linda, CA, USA

Navid Ezra, M.D. Department of Dermatology, Indiana University School of Medicine, New York, NY, USA

Elizabeth Farhat, M.D. Department of Dermatology, Henry Ford Health System, West Bloomfield, MI, USA

Patricia K. Farris, M.D. Department of Dermatology, Old Metairie Dermatology, Metairie, LA, USA

Steven R. Feldman, M.D., Ph.D. Department of Dermatology, Pathology, and Public Health Sciences, Wake Forest University Baptist Medical Center, Winston-Salem, NC, USA

Joseph F. Fowler Jr., M.D. Division of Dermatology, University of Louisville, Louisville, KY, USA

Adam Friedman, M.D. Department of Dermatology, Montefiore – Albert Einstein College of Medicine, Bronx, NY, USA

Bryan Gammon, M.D. Department of Dermatology, Northwestern University, Chicago, IL, USA

Marisa Kardos Garshick Department of Dermatology, Massachusetts General Hospital, Boston, MA, USA

Jessica Gjede, M.D. Department of Dermatology, Boston Medical Center, Boston, MA, USA

Bradely Glodny, M.D. Department of Dermatology, Mt. Sinai, New York, NY, USA

Alexandra Golant, M.D. Department of Dermatology, The Mt. Sinai Hospital, New York, NY, USA

Linda Stein Gold, M.D. Department of Dermatology, Henry Ford Health System, West Bloomfield, MI, USA

Gary Goldenberg, M.D. Department of Dermatology, The Mount Sinai Hospital, New York, NY, USA

Kristina Goldenberg, M.D. Department of Dermatology, Mt. Sinai School of Medicine, New York, NY, USA

Rachel Gordon, M.D. Department of Dermatology, The University of Texas Medical School at Houston, Houston, TX, USA

Emmy Graber, M.D. Department of Dermatology, Boston Medical Center & Boston University School of Medicine, Boston, MA, USA

Jeremy B. Green, M.D. Private Practice, Dr. Brandt Dermatology Associates, Coral Gables, FL, USA

Nicholas Gulati, B.A. Laboratory for Investigative Dermatology, The Rockefeller University, New York, NY, USA

Cheryl J. Gustafson, M.D. Department of Dermatology, Wake Forest University Baptist Medical Center, Winston-Salem, NC, USA

Emma Guttman-Yassky, M.D. Department of Dermatology, Mount Sinai NY, New York, NY, USA

Madelaine Haddican, M.D. Department of Dermatology, Mount Sinai School of Medicine, New York, NY, USA

Salar Hazany, M.D. Division of Dermatology, Harbor-UCLA Medical Center, Torrance, CA, USA

Adelaide A. Hebert, M.D. Department of Dermatology, University of Texas Health Science Center, Houston, Houston, TX, USA

Gillian Heinecke, M.D. Department of Dermatology, Mount Sinai, New York, NY, USA

Joely Kaufman, M.D. Private Practice, Dr. Brandt Dermatology Associates, Coral Gables, FL, USA

Mark D. Kaufmann, M.D. Department of Dermatology, Icahn School of Medicine at Mt. Sinai, New York, NY, USA

Jonette Keri, M.D., Ph.D. Department of Dermatology and Cutaneous Surgery, Veterans Hospital, University of Miami, Miami, FL, USA

Alexa Kimball, M.D., M.P.H. Department of Dermatology, Massachusetts General Hospital, Boston, MA, USA

Joslyn S. Kirby, M.D. Department of Dermatology, Penn State Hershey, Hershey, PA, USA

Leon H. Kircik, M.D. Department of Dermatology, Mt. Sinai School of Medicine, New York, NY, USA

Indiana University School of Medicine, Indianapolis, IN, USA

Mary-Margaret Kober, M.D. Department of Dermatology, SUNY Downstate Medical Center, Brooklyn, NY, USA

Lauren Kole, M.D. Department of Dermatology, University of Alabama, Birmingham, Birmingham, AL, USA

John Y.M. Koo, M.D. Psoriasis and Skin Treatment Center, University of California San Francisco, San Francisco, CA, USA

Angela Lamb, M.D. Department of Dermatology, Mount Sinai Hospital, New York, NY, USA

Whitney Lapolla, M.D. Department of Dermatology, The University of Texas at Houston, Houston, TX, USA

Caroline L. LaRosa, B.S. Department of Dermatology and Pediatrics, Penn State/ Milton S. Hershey Medical Center, Hershey, PA, USA

Mark G. Lebwohl, M.D. Department of Dermatology, Mt. Sinai School of Medicine, New York, NY, USA

Jacquelyn Levin, D.O. Department of Dermatology, Largo Medical Center, Largo, FL, USA

Moise L. Levy, M.D. Department of Pediatric Dermatology, Dell Children's Medical Center, Austin, TX, USA

Rita V. Linkner, M.D. Department of Dermatology, Mount Sinai School of Medicine, New York, NY, USA

Fan Liu, B.A. Department of Dermatology, University of California, San Francisco, San Francisco, CA, USA

Adam J. Luber, B.A. Department of Dermatology, Mount Sinai Hospital, New York, NY, USA

Joy Makdisi, B.S. Department of Medicine, Montefiore – Albert Einstein College of Medicine, Bronx, NY, USA

Paula S. Malhotra, B.A., M.D. Department of Dermatology, Northwestern University, Chicago, IL, USA

Rana Mays, M.D. Department of Dermatology, Baylor College of Medicine, Houston, TX, USA

Richard Miller, D.O. Nova Southeastern University College of Osteopathic Medicine, Tampa, FL, USA

Jillian Wong Millsop Department of Dermatology, Psoriasis and Skin Treatment Center, University of California San Francisco, San Francisco, CA, USA

Maria Elena Miyar, M.D. Department of Dermatology, UT Southwestern, Austin, TX, USA

Andrea Murina, M.D. Department of Dermatology, Tulane University, New Orleans, LA, USA

Rajiv I. Nijhawan, M.D. Department of Dermatology, St. Luke's-Roosevelt Hospital Center, New York, NY, USA

Oge Onwudiwe, M.D. Callender Dermatology and Cosmetic Center, Glenn Dale, MD, USA

Omar Pacha, M.D. Department of Dermatology, University of Texas Health Science Center, Houston, Houston, TX, USA

Kristen Pacific, B.A. Department of Dermatology, Mount Sinai School of Medicine, New York, NY, USA

Silvina Pugliese, M.D. Department of Dermatology, Loma Linda University, Loma Linda, CA, USA

Rachel Reynolds, M.D. Department of Dermatology, Beth Israel Deaconess Medical Center, Brookline, MA, USA

Libby Rhee, D.O., M.S. Department of Dermatology, St. Barnabas Hospital, Bronx, NY, USA

Sara Risner-Rumhor, M.D. Department of Dermatology, Baylor College of Medicine, Houston, TX, USA

Ted Rosen, M.D. Department of Dermatology, Baylor College of Medicine, Houston, TX, USA

Misha Rosenbach, M.D. Department of Dermatology, University of Pennsylvania, Philadelphia, PA, USA

Aman Samrao, M.D. Division of Dermatology, Harbor-UCLA Medical Center, Torrance, CA, USA

Bethanee J. Schlosser, M.D., Ph.D. Department of Dermatology, Northwestern University, Chicago, IL, USA

Alison Schram, B.S. School of Medicine, University of Pennsylvania, Philadelphia, PA, USA

Alan R. Shalita, M.D. Department of Dermatology, SUNY Downstate Medical Center, Brooklyn, NY, USA

Kanade Shinkai, M.D., Ph.D. Department of Dermatology, University of California, San Francisco, San Francisco, CA, USA

Deanna M. Sikorski, M.D. Department of Dermatology, The Cleveland Clinic Foundation, Cleveland, OH, USA

Andrea Smith, M.D. Department of Dermatology, Loma Linda University, Loma Linda, CA, USA

Rebecca L. Smith, M.D. Fort Mill Dermatology, LLC, Fort Mill, SC, USA

James Spencer, M.D. Department of Dermatology, Mt. Sinai School of Medicine, New York, NY, USA

Ani L. Tajirian, M.D. Fletcher Allen Health Care, University of Vermont College of Medicine, Burlington, VT, USA

Webster Management Inc., Oakland, CA, USA

Laura Thornsberry, M.D. Department of Internal Medicine, University of Pittsburgh, UPMC Montefiore Hospital, Pittsburgh, PA, USA

Kenneth J. Tomecki, M.D. Department of Dermatology, The Cleveland Clinic Foundation, Cleveland, OH, USA

Abel Torres, M.D. Department of Dermatology, Loma Linda University, Loma Linda, CA, USA

Stephen Tyring, M.D., Ph.D., M.B.A. Department of Dermatology, The University of Texas at Houston, Houston, TX, USA

Alejandra Vivas, M.D. Department of Dermatology, University of Miami, Miami, FL, USA

Guy F. Webster, M.D., Ph.D. Department of Dermatology, Jefferson Medical College, Hockessin, DE, USA

Jonathan S. Weiss, M.D. Department of Dermatology, Emory University, Atlanta, GA, USA

Elijah B. Wilder, D.O. Philadelphia College of Osteopathic Medicine, Georgia, Atlanta, GA, USA

Stephen E. Wolverton, M.D. Department of Dermatology, Indiana University School of Medicine, New York, NY, USA

Gregory N. Yañez, B.A. Icahn School of Medicine at Mount Sinai Class of 2015, New York, NY, USA

Andrea L. Zaenglein, M.D. Department of Dermatology and Pediatrics, Penn State/Milton S. Hershey Medical Center, Hershey, PA, USA

Joshua A. Zeichner, M.D. Department of Dermatology, Mt. Sinai School of Medicine, New York, NY, USA

Nick Zilieris, D.O., B.sc., M.D. Department of Internal Medicine, Baptist Hospital, Miami Beach, FL, USA

Part I
Acne Vulgaris

Chapter 1
Acne Pathophysiology

Shinjita Das and Rachel Reynolds

1.1 Introduction

Acne vulgaris is the result of multifactorial processes in and around the pilosebaceous unit. Currently, the major pathogenic factors are thought to be:

1. Androgens [1–3]
2. Sebum [4]
3. Abnormal keratinization [5]
4. *Propionibacterium acnes* (*P. acnes*) [6]
5. Innate immune system-mediated inflammation [6, 7]

The traditional notion that these factors contribute independently to acne development has been replaced by a more nuanced understanding of their complex interplay. Though the multifactorial nature of acne pathogenesis makes effective treatment challenging, research has shed light on both the mechanisms of action of current treatments and discovered new targets for acne therapy.

S. Das, M.D.
Department of Dermatology, Harvard Combined Dermatology Residency Program, Boston, MA, USA
e-mail: shinjita.das@gmail.com

R. Reynolds, M.D. (✉)
Department of Dermatology, Beth Israel Deaconess Medical Center, 330 Brookline Avenue, Brookline, MA 02215, USA
e-mail: rreynold@bidmc.harvard.edu

J.A. Zeichner (ed.), *Acneiform Eruptions in Dermatology: A Differential Diagnosis*, DOI 10.1007/978-1-4614-8344-1_1, © Springer Science+Business Media New York 2014

1.2 Overview of the Innate Immune System

The immune system consists of both innate (rapid response but no memory to pathogens) and adaptive (delayed, antigen-specific response forming memory) mechanisms against pathogens [8]. The skin is a first-line agent of the innate immune system. As an anatomic barrier, skin physically prevents invasion of external toxins and maintains an acidic stratum corneum (from free fatty acids generated by *P. acnes*) that limits bacterial colonization [9–11]. It can also generate soluble immune factors (antimicrobial peptides, complement factors, chemokines, and cytokines) and express pattern recognition receptors (PRRs) to mediate responses against pathogen-associated molecular patterns (PAMPs) via effector cells, such as monocytes/macrophages, natural killer (NK) cells, neutrophils, and dendritic cells (DCs) [12–15].

1.2.1 Toll-Like Receptors

Toll-like receptors (TLRs), a subtype of PRRs found on immune cells (such as neutrophils, monocytes/macrophages, and DCs), serve as potent initiators of innate immune responses. While nearly a dozen TLRs have been identified, TLR2 and TLR4 seem to play the greatest roles in acne pathogenesis (via *P. acnes* activation) [16, 17]. Stimulation of TLRs by microbial ligands activates various pathways that converge at the level of transcriptional regulation of inflammatory genes via nuclear factor κB (NF-κB). This results in release of inflammatory molecules (such as IL-1, IL-6, IL-8, IL-10, IL-12, and TNFα) and destruction of pathogens by effector cells like neutrophils and NK cells [18, 19].

1.2.2 Inflammation via Innate Immune System

Innate immunity-mediated inflammation is both a precipitating and propagating factor in acne pathogenesis. The key player appears to be IL-1α. There are multiple hypotheses about what stimuli promote IL-1α production. IL-1 upregulation may be mediated by increased sebum production and breakdown of the skin barrier from decreased linoleic acid in the follicle [20, 21]. *P. acnes* induction of TLR2 and oxidized squalene via NFkB-mediated transcription may also drive IL-1 expression. Damaged keratinocytes stimulate IL-1 production, and in a paracrine manner, lymphocytes, selectins, and fibroblasts are summoned to the pilosebaceous unit via IL-1 that also has autocrine function, in that it promotes keratinocyte migration, proliferation, and further production of IL-1. This in turn continues the cycle of hyperkeratinization, a driving factor in comedo formation [22, 23]. In vitro studies have demonstrated increased levels of perifollicular inflammatory markers even before hyperproliferation of keratinocytes [7, 22]. Furthermore, IL-1α receptor blockade mitigates hyperkeratinization and comedo formation, suggesting that the process is IL-1 specific [24]. Furthermore, follicular IL-1α can stimulate endothelial cells of surrounding vasculature to produce inflammatory vascular markers (E-selectin, vascular cell adhesion molecule-1 VCAM-1, intercellular adhesion molecule-1, ICAM-1, and human leukocyte antigen-DR HLA-DR) [22].

1.3 Development of Acne Lesions

Acne lesions start as microcomedones, which are present in clinically normal appearing skin and can mature into visible noninflammatory comedones or inflammatory papules. While the multifactorial and synergistic nature of acne pathogenesis has long been recognized, in vitro studies have shed light on the extensive cross talk that occurs among the various factors and the innate immune system. Under physiologic circumstances, the skin harnesses the innate immune response to protect the internal environment from extrinsic pathogens. However, collateral damage to adjacent tissues is an unavoidable consequence of this protective mechanism and manifests clinically as inflammatory conditions such as acne. It has become clear that acne is a disease of the innate immune response, as acne lesions have been shown to express higher levels of inflammatory components compared to normal skin. Studies have revealed that the initial microcomedo is a product of inflammation and hyperproliferation of the follicular epithelium [22, 24, 25].

1.3.1 Androgens

Androgens are involved in promoting growth of sebaceous glands and sebum secretion, inducing keratinocyte proliferation, stimulating hair growth, and inhibiting wound healing [26, 27]. They are produced by adrenal glands and gonads as well as locally within the sebaceous gland. Androgens from adrenal glands and the gonads are converted to testosterone and dihydrotestosterone in the skin via type 1 5α-reductase from the infrainfundibulum [28]. The rise in androgens during puberty stimulates sebum production by binding androgen receptors on pilosebaceous ducts and sebaceous glands. Acne-prone skin has higher androgen receptor density and higher 5α-reductase activity [28]. Androgens stimulate keratinocyte differentiation mediated by growth factors and IL-1α that can result in hyperkeratinization in the ductal and infundibular regions leading to comedogenesis [7]. Evidence for a hormonal component to acne stems from clinically higher acne rates seen in patients with androgen excess states, such as polycystic ovarian syndrome, congenital adrenal hyperplasia, and tumors [29–31]. In addition, castrated males and those with androgen insensitivity syndromes (from lack of functional androgen receptors) do not produce sebum and do not develop acne [32].

1.3.2 Sebum

Sebum is secreted by sebaceous glands through holocrine secretion (extrusion of the entire cell). The primary components of sebum include squalene, cholesterol, cholesterol esters, wax esters, and triglycerides [4]. As sebum passes through the follicular duct, lipases from *P. acnes* hydrolyze a portion of triglycerides into free fatty acids and mono- and diglycerides [33].

Androgens and retinoids regulate sebum production by sebaceous glands. Functional androgen receptors have been identified on the basal layer of sebaceous glands, and androgens stimulate sebaceous gland growth and secretion [34]. Retinoids (such as isotretinoin, 1-cis retinoic acid), on the other hand, arrest sebocyte differentiation. This causes sebaceous gland shrinkage and inhibits sebum secretion [35, 36]. Sebocytes are regulated at the transcriptional level by peroxisome proliferator-activated proteins (PPARs). PPARs are orphan receptors that heterodimerize with retinoid receptors to regulate sebum production and keratinocyte differentiation [37, 38]. Melanocortins (melanocyte-stimulating hormone, MSH, and adrenocorticotropic hormone, ACTH) have been found to increase sebum production by binding to their receptors on sebaceous glands [39–41]. Corticotropin-releasing hormone (released in response to physiologic stress) and CRH receptors are expressed by sebaceous glands; in vitro studies have demonstrated increased sebocyte lipid production in response to CRH exposure [42, 43]. More recently, it has been found that insulin-like growth factor-1 (IGF-1)-induced sterol response element-binding protein-1 (SREBP-1) regulates lipogenesis by sebocytes [44]. These findings suggest a role of the sebaceous gland in neuroendocrine function and the stress response.

In addition to lubricating skin and hair, sebum also plays a role within the innate immune system through multiple pathways. Increased production of sebum is necessary but not sufficient for acne pathogenesis; the composition of sebum lipids also has an impact on inflammation. There are increased free fatty acids, squalene, and squalene oxidase and decreased linoleic acid, conditions which promote hypercornification of the follicle through direct and indirect modulation of the innate immune system [38, 45–48]. Sebum lipids activate neutrophil degranulation and increase leukocyte recruitment. Furthermore, oxidized squalene upregulates 5-lipoxygenase (5-LOX), which catalyzes conversion of arachidonic acid to leukotriene B4 (LTB4), a potent recruiter of inflammatory cells via PPARα. 5-LOX is increased in acne patients and stimulates inflammatory cytokine production. Oxidized squalene can also stimulate hyperproliferation of keratinocytes via IL-1α upregulation [49–51]. PPARs also activate T-cell signaling via AP-1- and NFkB-mediated transcriptional regulation [52]. Lower levels of linoleic acid within sphingolipids of the follicle may also lead to hyperkeratinization [21, 48].

Sebum-mediated acne pathogenesis occurs in concert with *P. acnes*. The anaerobic environment of sebaceous glands and sebum lipids allows proliferation of *P. acnes*, which expresses lipases that break down triglycerides into proinflammatory free fatty acids [9–11]. When stimulated by *P. acnes* binding to TLR2 and TLR4 on sebaceous

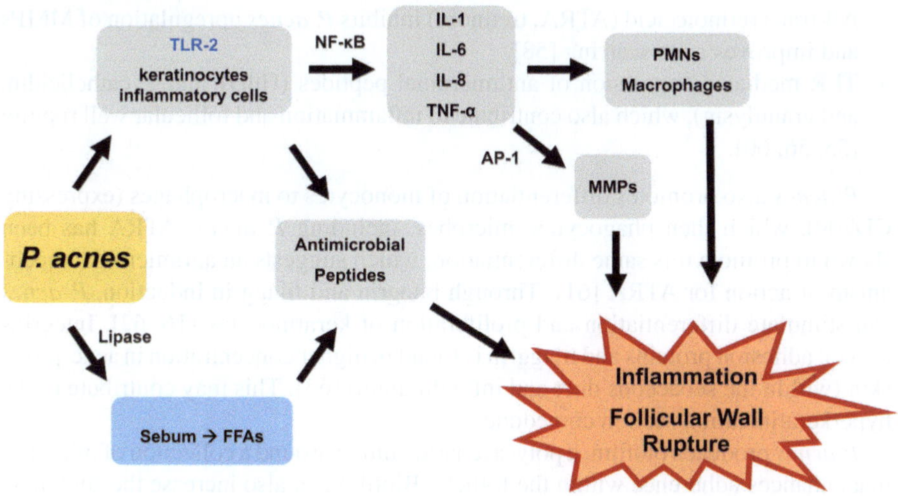

Fig. 1.1 *P. acnes* promotes acne pathogenesis through multiple pathways involving the innate immune system

glands, sebocytes also direct innate immunity by producing antimicrobial peptides (such as HβD1 and HβD2) and inflammatory molecules, such as TNFα, IL-1α, and IL-8 [53–56]. This complement of findings suggests the important role of sebaceous glands in pathogen recognition and in regulation of the innate immune system on the skin surface.

1.3.3 Propionibacterium acnes *(*P. acnes*)*

P. acnes is a commensal anaerobic, gram-positive rod whose interaction with the innate immune systems plays a significant role in acne development. This bacteria expresses lipases that convert sebum triglycerides into free fatty acids, which stimulate release of antimicrobial peptides and therefore inflammation and comedogenesis [57]. By activating TLR2 (via peptidoglycan as the PAMP) and TLR4 on keratinocytes and inflammatory cells (e.g., monocytes and macrophages) [16, 53], *P. acnes* can stimulate the following (Fig. 1.1):

1. TLR-mediated release of cytokines and chemokines (IL-1β, IL-6, IL-8, and TNFα), which then recruit neutrophils (via IL-8) and macrophages to the pilosebaceous unit and promote inflammation and rupture of the follicular wall. Macrophages propagate the cycle by releasing IL-8 (more neutrophil recruitment) and IL-12 (promotes Th1 response) [6, 53–55].
2. TLR-mediated release of cytokines and chemokines that also amplifies the AP-1 transcription factor, which induces production of matrix metalloproteinases (MMPs) [58, 59]. MMPs are involved in tissue destruction and scar formation.

All-trans retinoic acid (ATRA, tretinoin) inhibits *P. acnes* upregulation of MMPs and improves acne scarring [58].

3. TLR-mediated expression of antimicrobial peptides (HβD1 and 2, cathelicidin, and granulysin), which also contribute to inflammation and follicular wall rupture [55, 56, 60].

P. acnes also promotes differentiation of monocytes to macrophages (expressing CD209), which then phagocytize microbes, including *P. acnes*. ATRA has been shown to promote this same differentiation, which suggests an antimicrobial mechanism of action for ATRA [61]. Through integrin and filaggrin induction, *P. acnes* can stimulate differentiation and proliferation of keratinocytes [16, 62]. Integrins are cell adhesion proteins and filaggrin is found in higher concentration in acne-prone skin (within the sebaceous duct and infundibulum) [63]. This may contribute to the hyperkeratinization seen in comedones.

P. acnes produces biofilm, a polysaccharide lining around a collection of microbes that enhances adherence within the follicle. Biofilm can also increase the stickiness of sebum and impede keratinocyte desquamation, leading to the keratin plug seen in comedones. Biofilm also enhances *P. acnes* resistance to antibiotics [64].

1.3.4 Abnormal Keratinization

The microcomedo is the initial lesion of acne development. Previously, abnormal keratinization was thought to precede inflammation associated with acne. However, it has become clear that IL-1α-mediated inflammation precedes hyperkeratinization. In fact, IL-1α has been localized to open comedones [17, 22]. Hyperkeratinization is the result of both hyperproliferation and retention of keratinocytes within the follicle [65]. Factors that promote hyperproliferation include changes in lipid composition of sebum, response to androgens, inflammation from local cytokines, and *P. acnes*. Normally, flow of sebum out of the pilosebaceous duct carries with it old keratinocytes. However, normal sebum flow is impeded by factors such as *P. acnes* biofilm adhering to follicular lining and the "bottleneck" effect of microcomedo that limits extrusion of sebaceous material. This, in turn, leads to decreased ductal keratinocyte desquamation and increased keratinocyte cohesion [22, 64].

1.4 Conclusions

Acne is a disease of inflammation mediated by the innate immune system at the level of the pilosebaceous unit. Multiple factors share an intertwined and synergistic dynamic within the greater context of the innate immune responses that underlie acne pathogenesis. As discussed in this section, the overarching concepts of acne development are the following (Fig. 1.2):

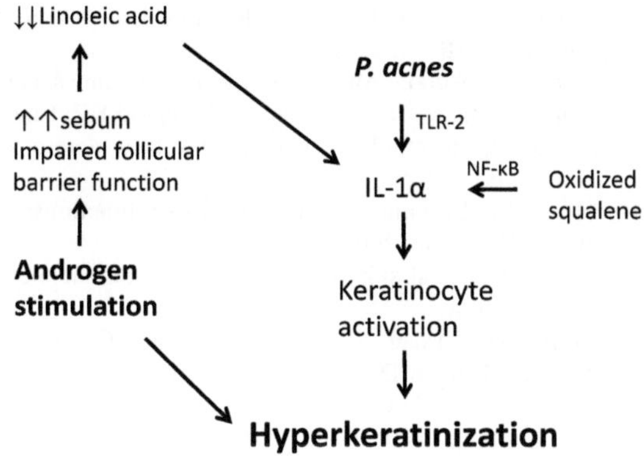

Fig. 1.2 Abnormal hyperkeratinization (leading to microcomedo formation) is mediated by androgen stimulation, sebum, and *P. acnes* through innate immune mechanisms

- Androgen production drives sebum secretion.
- Sebum lipids activate the innate immune system.
- Abnormal keratinization is driven by IL-1-mediated inflammation and androgen production.
- *P. acnes* activates innate immune response via TLRs, activates MMPs, stimulates production of AMPs, and stimulates sebum secretion.

Recent insights into the pathogenesis of acne may facilitate development of novel therapeutics. For example, there may be a role for 5-LOX inhibitors in reducing inflammatory acne lesions in vivo (zileuton is already approved for asthma). Topical linoleic acid (a lipid that is decreased in acne lesions) or melanocortin receptor antagonists may serve as an anti-inflammatory treatment. Blocking physiologic stress responses may also provide benefit. Further studies will allow us to finesse our understanding of the immunologic underpinnings of acne pathophysiology and develop more targeted treatments for acne.

References

1. Thiboutot D. Hormones and acne: pathophysiology, clinical evaluation, and therapies. Semin Cutan Med Surg. 2001;20(3):144–53.
2. Thiboutot D, Jabara S, McAllister JM, Sivarajah A, Gilliland K, Cong Z, Clawson G. Human skin is a steroidogenic tissue: steroidogenic enzymes and cofactors are expressed in epidermis, normal sebocytes, and an immortalized sebocyte cell line (SEB-1). J Invest Dermatol. 2003;120(6):905–14.
3. Thiboutot D. Acne: hormonal concepts and therapy. Clin Dermatol. 2004;22(5):419–28. Review.
4. Thiboutot D. Regulation of human sebaceous glands. J Invest Dermatol. 2004;123(1):1–12. Review.
5. Plewig G, Fulton JE, Kligman AM. Cellular dynamics of comedo formation in acne vulgaris. Arch Dermatol Forsch. 1971;242(1):12–29.
6. Vowels BR, Yang S, Leyden JJ. Induction of proinflammatory cytokines by a soluble factor of Propionibacterium acnes: implications for chronic inflammatory acne. Infect Immun. 1995; 63(8):3158–65.

7. Guy R, Green MR, Kealey T. Modeling acne in vitro. J Invest Dermatol. 1996;106(1):176–82. PubMed PMID: 8592071.
8. Parkin J, Cohen B. An overview of the immune system. Lancet. 2001;357:1777–89.
9. Fluhr JW, Kao J, Jain M, Ahn SK, Feingold KR, Elias PM. Generation of free fatty acids from phospholipids regulates stratum corneum acidification and integrity. J Invest Dermatol. 2001;117(1):44–51.
10. Elias PM. Stratum corneum defensive functions: an integrated view. J Invest Dermatol. 2005;125(2):183–200. Review.
11. Elias PM. The skin barrier as an innate immune element. Semin Immunopathol. 2007;29(1): 3–14. Review.
12. Braff MH, Bardan A, Nizet V, Gallo RL. Cutaneous defense mechanisms by antimicrobial peptides. J Invest Dermatol. 2005;125(1):9–13. Review.
13. Schauber J, Gallo RL. Antimicrobial peptides and the skin immune defense system. J Allergy Clin Immunol. 2008;122(2):261–6.
14. Walport MJ. Complement. First of two parts. N Engl J Med. 2001;344(14):1058–66. Review.
15. Modlin RL, Miller LS, Bangert C, Stingl G. Innate and Adaptive Immunity in the Skin. In: Goldsmith LA, Katz SI, et al., editors. Fitzpatrick's dermatology in general medicine. 8th ed. New York, NY: McGraw-Hill; 2012.
16. Jugeau S, Tenaud I, Knol AC, Jarrousse V, Quereux G, Khammari A, Dreno B. Induction of toll-like receptors by Propionibacterium acnes. Br J Dermatol. 2005;153(6):1105–13.
17. Kim J. Review of the innate immune response in acne vulgaris: activation of Toll-like receptor 2 in acne triggers inflammatory cytokine responses. Dermatology. 2005;211(3):193–8. Review.
18. McInturff JE, Kim J. The role of toll-like receptors in the pathophysiology of acne. Semin Cutan Med Surg. 2005;24(2):73–8. Review.
19. McInturff JE, Modlin RL, Kim J. The role of toll-like receptors in the pathogenesis and treatment of dermatological disease. J Invest Dermatol. 2005;125(1):1–8. Review.
20. Perisho K, Wertz PW, Madison KC, Stewart ME, Downing DT. Fatty acids of acylceramides from comedones and from the skin surface of acne patients and control subjects. J Invest Dermatol. 1988;90(3):350–3.
21. Elias PM, Brown BE, Ziboh VA. The permeability barrier in essential fatty acid deficiency: evidence for a direct role for linoleic acid in barrier function. J Invest Dermatol. 1980; 74(4):230–3.
22. Jeremy AH, Holland DB, Roberts SG, Thomson KF, Cunliffe WJ. Inflammatory events are involved in acne lesion initiation. J Invest Dermatol. 2003;121(1):20–7.
23. Freedberg IM, Tomic-Canic M, Komine M, Blumenberg M. Keratins and the keratinocyte activation cycle. J Invest Dermatol. 2001;116(5):633–40. Review.
24. Guy R, Kealey T. Modelling the infundibulum in acne. Dermatology. 1998;196(1):32–7.
25. Guy R, Kealey T. The effects of inflammatory cytokines on the isolated human sebaceous infundibulum. J Invest Dermatol. 1998;110(4):410–5.
26. Deplewski D, Rosenfield RL. Role of hormones in pilosebaceous unit development. Endocr Rev. 2000;21(4):363–92. Review.
27. Gilliver SC, Ashworth JJ, Ashcroft GS. The hormonal regulation of cutaneous wound healing. Clin Dermatol. 2007;25(1):56–62. Review.
28. Thiboutot D, Harris G, Iles V, Cimis G, Gilliland K, Hagari S. Activity of the type 1 5 alpha-reductase exhibits regional differences in isolated sebaceous glands and whole skin. J Invest Dermatol. 1995;105(2):209–14.
29. Merke DP, Bornstein SR. Congenital adrenal hyperplasia. Lancet. 2005;365(9477):2125–36. Review.
30. Lolis MS, Bowe WP, Shalita AR. Acne and systemic disease. Med Clin North Am. 2009; 93(6):1161–81.
31. Maluki AH. The frequency of polycystic ovary syndrome in females with resistant acne vulgaris. J Cosmet Dermatol. 2010;9(2):142–8.
32. Imperato-McGinley J, Gautier T, Cai LQ, Yee B, Epstein J, Pochi P. The androgen control of sebum production. Studies of subjects with dihydrotestosterone deficiency and complete androgen insensitivity. J Clin Endocrinol Metab. 1993;76(2):524–8.

33. Patil V, Bandivadekar A, Debjani D. Inhibition of Propionibacterium acnes lipase by extracts of Indian medicinal plants. Int J Cosmet Sci. 2012;34(3):234–9.
34. Kariya Y, Moriya T, Suzuki T, Chiba M, Ishida K, Takeyama J, Endoh M, Watanabe M, Sasano H. Sex steroid hormone receptors in human skin appendage and its neoplasms. Endocr J. 2005;52(3):317–25.
35. Zouboulis CC, Korge B, Akamatsu H, Xia LQ, Schiller S, Gollnick H, Orfanos CE. Effects of 13-cis-retinoic acid, all-trans-retinoic acid, and acitretin on the proliferation, lipid synthesis and keratin expression of cultured human sebocytes in vitro. J Invest Dermatol. 1991; 96(5):792–7.
36. Nelson AM, Gilliland KL, Cong Z, Thiboutot DM. 13-cis Retinoic acid induces apoptosis and cell cycle arrest in human SEB-1 sebocytes. J Invest Dermatol. 2006;126(10):2178–89.
37. Schoonjans K, Staels B, Auwerx J. The peroxisome proliferator activated receptors (PPARS) and their effects on lipid metabolism and adipocyte differentiation. Biochim Biophys Acta. 1996;1302(2):93–109.
38. Ottaviani M, Camera E, Picardo M. Lipid mediators in acne. Mediators Inflamm 2010; 2010: 858176.
39. Zhang L, Anthonavage M, Huang Q, Li WH, Eisinger M. Proopiomelanocortin peptides and sebogenesis. Ann N Y Acad Sci. 2003;994:154–61.
40. Ganceviciene R, Graziene V, Böhm M, Zouboulis CC. Increased in situ expression of melanocortin-1 receptor in sebaceous glands of lesional skin of patients with acne vulgaris. Exp Dermatol. 2007;16(7):547–52.
41. Thiboutot D, Sivarajah A, Gilliland K, Cong Z, Clawson G. The melanocortin 5 receptor is expressed in human sebaceous glands and rat preputial cells. J Invest Dermatol. 2000;115(4):614–9.
42. Zouboulis CC, Seltmann H, Hiroi N, Chen W, Young M, Oeff M, Scherbaum WA, Orfanos CE, McCann SM, Bornstein SR. Corticotropin-releasing hormone: an autocrine hormone that promotes lipogenesis in human sebocytes. Proc Natl Acad Sci U S A. 2002;99(10):7148–53.
43. Ganceviciene R, Graziene V, Fimmel S, Zouboulis CC. Involvement of the corticotropin-releasing hormone system in the pathogenesis of acne vulgaris. Br J Dermatol. 2009; 160(2):345–52.
44. Smith TM, Gilliland K, Clawson GA, Thiboutot D. IGF-1 induces SREBP-1 expression and lipogenesis in SEB-1 sebocytes via activation of the phosphoinositide 3-kinase/Akt pathway. J Invest Dermatol. 2008;128(5):1286–93.
45. Kligman AM, Katz AG. Pathogenesis of acne vulgaris. I. Comedogenic properties of human sebum in external ear canal of the rabbit. Arch Dermatol. 1968;98(1):53–7.
46. Mills Jr OH, Kligman AM. A human model for assessing comedogenic substances. Arch Dermatol. 1982;118(11):903–5.
47. Motoyoshi K. Enhanced comedo formation in rabbit ear skin by squalene and oleic acid peroxides. Br J Dermatol. 1983;109(2):191–8.
48. Downing DT, Stewart ME, Wertz PW, Strauss JS. Essential fatty acids and acne. J Am Acad Dermatol. 1986;14(2 Pt 1):221–5.
49. Zouboulis CC. Acne and sebaceous gland function. Clin Dermatol. 2004;22(5):360–6. Review.
50. Ottaviani M, Alestas T, Flori E, Mastrofrancesco A, Zouboulis CC, Picardo M. Peroxidated squalene induces the production of inflammatory mediators in HaCaT keratinocytes: a possible role in acne vulgaris. J Invest Dermatol. 2006;126(11):2430–7.
51. Alestas T, Ganceviciene R, Fimmel S, Müller-Decker K, Zouboulis CC. Enzymes involved in the biosynthesis of leukotriene B4 and prostaglandin E2 are active in sebaceous glands. J Mol Med (Berl). 2006;84(1):75–87.
52. Weindl G, Schäfer-Korting M, Schaller M, Korting HC. Peroxisome proliferator-activated receptors and their ligands: entry into the post-glucocorticoid era of skin treatment? Drugs. 2005;65(14):1919–34.
53. Kim J, Ochoa MT, Krutzik SR, Takeuchi O, Uematsu S, Legaspi AJ, Brightbill HD, Holland D, Cunliffe WJ, Akira S, Sieling PA, Godowski PJ, Modlin RL. Activation of toll-like receptor 2 in acne triggers inflammatory cytokine responses. J Immunol. 2002;169(3):1535–41.
54. Kuwahara K, Kitazawa T, Kitagaki H, Tsukamoto T, Kikuchi M. Nadifloxacin, an antiacne quinolone antimicrobial, inhibits the production of proinflammatory cytokines by human

peripheral blood mononuclear cells and normal human keratinocytes. J Dermatol Sci. 2005;38(1):47–55.
55. Nagy I, Pivarcsi A, Koreck A, Széll M, Urbán E, Kemény L. Distinct strains of Propionibacterium acnes induce selective human beta-defensin-2 and interleukin-8 expression in human keratinocytes through toll-like receptors. J Invest Dermatol. 2005;124(5):931–8.
56. Nagy I, Pivarcsi A, Kis K, Koreck A, Bodai L, McDowell A, Seltmann H, Patrick S, Zouboulis CC, Kemény L. Propionibacterium acnes and lipopolysaccharide induce the expression of antimicrobial peptides and proinflammatory cytokines/chemokines in human sebocytes. Microbes Infect. 2006;8(8):2195–205.
57. Dessinioti C, Katsambas AD. The role of Propionibacterium acnes in acne pathogenesis: facts and controversies. Clin Dermatol. 2010;28(1):2–7.
58. Jalian HR, Liu PT, Kanchanapoomi M, Phan JN, Legaspi AJ, Kim J. All-trans retinoic acid shifts Propionibacterium acnes-induced matrix degradation expression profile toward matrix preservation in human monocytes. J Invest Dermatol. 2008;128(12):2777–82.
59. Choi JY, Piao MS, Lee JB, Oh JS, Kim IG, Lee SC. Propionibacterium acnes stimulates pro-matrix metalloproteinase-2 expression through tumor necrosis factor-alpha in human dermal fibroblasts. J Invest Dermatol. 2008;128(4):846–54.
60. Chronnell CM, Ghali LR, Ali RS, Quinn AG, Holland DB, Bull JJ, Cunliffe WJ, McKay IA, Philpott MP, Müller-Röver S. Human beta defensin-1 and -2 expression in human pilosebaceous units: upregulation in acne vulgaris lesions. J Invest Dermatol. 2001;117(5):1120–5.
61. Lu PT, Phan J, Tang D, Kanchanapoomi M, Hall B, Krutzik SR, Kim J. CD209(+) macrophages mediate host defense against Propionibacterium acnes. J Immunol. 2008;180(7): 4919–23.
62. Jarrousse V, Castex-Rizzi N, Khammari A, Charveron M, Dréno B. Modulation of integrins and filaggrin expression by Propionibacterium acnes extracts on keratinocytes. Arch Dermatol Res. 2007;299(9):441–7.
63. Kurokawa I, Mayer-da-Silva A, Gollnick H, Orfanos CE. Monoclonal antibody labeling for cytokeratins and filaggrin in the human pilosebaceous unit of normal, seborrhoeic and acne skin. J Invest Dermatol. 1988;91(6):566–71.
64. Burkhart CG, Burkhart CN. Expanding the microcomedone theory and acne therapeutics: propionibacterium acnes biofilm produces biological glue that holds corneocytes together to form plug. J Am Acad Dermatol. 2007;57(4):722–4.
65. Holmes RL, Williams M, Cunliffe WJ. Pilo-sebaceous duct obstruction and acne. Br J Dermatol. 1972;87(4):327–32.

Chapter 2
Clinical Presentation of Acne

Guy F. Webster

2.1 Introduction

Acne is a disease of the pilosebaceous unit that typically begins on the face and has a spectrum of lesions and severity (Table 2.1). The classic lesion is a pustule, but inflammatory papules and nodules are common. The primary lesion, from which all others develop, is the microcomedo, an impaction and distention of the follicle with sebum and improperly desquamated keratinocytes from the follicular epithelium. When microcomedones become visible, they are described as open or closed comedones. An open comedo has a visible pore that appears as a dark spot (Fig. 2.1). The pigment is not dirt, but is oxidized lipid and melanin. Closed comedones have a pore too small to see and appear as white bumps (Fig. 2.2).

In patients who are hypersensitive to *Propionibacterium acnes* that colonizes follicles, [1] inflammatory lesions may develop from the microcomedones. Papules and pustules may be superficial or deep and scarring depending on the vigor of hypersensitivity (Fig. 2.3). Nodules are inflammatory lesions >0.5–1 cm in size. Nodules may develop into abscesses, which have incorrectly been termed "cysts" (Fig. 2.4). The term "nodulocystic acne" is incorrect, but probably too deeply ensconced to readily fall from use. *Conglobate* lesions are intensely inflamed neighboring nodules that merge into a loculated abscess. Secondary lesions such as scars, keloids, sinus tracts, and true cysts may follow in the most inflammatory disease.

G.F. Webster, M.D., Ph.D. (✉)
Department of Dermatology, Jefferson Medical College, Hockessin, DE, USA

J.A. Zeichner (ed.), *Acneiform Eruptions in Dermatology: A Differential Diagnosis*,
DOI 10.1007/978-1-4614-8344-1_2, © Springer Science+Business Media New York 2014

Table 2.1 The spectrum of acne lesions

Noninflammatory
Microcomedo
Open comedo
Closed comedo
Inflammatory
Papule
Pustule
Nodule/abscess
Conglobate lesions
Secondary lesions
Scars, keloids, hypertrophic scars
True cysts
Sinus tracts

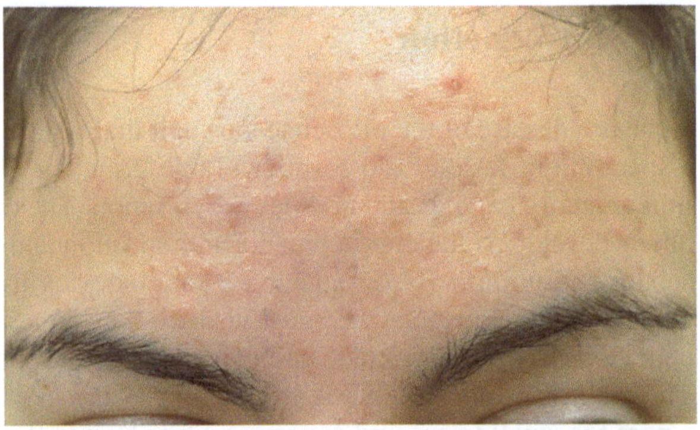

Fig. 2.1 Mixed open comedones (blackheads) and closed comedones (whiteheads) on the forehead of a teenage girl (Photo credit: Joshua A. Zeichner, M.D.)

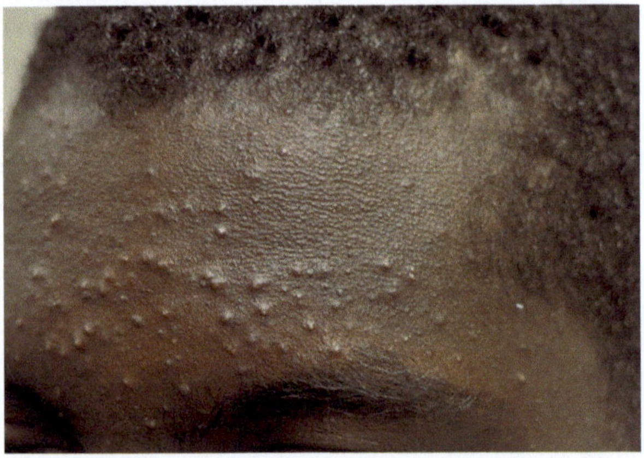

Fig. 2.2 Closed comedones (whiteheads) on the forehead of a teenage boy (Photo credit: Joshua A. Zeichner, M.D.)

2.2 The Onset of Acne

Acne usually begins with the onset of puberty [2, 3]. Androgens stimulate sebaceous secretion and microcomedones inflate with sebum and become visible. Typically initial lesions are noninflammatory and centrofacial (Fig. 2.5). As maturation progresses

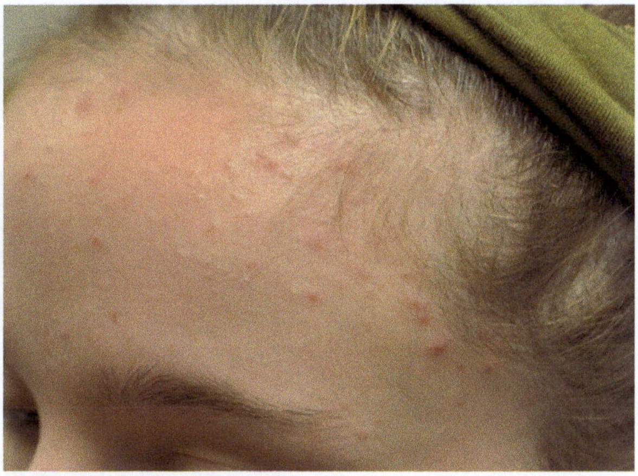

Fig. 2.3 Mixed comedonal acne with inflammatory papules and scattered pustules on the forehead of a teenage girl (Photo credit: Joshua A. Zeichner, M.D.)

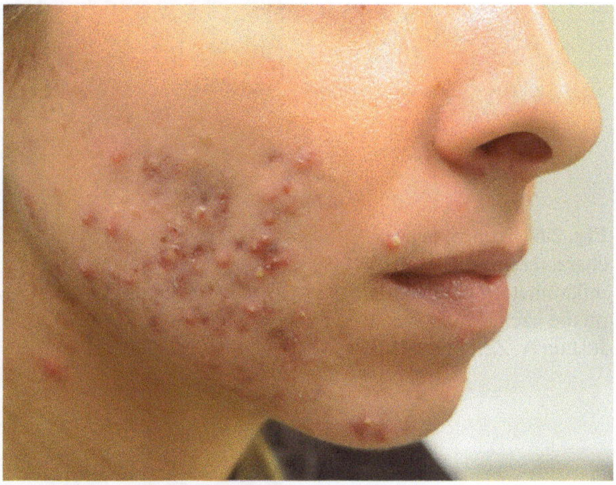

Fig. 2.4 Severe, inflammatory acne on the cheeks of an adult woman. Pustules, papules, nodules, and scars are clinically apparent (Photo credit: Joshua A. Zeichner, M.D.)

inflammatory lesions may appear, and the distribution spreads across the face and perhaps to the trunk (Fig. 2.6). Severity of acne is clearly correlated with the stage of puberty. Lucky et al. [4] has shown that early in puberty comedonal acne is common, but inflammatory acne is rare. In later stages of puberty, inflammatory acne may reach a 50 % incidence in boys [5]. Mourlatos and colleagues [6] demonstrated that both sebaceous secretion and follicular *P. acnes* colonization are elevated early in those children destined to develop acne.

In some patients, adrenarche is a sufficient stimulus and acne may appear in 7–11-year-olds. Lucky [4] has shown that early acne in girls reflects rising levels of adrenal dehydroepiandrosterone sulfate (DHEAS). She also found that such patients tended to have more severe acne as teens, though a sign of difficult acne to come, such as *preadolescent acne*, is not a cause for medical concern. However, acne that occurs between 1 and 7 years, termed *mid-childhood acne*, is much more unusual and may reflect an underlying medical condition such as endocrinopathy or tumor. Work-up by a pediatric endocrinologist is indicated [3].

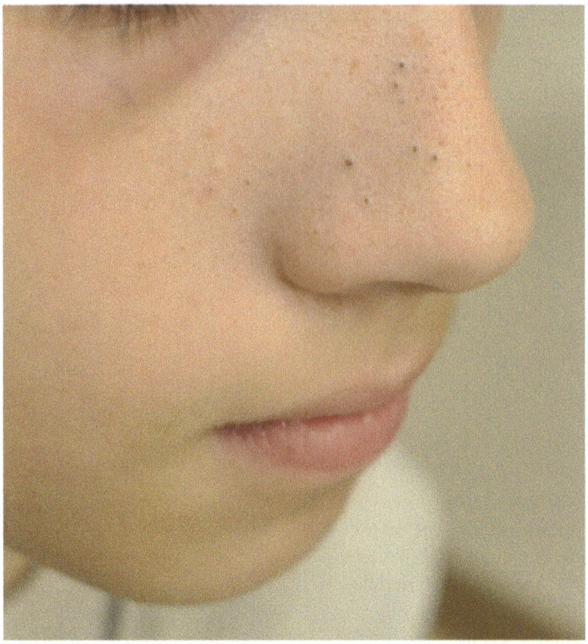

Fig. 2.5 Open comedones (blackheads) on the nose of an adolescent boy. This acne was one of the first signs of puberty (Photo credit: Joshua A. Zeichner, M.D.)

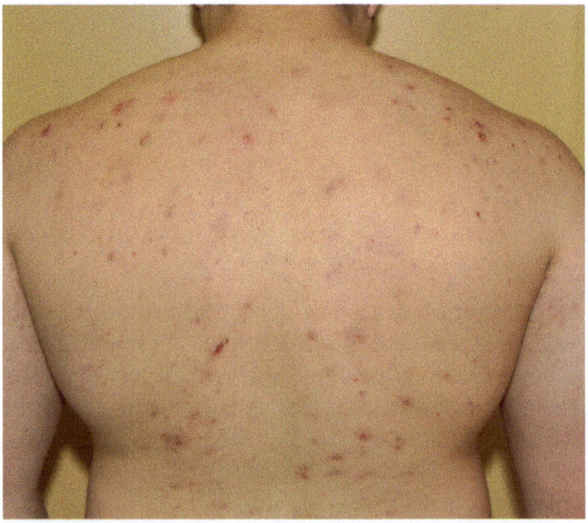

Fig. 2.6 Truncal acne characterized by inflammatory papules on the back (Photo credit: Joshua A. Zeichner, M.D.)

2.3 Grading Acne Severity

Grading acne is a surprisingly difficult task. The severity of acne varies widely among patients and even during the course of disease in a single patient. The traditional grading method in clinical trials involves counting inflammatory and noninflammatory lesions, but this is confounded by the variable severity of inflammatory lesions. Papules may be barely visible, or deep, scarring, or just short of a nodule, and still be counted as equivalent lesions.

Determination of acne severity in clinical trials is problematic. Tan and colleagues [7] have analyzed the gradable aspects of acne and list lesion type, number of lesions, extent of lesions, regional involvement, secondary lesions, and patient experiences as important considerations. Cunliffe and colleagues [8] and more recently Dreno and coworkers [9] have developed grading systems based on comparison of the patient with standardized photos of acne of varying severity that in some measure answers this problem. A limitation of these systems is that they are not as quantifiable as lesion counting. Clinical trials typically rely on a combination of lesion counting and severity grading in order to generate both quantifiable and comparable data. The situation is not yet ideal.

Judging severity in day-to-day practice is much less complex. At the initial visit, experienced clinicians look at the type and number of lesions, the severity of inflammation, the presence of pigmentary disturbance and scarring, and the distribution of lesions and quickly have a grasp of the severity and likely response to different treatments. The presence of deep inflammation, nodules, scarring, and trunk lesions all point toward more severe acne. A second but important factor in judging acne severity is the effect of the disease on the patient. If each pimple is a tragedy, then even mild disease is severe.

References

1. Webster GF. Inflammation in acne vulgaris. J Am Acad Dermatol. 1995;33:247–53.
2. Friedlander SF, Eichenfield LF, Fowler JF, Fried RG, Levy ML, Webster GF. Acne epidemiology and pathophysiology. Semin Cutan Med Surg. 2010;29:2–4.
3. Mancini AJ, Baldwin HE, Eichenfield LF, Friedlander SF, Yan AC. Acne life cycle: the spectrum of pediatric disease. Semin Cutan Med Surg. 2011;30:S2–5.
4. Lucky AW, Biro FM, Simbarti LA, Morrisson JA, Sorg NW. Predictors of severity of acne vulgaris in young adolescent girls: results of a five year longitudinal study. J Pediatr. 1997;130:30–9.
5. Lucky AW, Biro FM, Huster GA, Morrison JA, Elder N. Acne vulgaris in early adolescent boys. Correlations wit pubertal maturation and age. Arch Dermatol. 1991;127:210–6.
6. Mourlatos K, Eady EA, Cunliffe WJ. Temporal changes in sebum excretion and propionibacterial colonization in preadolescent children with and without acne. Br J Dermatol. 2007; 156:22–31.
7. Tan J, Wolfe B, Weiss J, Stein-Gold L, Bikowski J, Delrosso J, Webster GF, Lucky A, Thiboutot D, Wilkin J, Leyden J, Chren MM. Acne severity grading: determining essential clinical components and features using Delphi consensus. J Am Acad Dermatol. 2012;67:187–93.
8. O'Brien SC, Lewis JB, Cunliffe WJ. The Leeds revised acne grading system. J Dermatol Treat. 1998;9:215–20.
9. Dreno B, Poli F, Pawin H, Beylot C, Faure M, et al. Development and evaluation of a global acne severity scale (GEA scale) suitable for France and Europe. J Eur Acad Dermato Venereol. 2011;25:43–8.

Chapter 3
Topical Therapies for Acne

Mary-Margaret Kober, Whitney P. Bowe, and Alan R. Shalita

3.1 Introduction

Topical treatment is a key component of acne therapy. Acne treatments target factors contributing to acne formation and act to normalize follicular keratinization and decrease sebaceous gland activity and follicular bacterial populations [1]. With early treatment, acne scarring, post-inflammatory hyperpigmentation, and psychological distress may be reduced or prevented [2]. Topical therapies for acne come in prescription and over-the-counter formulations. This chapter will focus on prescription products only.

3.2 Topical Retinoids

Biologically active molecules derived from vitamin A, topical retinoids have become a mainstay in acne therapy. Retinoids bind retinoic acid receptors (RARs) and retinoic X receptors (RXRs). Three subgroups of RARs exist: RAR-α (alpha), RAR-β (beta), and RAR-γ (gamma). RAR-α (alpha) is expressed throughout adult and embryonic tissue. RAR-β (beta) resides in dermal fibroblasts, and RAR-γ (gamma), present throughout the epidermis, is likely the receptor responsible for the positive effects retinoids exert on keratinocytes [3].

Once bound to their receptor, retinoids promote proliferation of basal keratinocytes, block the terminal stages of epithelial differentiation, and reduce filaggrin expression and proteolysis of keratins 1 and 14 [4]; these changes normalize keratinization and prevent the hyperproliferative state associated with comedo formation [5, 6]

M.-M. Kober, M.D. (✉) • W.P. Bowe, M.D. • A.R. Shalita, M.D.
Department of Dermatology, SUNY Downstate Medical Center,
450 Clarkson Road, Brooklyn, NY, USA
e-mail: mmkober@gmail.com; wpbowe@gmail.com; alan.shalita@downstate.edu

J.A. Zeichner (ed.), *Acneiform Eruptions in Dermatology: A Differential Diagnosis*,
DOI 10.1007/978-1-4614-8344-1_3, © Springer Science+Business Media New York 2014

Currently, four topical retinoids are available: tretinoin, isotretinoin, tazarotene, and adapalene. However, only tretinoin, tazarotene, and adapalene are available in the United States.

3.2.1 Tretinoin (First-Generation Retinoids)

Tretinoin is the oldest of the retinoids and binds with equal affinity to all RAR receptors. Tretinoin demonstrates superiority to benzoyl peroxide (BP), sulfur-resorcinol, and vehicle in the reduction of inflammatory and noninflammatory acne lesions as well as the global severity of acne [7, 8].

Although there may be some improvement noted after 2–3 weeks, the most significant reduction in acne lesions is noted after 3–4 months of consistent use [9]. The histopathologic findings seen in skin receiving tretinoin include acanthosis, parakeratosis, and thinning of the stratum corneum [8], which correlates with the observation that the tretinoin-induced thinning of the stratum corneum allows for improved efficacy of topical antimicrobial products [10].

Ultraviolet light and oxidants such as benzoyl peroxide degrade tretinoin upon exposure [9]. Advances in formulation technology have allowed for the development of new tretinoin containing topicals that combat these limitations. One such example is the development of microsphere formations (Retin-A Micro®) that significantly decreases degradation [11]. Microsphere formulations also provide a gradual time release of tretinoin, increasing transdermal penetration and decreasing the irritation [12].

3.2.2 Tazarotene and Adapalene (Third-Generation Retinoids)

Tazarotene and adapalene only bind to RAR-β (beta) and RAR-γ (gamma) receptor subtypes, leading to reduced side effects compared to tretinoin.

Although similar in efficacy to tretinoin in the reduction of inflammatory lesions, tazarotene has proven to be superior to tretinoin in reducing the number of noninflammatory lesions [13]. Tazarotene also shows superiority compared to adapalene in clearing post-inflammatory hyperpigmentation caused by acne [13].

Adapalene shows similar efficacy to tretinoin in reducing inflammatory and noninflammatory lesions and the global severity of acne [14]. However, when compared to tazarotene, adapalene is less effective in decreasing the number of inflammatory and noninflammatory lesions [15]. In general, adapalene demonstrates the best tolerability profile of the topical retinoids [16, 17].

Both tazarotene and adapalene have increased stability in the presence of ultraviolet light and BP as a result of replacing the labile, light sensitive double bonds of tretinoin with naphthoic acid rings [18]. This allows for the development of stable combination products containing third-generation retinoids with other active ingredients, such as BP.

Combination products are now available on the market, including adapalene/BP, tretinoin/clindamycin, and erythromycin/BP or clindamycin/BP. In addition to the comedolytic effects of retinoids, these products decrease *P. acnes* counts. Combination products often have faster results than monotherapy and improved patient compliance [19, 20].

The most common adverse reactions to topical retinoids include localized dry skin, erythema, and scaling. Compared to the newer formulations of retinoids, older forms of tretinoin caused more burning, erythema, and desquamation. Tolerance typically develops with continued exposure. Unlike systemic retinoids, studies have not demonstrated a teratogenic effect of topical retinoids; however, given the theoretical risk, many dermatologists advise patients to stop application during pregnancy [21].

Given the chronic nature of acne and its tendency to recur upon cessation of treatment, maintenance therapy is often required; first-line maintenance therapy is a topical retinoid. In one study of patients with moderate acne who had initial treatment with a topical retinoid and antimicrobial, those continued on topical retinoid therapy had significant less rebound and maintained few acne lesions compared to those who did not receive maintenance therapy [22].

3.3 Topical Antimicrobials

3.3.1 Antibiotics

Clindamycin and erythromycin represent the topical antibiotics most commonly used for acne treatment, although recent trends suggest that clindamycin is the most commonly prescribed [23]. Their mechanism of action is based on the reduction of *P. acnes* organisms present on the skin, leading to a reduction in inflammatory pathways and consequently a decrease in the number of inflammatory and noninflammatory acne lesions [24–26].

Several concerns have developed regarding the use of topical antibiotics, specifically surrounding the emergence of resistant strains of *P. acnes*. Rates of erythromycin and clindamycin resistant *P. acnes* have increased to 40 % globally, leading to a decrease in treatment efficacy of topical antibiotics [27–29]. Although resistance has emerged to both erythromycin and clindamycin, the clinical efficacy of clindamycin has been preserved relative to erythromycin [23].

Perhaps more concerning is the data suggesting pharyngeal colonization with *Streptococcus pyogenes* with chronic use of topical antibiotics [14]. Long-term antibiotic use has also shown the development of bacterial resistance in coagulase-negative staphylococci [30]. Although coagulase-negative staphylococci are rarely pathogenic, it may serve as a reservoir of bacterial resistant genes, spreading resistant genes to other organisms, such as *Staphylococcus aureus* [31].

Combining BP with a topical antibiotic reduces the emergence of resistant strains and improves efficacy [32]. Given the occurrence of antibiotic resistance with monotherapy of topical antibiotics, it is only recommended to use topical antibiotics as part of combination therapy [33]. Several combination products are available that combine a topical antibiotic with BP into a single product. Combination gels have reduced antibiotic-resistant strains of *P. acnes* by 97 % [34] and have shown to improve patient adherence to treatment regimens [35].

Side effects of topical antibiotics are limited. The most common adverse effects include reactions at the site of application (erythema, scaling, stinging, or burning); these reactions have been shown to be at least in part dependent on the vehicle formulation [23, 24].

3.3.2 Azelaic Acid

The antimicrobial properties of azelaic acid make it another topical treatment option for acne [33]. Trials comparing azelaic acid to BP or topical clindamycin show similar reductions in the number or acne lesions [36]. Reduction in the number of lesions can be seen as early as 4–8 weeks; however, maximum benefit typically occurs after 16 weeks. Cutaneous side effects of stinging or burning may occur in 10–20 % of patients upon initial use; however, these side effects typically resolve with continued use and rarely necessitate the cessation of treatment [37, 38]. It should be noted, however, that one of the authors found little or no efficacy with the original formulation of azelaic acid and one laboratory found no antibacterial effect on *P. acnes*.

Topical clindamycin, erythromycin, and azelaic acid appear to be safe during pregnancy (Category B), with no reports of teratogenicity to date.

3.3.3 Dapsone

Topical dapsone has been approved for the treatment of acne vulgaris, although it may result in a more modest reduction in acne lesions compared to other therapies. It has an excellent tolerability profile, but may result in a temporary yellow discoloration of the skin when combined with BP [34]. Topical dapsone appears to work well as an adjuvant to topical retinoids, reducing the irritation and desquamation commonly associated with topical retinoids as well as significantly increasing their efficacy [34].

3.4 New Developments in Topical Acne Therapy

Novel topical acne therapies focus on targeting drug delivery to the follicle.

3.4.1 *Liposomes*

Liposomes are phospholipid bilayers that create a spherical vesicle with a central aqueous cavity and possess both hydrophobic and lipophilic properties. Clindamycin in liposomes has shown a statistically significant decrease in acne lesions compared to liposome-free clindamycin products [39]; similar efficacy has been seen with liposome-derived tea tree oil, salicylic acid, retinoids, and BP [40].

3.4.2 *Micronization*

Smaller particles permit deeper penetration into the pilosebaceous unit. Micronizing formulations create products of smaller particle sizes, with particles frequently less than 10 μm. A micronized formulation of tretinoin gel, Atralin®, has demonstrated enhanced moisture capacity and tolerability with similar lesion reduction compared to generic tretinoin gel [41].

3.5 Treatment Guidelines

Mild acne responds to treatment with a topical retinoid with possible addition of BP and/or a topical antibiotic if inflammatory lesions are present. Mild-to-moderate acne typically requires combination therapy using one of the following regimens: a topical retinoid combined with BP and an oral antibiotic or a topical retinoid combined with a topical BP/antibiotic product [42]. Moderate-to-severe acne may be treated with topical retinoids in combination with BP, topical, and/or oral antibiotics; however, acne this severe may require systemic isotretinoin, discussed elsewhere.

3.6 Conclusion

Acne vulgaris is a chronic disease that requires a patient-centered approach. The most common topical treatments include retinoids and antibiotics with the addition of BP to reduce the development of antibiotic resistant strains of *P. acnes*. New products and novel formulation of existing drugs continue to expand the arsenal of available treatments and reduce adverse effects such as irritation and erythema. Maintenance therapy with topical retinoids is often recommended after initial treatment to prevent relapses.

References

1. Gong P, Gasparrini P, Rho D, et al. An in situ respirometric technique to measure pollution-inducted microbial community tolerance in soils contaminated with 2,4,6-trinitrotoulene. Ecotoxicol Environ Saf. 2000;47(1):96–103.
2. Thiboutot D, Gollnick H, Bettoli V, et al. New insights into the management of acne: an update form the Global Alliance to Improve Outcomes in Acne. J Am Acad Dermatol. 2009; 60(5 suppl 1):S1–50.
3. Czernielewski J, Michel S, Bouclier M, et al. Adapalene biochemistry and the evolution of a new topical retinoid for treatment of acne (review). J Eur Acad Dermatol Venereol. 2001;15 suppl 3:5–12.
4. Eichner R. Epidermal effects of retinoids: in vitro studies. J Am Acad Dermatol. 1986;15 (4 pt 2):789–97.
5. Eichner R, Kahn M, Capetola RJ, et al. Effects of topical retinoids on cytoskeletal proteins: implications for retinoid effects on epidermal differentiation. J Invest Dermatol. 1992; 98(2):154–61.
6. Papa CM. The cutaneous safety of topical tretinoin. Acta Derm Venereol Suppl (Stockh). 1975;74:128–32.
7. Krautheim A, Gollnick H. Acne: topical treatment (review). Clin Dermatol. 2004;22(5): 398–407.
8. Kligman AM, Fulton Jr JE, Plewig G. Topical vitamin A acid in acne vulgaris. Arch Dermatol. 1969;99(4):469–76.
9. Hui AM, Shalita AR. Topical retinoids. In: Shalita AR, Del Rosso JQ, Webster GF, editors. Acne vulgaris. New York, NY: Informa Healthcare; 2011. p. 86–94.
10. Leyden JJ, Marples RR, Mills OH, et al. Tretinoin and antibiotic therapy in acne vulgaris. South Med J. 1974;67(1):20–5.
11. Nyirady J, Lucas C, Yusuf M, et al. The stability of tretinoin in tretinoin gel microsphere 0.1%. Cutis. 2002;70(5):295–8.
12. Leyden JJ, Tanghetti EA, Miller B, et al. Once-daily tazarotene 0.1% gel versus once daily tretinoin 0.1% microsponge gel for the treatment of facial acne vulgaris: a double bind randomized control trial. Cutis. 2002;69(2 suppl):12–9.
13. Tanghetti E, Dhawan S, Green L, et al. Randomized comparison of the safety and efficacy of tazarotene 0.1% cream and adapalene 0.3% gel in the treatment of patients with at least moderate facial acne vulgaris. J Drugs Dermatol. 2009;9(5):549–58.
14. Ellis CN, Milikan LE, Smith EB, et al. Comparison of adapalene 0.1% solution and tretinoin 0.025% gel in the topical treatment of acne vulgaris. Br J Dermatol. 1998;139 suppl 52:41–7.
15. Webster GF, Guenther L, Poulin YP, et al. A multicenter, double-blind, randomized comparison study of the efficacy and tolerability of once-daily tazarotene 0.1% gel and adapalene 0.1% gel for the treatment of facial acne vulgaris. Cutis. 2002;69(2 suppl):20–9.
16. Galvin SA, Gilbert R, Baker M, et al. Comparative tolerance of adapalene 0.1% gel and six different tretinoin formulations. Br J Dermatol. 1998;139 suppl 52:34–40.
17. Caron D, Sorba V, Clucas A, et al. Skin tolerance of adapalene 0.1% gel in combination with other topical antiacne treatments. J Am Acad Dermatol. 1997;35(6 pt 2):S113–5.
18. Martin B, Meunier C, Montels D, et al. Chemical stability of adapalene and tretinoin when combined with benzoyl peroxide in presence and in absence of visible light and ultraviolet radiation. Br J Dermatol. 1998;139 suppl 52:8–11.
19. Thiboutot DM, Weiss J, Bucko A, Adapalene-BPO Study Group, et al. Adapalene-benzoyl peroxide, a fixed-dose combination for treatment of acne vulgaris: results of a multicenter, randomized double-blind, controlled study. J Am Acad Dermatol. 2007;57(5):791–9.
20. Eichenfield LF, Wortzman M. A novel gel formulation of 0.025% tretinoin and 1.2% clindamycin phosphate: efficacy in acne vulgaris patients aged 12 to 18 years. Pediatr Dermatol. 2009; 26(3):257–61.

21. Loureiro KD, Kao KK, Jones KL, et al. Minor malformations characteristic of the retinoic acid embryopathy and other birth outcomes in children of women exposed to topical tretinoin during early pregnancy. Am J Med Genet A. 2005;136(2):117–21.
22. Zhang JZ, Li LF, Tu YT, et al. A successful maintenance approach in inflammatory acne with adapalene gel 0.1% after an initial treatment in combination with clindamycin topical solution 1% or after monotherapy with clindamycin topical solution 1%. J Dermatol Treat. 2004; 15(6):372–8.
23. Leyden JJ, Del Rosso JQ, Webster GF. Clinical considerations in the treatment of acne vulgaris and other inflammatory skin disorders: focus on antibiotic resistance. Cutis. 2007;79 suppl 6:9–25.
24. Gollnick H, Cunliffe W, Berson D, et al. Management of acne: a report from the global alliance to improve outcomes in acne. J Am Acad Dermatol. 2003;49 suppl 1:S1–38.
25. Leyden JJ. The evolving role of *Propionibacterium acne*s in acne. Semim Cutan Med Surg. 2001;20:139–43.
26. Shalita AR, Myers JA, Krochman L, et al. The safety and efficacy of clindamycin phosphate foam 1% versus clindamycin phosphate topical gel 1% for the treatment of acne vulgaris. J Drugs Dermatol. 2005;4:46–8.
27. Ross JL, Snelling AM, Carneige E, et al. Antibiotic resistant acne lesions: lessons from Europe. Br J Dermatol. 2003;148:467–78.
28. Dreno B, Reynaud A, Moyse D, et al. Erythromycin-resistance of cutaneous bacterial flora in acne. Eur J Dermatol. 2001;11:549–53.
29. Esperson F. Resistance to antibiotics used in dermatologic practice. Br J Dermatol. 1998; 139:4–8.
30. Vowels BR, Feingold DS, Sloughfy C, et al. Effects of topical erythromycin on ecology of aerobic cutaneous bacterial flora. Antimicrob Agents Chemother. 1996;40:2598–604.
31. Naidoo J. Interspecific co-transfer of antibiotic resistance plasmids in staphylococci in vivo. J Hyg (Lond). 1984;93:59–66.
32. Del Rosso JQ, Leyden JJ, Thiboutot D, et al. Antibiotic use in acne vulgaris and rosacea: clinical considerations and resistance issues of significance to dermatologist. Cutis. 2008; 82(2S[ii]):5–12.
33. Del Rosso JQ. Topical antibiotics. In: Shalita AR, Del Rosso JQ, Webster GF, editors. Acne vulgaris. New York, NY: Informa Healthcare; 2011. p. 95–104.
34. Bowe WP, Glick JB, Shalita AR. Solodyn and updates on topical and oral therapies for acne. Solodyn and updates on topical and oral acne therapies for acne. Curr Dermatol Rep. 2012; 1(3):97–107.
35. Yentzer BA, Ade RA, Fountain JM, et al. Simplifying regimens promotes greater adherence and outcomes with topical acne medications: a randomized controlled trial. Cutis. 2010; 86:103–8.
36. Thiboutot D. Versatility of azelaic acid 15% gel in the treatment of inflammatory acne vulgaris. J Drugs Dermatol. 2008;7:13–6.
37. Cunliffe WJ, Hollan KT. Clinical and laboratory studies on treatment with 20% azelaic acid cream for acne. Acta Derm Venereol Suppl (Stockh). 1989;143:45–8.
38. Katsambas A, Graupe K. Azelaic acid for the treatment of acne vulgaris- a clinical comparison with vehicle and topical tretinoin. Acta Derm Venereol Suppl (Stockh). 1989;143:35–9.
39. Honzak L, Sentjurc M. Development of liposome encapsulated clindamycin for treatment of acne vulgaris. Pflugers Arch. 2000;440:44–5.
40. Castro GA, Ferreira LA. Novel vesicular and particular drug delivery systems for topical treatment of acne. Expert Opin Drug Deliv. 2008;5:665–79.
41. Torok HM, Pillai R. Safety and efficacy of micronized tretinoin gel (0.05%) in treating adolescent acne. J Drug Dermatol. 2011;10:647–51.
42. Villasenor J, Berson DS, Kroshinsky D. Combination therapy. In: Shalita AR, Del Rosso JQ, Webster GF, editors. Acne vulgaris. New York, NY: Informa Healthcare; 2011. p. 105–12.

Chapter 4
Systemic Therapies for Acne

Marisa Kardos Garshick, Alexa Kimball, and Lynn Drake

4.1 Introduction

Individuals with moderate-to-severe inflammatory acne may warrant systemic therapies, especially if they are unresponsive to topical treatments, or have significant quality of life decrements, which is not uncommon in this population. Specific clinical features, including the type and severity of acne, the presence of scarring, and the association with abnormal menses, can help guide the appropriate course of treatment. All dosages mentioned in this section must be adjusted according to the individual patient.

4.2 Oral Antibiotics

Oral antibiotics used for the treatment of moderate-to-severe inflammatory acne work by inhibiting the growth of *P. acnes*, or by anti-inflammatory effects [1]. Due to the widespread use of antibiotics, there is an increasing concern about antibiotic resistance. Given this, antibiotics are initially prescribed for a limited course. In the absence of clinical improvement after 6–8 weeks, a change in the antibiotic or other treatments may be considered. If partial improvement is observed, response to therapy should be reassessed after 6–8 weeks [2]. Using topical benzoyl peroxide or other topicals in combination with antibiotics may decrease the emergence of resistance [3]. Once acne is improved, oral antibiotics are often discontinued and patients should continue topical therapies for long-term maintenance as acne tends to flare in the absence of treatment.

M.K. Garshick, B.S. (✉) • A. Kimball, M.D., M.P.H. • L. Drake, M.D.
Department of Dermatology, Massachusetts General Hospital, 50 Staniford Street Suite 240, Boston, MA 02114, USA
e-mail: marisa.kardos@gmail.com

J.A. Zeichner (ed.), *Acneiform Eruptions in Dermatology: A Differential Diagnosis*, DOI 10.1007/978-1-4614-8344-1_4, © Springer Science+Business Media New York 2014

4.2.1 Macrolides

Erythromycin is not commonly used given the incidence of treatment failure perhaps due to the development of *P. acnes* antibiotic resistance or the low level of anti-inflammatory activity. Erythromycin is usually recommended when tetracycline derivatives are contraindicated [4]. A common acne dose is 500 mg twice daily. Side effects may include gastrointestinal (GI) distress, which might be reduced if administered with food.

Azithromycin has been reported as effective in the treatment of acne, though there is little consensus for its use and optimum dosing [5–7]. Given its role in the treatment of respiratory infections and as an alternative treatment for patients allergic to beta-lactam antibiotics, there is concern with increasing resistance. Azithromycin does not usually cause GI upset and should be taken on an empty stomach to enhance GI absorption.

4.2.2 Tetracyclines

The tetracyclines are probably the most commonly used antibiotics, and they have both antibiotic and anti-inflammatory properties. The newer generation tetracyclines (doxycycline and minocycline) are often preferred over tetracycline, due to decreased rates of resistance and better tolerability [8]. Evidence suggests a reduced incidence of bacterial resistance with minocycline- and tetracycline-resistant *P. acnes* cross-resistant to doxycycline, but sensitive to minocycline [9, 10]. Despite this, minocycline may be used as first-line therapy due to cost, toxicities, and no clear evidence of superior efficacy [11, 12].

Tetracycline is typically dosed at 500 mg twice daily, although 250 mg once or twice daily may also be effective. Patients should be advised to take tetracycline on an empty stomach as absorption is inhibited by food and with concurrent ingestion of calcium, magnesium, and aluminum. The absorption of doxycycline and minocycline is not inhibited by food, though concomitant administration with iron supplements may decrease absorption. Doxycycline is commonly prescribed at 50–100 mg once or twice daily. Although the data is limited, there may be a role for subantimicrobial dosing of doxycycline (20 mg twice daily) by which the anti-inflammatory mechanism is maintained, but the antibacterial properties are lost [13]. Until more data becomes available, subantimicrobial doses are usually only recommended when deemed to be in the best interest of the patient. While dosing of minocycline is usually 50–100 mg twice daily, an extended-release, once daily formulation of minocycline is FDA-approved at 1 mg/kg/day [14, 15].

The class-related side effects may include GI distress, including esophagitis; photosensitivity, particularly with doxycycline and tetracycline; and idiopathic intracranial hypertension (pseudotumor cerebri). To minimize GI side effects, doxycycline and minocycline can be administered with food and water. All tetracyclines should be avoided in pregnant women and children due to the potential for reduced bone growth and discoloration of developing teeth. Minocycline has been associated with acute vestibular adverse events; brown, gray, or blue pigmentation of the skin; lupus-like syndrome; and drug hypersensitivity syndrome [16]. Although it has been thought that continued use of systemic tetracycline antibiotics results in colonization with tetracycline-resistant *Staphylococcus aureus*, this may not be the case. Evidence suggests that *S. aureus* may remain sensitive to tetracycline even after prolonged use [17].

4.2.3 Other Antibiotics

Trimethoprim-sulfamethoxazole has been reported in the treatment of acne [18]. Severe, but rare, adverse effects may include drug hypersensitivity and hematologic reactions. Given the need to use trimethoprim-sulfamethoxazole in the treatment of methicillin-resistant *S. Aureus* infections and the potential side effects, trimethoprim-sulfamethoxazole should probably be used only in selected cases.

4.3 Isotretinoin

Isotretinoin, a vitamin A analogue, inhibits sebaceous gland activity and promotes normalization of epidermal differentiation. Additional properties that contribute to its efficacy include its anti-inflammatory and antibacterial effects. Isotretinoin is FDA-approved for use in patients with severe, recalcitrant, nodular acne [19] and may also be used in individuals with acne scarring.

Dosing is 0.5–1 mg/kg/day divided twice daily [19]. It is frequently initiated at 0.5 mg/kg/day to minimize the initial inflammatory response. If after the first 4 weeks, no adverse events occur, the dose may be increased as tolerated to 1 mg/kg/day to ultimately achieve a cumulative dose of 120–150 mg/kg [20]. A short course of prednisone may be considered prior to initial treatment or co-administered with isotretinoin in individuals at risk of a severe inflammatory reaction [21].

Isotretinoin can approach a cure in approximately 40 % of treated patients and improves many others [22]. Relapses may occur, especially in younger patients, males, and those with truncal acne. However, they can often be managed with topical agents or oral antibiotics. If acne remains severe, a repeat course of isotretinoin may be considered [23].

A number of adverse effects are associated with isotretinoin, some of which are dose dependent, and many are reversible. Cheilitis and mucocutaneous dryness are the most common and serve as an indicator of compliance and appropriate dosing. Dyslipidemia, specifically hypertriglyceridemia, is another common and reversible side effect [24]. Typically, the alteration in blood lipids occurs during the first 2 months of treatment and then stabilizes. Other less common side effects include increased transaminase levels, pancytopenia, nausea, diarrhea, idiopathic intracranial hypertension, arthralgias, and myalgias.

Isotretinoin is teratogenic and contraindicated during pregnancy. It poses the greatest risk in the first trimester and can result in spontaneous abortion, birth defects, and impaired neurological functioning [25, 26]. To minimize the risk of pregnancy, all US patients must be enrolled in the iPLEDGE program, which is an Internet-based registry to ensure that medication is only dispensed after proper counseling, documentation of two methods of contraception, and negative urinary pregnancy tests. Patients should not get pregnant for at least 1 month after discontinuing isotretinoin to guarantee clearance [19].

Some controversial side effects may exist for which the evidence is not clear. These include altered bone mineralization, diffuse idiopathic skeletal hyperostosis (DISH), the development of inflammatory bowel disease (IBD), and mood disturbances [27–29]. Although there is insufficient evidence to prove a causal relationship between isotretinoin and IBD, it may be important to inform patients of this potential effect [30]. While some studies show no increased risk of depression or suicidal ideation, physicians and patients may wish to continue to monitor for mood changes [31–33].

4.4 Hormonal Therapies

Androgens stimulate sebaceous glands to produce sebum and may also affect follicular hyperkeratinization. As a result, increased levels of serum androgens and heightened sensitivity of sebaceous glands to circulating androgens may increase the risk of acne [34]. Even in the absence of androgen excess, hormonal therapies may be effective through inhibition of androgen action on the pilosebaceous units [35]. Hormonal therapies are typically reserved for adolescent and adult females with moderate-to-severe acne and should be considered in those with inflammatory lesions along jaw line and neck that flare prior to menses, concomitant hirsutism, or menstrual irregularity.

4.4.1 Oral Contraceptives

The estrogen in certain oral contraceptives suppresses ovarian androgen production and increases sex hormone-binding globulin (SHBG), resulting in an overall decrease in testosterone bioavailability [36]. The FDA-approved oral contraceptive pills (OCPs) for the treatment of acne include ethinyl estradiol with different progestins: norgestimate, norethindrone, and drospirenone [37]. Although a Cochrane review in 2009 concluded that combined OCPs were more effective than placebo in controlling acne vulgaris, it has yet to be determined which combined OCPs are superior [38]. There was a slightly greater improvement in acne with ethinyl estradiol/drospirenone versus ethinyl estradiol/norgestimate in one clinical trial, perhaps related to the antiandrogenic progestin [39].

The risks associated with OCPs should be considered prior to initiating therapy. Individuals with a history of thromboembolic disease should not be placed on an OCP, and female smokers greater than 35 years of age should be counseled prior to treatment with an OCP due to the increased risk of thrombosis [40, 41]. Other reported side effects include nausea, decreased libido, breast tenderness, headache, breakthrough bleeding, mood disturbances, and potential for weight gain. Due to the risk of hyperkalemia with drospirenone-containing OCPs, these medications are contraindicated in patients with renal or adrenal insufficiency and hepatic dysfunction [40]. Other than for rifampin, there is no definitive evidence to suggest that antibiotics increase OCP failure rate [42]. Despite this, some individuals have large decreases in ethinyl estradiol concentrations when they take tetracycline and penicillin derivatives [43]. If acne does not improve within 6 months of OCP use, it typically will not improve [44].

4.4.2 Spironolactone

Spironolactone is an antiandrogen that inhibits androgen biosynthesis by inhibiting 5-α(alpha) reductase and blocks the androgen receptor [45]. Spironolactone may be considered in females with refractory acne or who prefer to avoid isotretinoin. Although several studies have demonstrated efficacy, a 2009 Cochrane review found insufficient evidence to confirm the effectiveness of spironolactone versus placebo in the treatment of acne [46–49]. While benefits may be observed at 25–200 mg/day, doses ranging from 50 to 100 mg/day are often recommended as lower doses may reduce the risk of side effects [50, 51]. Doses of 25 mg daily might be sufficient for some women with sporadic outbreaks or isolated cysts [52]. Absorption may be increased when administered with food.

Side effects may include hyperkalemia, orthostatic hypotension, menstrual irregularities, gynecomastia, headaches, fatigue, and GI symptoms. The most concerning is the risk of hyperkalemia, which is greater with higher doses, in older women, those taking chronic nonsteroidal anti-inflammatory agents and angiotensin-converting enzyme inhibitors, and those with renal insufficiency or severe cardiac disease. Potassium levels should be checked in the first month of treatment and monitored thereafter to determine if any dose adjustments need to be made, and patients should avoid potassium in their diet. Although breast tumors have been reported in mice treated with spironolactone, there is no definitive human evidence [51]. Despite this, some prefer to avoid this medication in women with a personal or family history of breast cancer. Spironolactone is a pregnancy category C medication due to the risk of feminization on male fetuses, so co-administration with an oral contraceptive is recommended.

4.4.3 Other Antiandrogens

Other antiandrogens have been used including cyproterone acetate and flutamide but only in selected cases [2, 52]. Oral corticosteroids may be used at low doses to suppress adrenal hyperactivity in individuals with adrenal androgen overproduction, seen in late-onset CAH. Frequently recommended doses are 2.5–5 mg of prednisone daily or 0.25–0.75 mg of dexamethasone [53]. Careful monitoring is always recommended.

4.5 Conclusion

Systemic therapies are an essential part of the management of moderate-to-severe acne. While systemic medications are effective in the treatment of acne, often they have associated side effects. As such, it is important to recognize which patients may benefit and to only use systemic treatment when it is clinically indicated.

References

1. Del Rosso JQ, Kim G. Optimizing use of oral antibiotics in acne vulgaris. Dermatol Clin. 2009;27:33–42.
2. Gollnick H, Cunliffe W, Berson D, et al. Management of acne: a report from a Global Alliance to Improve Outcomes in Acne. J Am Acad Dermatol. 2003;49:S1–37.
3. Leyden JJ. A review of the use of combination therapies for the treatment of acne vulgaris. J Am Acad Dermatol. 2003;49(3):S200–10.
4. Strauss JS, Krowchuk DP, Leyden JJ, et al. Guidelines of care for acne vulgaris management. J Am Acad Dermatol. 2007;56:651–63.
5. Rafiei R, Yaghoobi R. Azithromycin versus tetracycline in the treatment of acne vulgaris. J Dermatolog Treat. 2006;17:217–21.
6. Kus S, Yucelten D, Aytug A. Comparison of efficacy of azithromycin vs. doxycycline in the treatment of acne vulgaris. Clin Exp Dermatol. 2005;30:215–20.
7. Antonio JR, Pegas JR, Cestari T, Do Nascimento LV. Azithromycin pulses in the treatment of inflammatory and pustular acne: efficacy, tolerability and safety. J Dermatolog Treat. 2008; 19:210–5.
8. Leyden JJ, Del Rosso JQ, Webster GF. Clinical considerations in the treatment of acne vulgaris and other inflammatory skin disorders: focus on antibiotic resistance. Cutis. 2007;79:9–25.
9. Eady EA, Cove JH, Holland KT, Cunliffe WJ. Superior antibacterial action and reduced incidence of bacterial resistance in minocycline compared to tetracycline-treated acne patients. Br J Dermatol. 1990;122:233–44.
10. Eady EA, Jones CE, Gardner KJ, et al. Tetracycline-resistant propionibacteria from acne patients are cross-resistant to doxycycline but sensitive to minocycline. Br J Dermatol. 1993; 128:556–60.
11. Garner SE, Eady EA, Popescu C, et al. Minocycline for acne vulgaris: efficacy and safety. Coch Data Syst Rev. 2003; Issue 1: CD002086.
12. McManus P, Iheanacho I. Don't use minocycline as first line oral antibiotic in acne. BMJ. 2007;334:154.
13. Skidmore R, Kovach R, Walker C, et al. Effects of subantimicrobial-dose doxycycline in the treatment of moderate acne. Arch Dermatol. 2003;139:459–64.

14. Stewart DM, Torok HM, Weiss JS, et al. Dose-ranging efficacy of new once-daily extended-release minocycline for acne vulgaris. Cutis. 2006;78:11–20.
15. Fleischer Jr AB, Dinehart S, Stough D, et al. Safety and efficacy of a new extended-release formulation of minocycline for acne vulgaris. Cutis. 2006;78:21–31.
16. Sturkenboom MC, Meier CR, Jick H, Striker BH. Minocycline and lupus-like syndrome in acne patients. Arch Intern Med. 1999;159:493–7.
17. Fanelli M, Kupperman E, Lautenbach E, Edelstein PH, Margolis DJ. Antibiotics, acne, and staphylococcus aureus colonization. Arch Dermatol. 2011;147:917–21.
18. Bhambri S, Del Rosso JQ, Desai A. Oral trimethoprim/sulfamethoxazole in the treatment of acne vulgaris. Cutis. 2007;79(6):430–4.
19. Amnesteem® (Isotretinoin Capsules USP) [package insert]. Morgantown, WV: Mylan Pharmaceuticals, Inc. 2010.
20. Strauss JS, Rapini RP, Shalita AR, et al. Isotretinoin therapy for acne: results of a multicenter dose-response study. J Am Acad Dermatol. 1984;10:490–6.
21. Ellis CN, Krach KJ. Uses and complications of isotretinoin therapy. J Am Acad Dermatol. 2001;45(5):S150–7.
22. White GM, Chen W, Yao J, Wolde-Tsadik G. Recurrence rates after the first course of isotretinoin. Arch Dermatol. 1998;134:376–8.
23. Azoulay L, Oraichi D, Bérard A. Isotretinoin therapy and the incidence of acne relapse: a nested case-control study. Br J Dermatol. 2007;157(6):1240–8.
24. Bershad S, Rubinstein A, Paterniti JR, et al. Changes in plasma lipids and lipoproteins during isotretinoin therapy for acne. N Engl J Med. 1985;313:981–5.
25. Lammer EJ, Chen DT, Hoar RM, et al. Retinoic acid embryopathy. N Engl J Med. 1985; 313:837–41.
26. Adams J, Lammer EJ. Neurobehavioral teratology of isotretinoin. Reprod Toxicol. 1993; 7:175–7.
27. Margolis DJ, Attie M, Leyden JJ. Effects of isotretinoin on bone mineralization during routine therapy with isotretinoin therapy for acne vulgaris. Arch Dermatol. 1996;132:769–74.
28. Reddy D, Siegel CA, Sands BE, et al. Possible association between isotretinoin and inflammatory bowel disease. Am J Gastroenterol. 2006;101:1569–73.
29. Azoulay L, Blais L, Koren G, et al. Isotretinoin and the risk of depression in patients with acne vulgaris: a case-crossover study. J Clin Psychiatry. 2008;69:526–32.
30. Crockett SD, Gulati A, Sandler RS, et al. A causal association between isotretinoin and inflammatory bowel disease has yet to be established. Am J Gastroenterol. 2009;104: 2387–93.
31. Bigby M. Does isotretinoin increase the risk of depression? Arch Dermatol. 2008;144: 1197–9.
32. Marqueling AL, Zane LT. Depression and suicidal behavior in acne patients treated with isotretinoin: a systematic review. Semin Cutan Med Surg. 2007;26:210–20.
33. Chia CY, Lane W, Chibnall J, et al. Isotretinoin therapy and mood changes in adolescents with moderate to severe acne: a cohort study. Arch Dermatol. 2005;141:557–60.
34. Lolis MS, Bowe WP, Shalita AR. Acne and systemic disease. Med Clin North Am. 2009; 93:1161–81.
35. Kelekci KH, Kelekci S, Incki K, et al. Ovarian morphology and prevalence of polycystic ovary syndrome in reproductive aged women with or without mild acne. Int J Dermatol. 2010; 49:775–9.
36. Haider A, Shaw JC. Treatment of acne vulgaris. JAMA. 2004;292:726–35.
37. Junkins-Hopkins JM. Hormone therapy for acne. J Am Acad Dermatol. 2010;62(3):486–8.
38. Arowojolu AO, Gallo MF, Lopez LM, Grimes DA, Garner SE. Combined oral contraceptive pills for treatment of acne. Coch Data Syst Rev. 2009; Issue 3: CD004425.
39. Thorneycroft H, Gollnick H, Schellschmidt I. Superiority of a combined contraceptive containing drospirenone to a triphasic preparation containing norgestimate in acne treatment. Cutis. 2004;74:123–30.
40. Yaz® (Drospirenone/Ethinyl estradiol) [package insert]. Wayne, NJ: Bayer HealthCare Pharmaceuticals, Inc.: 2011.

41. Castelli WP. Cardiovascular disease: pathogenesis, epidemiology, and risk among users of oral contraceptives who smoke. Am J Obstet Gynecol. 1999;180:S349–56.
42. Helms SE, Bredle DL, Zajic J, Jatjoura D, Brodell RT, Krishnarao I. Oral contraceptive failure rates and oral antibiotics. J Am Acad Dermatol. 1997;36:705–10.
43. Dickinson BD, Altman RD, Nielsen NH, Sterling ML, Council on Scientific Affairs, American Medical Association. Interactions between oral contraceptives and antibiotics. Obstet Gynecol. 2001;98:853–60.
44. Berenson AB, Odom SD, Breitkopf CR, Rahman M. Physiologic and psychologic symptoms associated with use of injectable contraception and 20 microg oral contraceptive pills. Am J Obstet Gynecol. 2008;199:351.e1–e12.
45. Goodfellow A, Alaghband-Zadeh J, Carter G, et al. Oral spironolactone improves acne vulgaris and reduces sebum excretion. Br J Dermatol. 1984;111:209–14.
46. Brown J, Farquhar C, Lee O, et al. Spironolactone versus placebo or in combination with steroids for hirsutism and/or acne. Coch Data Syst Rev. 2009; Issue 2:CD000194.
47. Saint-Jean M, Ballanger F, Nguyen J, Khammari A, Dréno B. Importance of spironolactone in the treatment of acne in adult women. J Eur Acad Dermatol Venereol. 2010;25:1480–1. doi:10.1111/j.1468-3083.2010.03926.x.
48. Muhlemann MF, Carter GD, Cream JJ, Wise P. Oral spironolactone: an effective treatment for acne vulgaris in women. Br J Dermatol. 1986;115:227–32.
49. Burke BM, Cunliffe WJ. Oral spironolactone therapy for female patients with acne, hirsutism or androgenic alopecia. Br J Dermatol. 1985;112:124–5.
50. Shaw JC. Low-dose adjunctive spironolactone in the treatment of acne in women: a retrospective analysis of 85 consecutively treated patients. J Am Acad Dermatol. 2000;43:498–502.
51. Katsambas AD, Dessinioti C. Hormonal therapy for acne: why not as first line therapy? Facts and controversies. Clin Dermatol. 2010;28:17–23.
52. Van Wayjen R, van den Ende A. Experience in the long term treatment of patients with hirsutism and/or acne with cyproterone acetate-containing preparations: efficacy, metabolic, and endocrine effects. Exp Clin Endocrinol Diabetes. 1995;103:241–51.
53. Thiboutot D. Acne: hormonal concepts and therapy. Clin Dermatol. 2004;22:419–28.

Chapter 5
Laser and Light Based Therapies for Acne

Jeremy B. Green, Annelyse Ballin, and Joely Kaufman

5.1 Introduction

Conventional topical and systemic therapeutics are effective for treating acne vulgaris, but are not perfect solutions. Topical salicylic acid, benzoyl peroxide, and retinoid preparations can be irritating and present challenges with compliance. Systemic antibiotics also have issues with tolerability and increasing bacterial resistance, and isotretinoin has attracted negative attention due to its purported links to inflammatory bowel disease and depression. Laser and light-based treatments can potentially offer a viable adjunct or even alternative to these conventional options.

5.2 Light/Photodynamic Therapy

Light is thought to treat acne by taking advantage of the endogenous porphyrins produced by the pathogenic *Propionibacterium acnes* bacteria in sebaceous skin, coproporphyrin III and protoporphyrin IX. Porphyrin photoexcitation occurs maximally within the Soret band, with a peak in the blue light spectrum at approximately 410 nm, and additional smaller absorption peaks in the Q bands (500–635 nm) [1, 2]. Porphyrin excitation initiates a cascade of events that leads to the production of reactive oxygen species and destruction of *P. acnes*. This reaction can be potentiated by the addition of aminolevulinic acid (ALA), an exogenous photosensitizer that preferentially localizes to sebaceous glands and enhances intracellular porphyrin synthesis, the so-called photodynamic therapy (PDT).

J.B. Green, M.D. (✉) • A. Ballin, M.D. • J. Kaufman, M.D.
Private Practice, Dr. Brandt Dermatology Associates,
4425 Ponce De Leon Blvd, Suite 200, Coral Gables, FL 33146, USA
e-mail: jgreen@drfredricbrant.com

J.A. Zeichner (ed.), *Acneiform Eruptions in Dermatology: A Differential Diagnosis*,
DOI 10.1007/978-1-4614-8344-1_5, © Springer Science+Business Media New York 2014

There is a dearth of large, randomized controlled trials of lasers and lights for acne [3]. One exception was an industry-sponsored evaluation of 266 severe acne patients treated with blue light (417 ± 5 nm) and 20 % aminolevulinic acid (ALA) (BLU-U® and Levulan® Kerastick, DUSA Pharmaceuticals, Inc.) versus blue light and vehicle alone [4]. In this study, vehicle or ALA was applied for 45 min incubation followed by 16 min and 40 s of blue light (10 J/cm^2 total dose), one treatment every 3 weeks for four treatments. Interestingly the investigators found a decrease in inflammatory lesions of 37.5 % for the ALA group versus 41.7 % reduction in the vehicle group. Noninflammatory lesion counts were not performed. The study indicates that blue light alone is as effective as blue light plus ALA.

Blue light penetrates to a depth of approximately 90–150 μm. Although it is unlikely that significant amount of this wavelength reaches the sebaceous gland, exposure to blue light at a wavelength of 405–420 nm destroys *P. acnes*. Furthermore, blue light may inhibit the production of interleukin-1 alpha and intercellular adhesion molecule-1 [5], as well as tumor necrosis factor alpha and matrix metalloproteinase 2, all inflammatory mediators implicated in the pathogenesis of acne [6].

Within the visible light spectrum, a longer wavelength of light correlates with deeper skin penetration, as there is less melanin absorption and less scattering by connective tissue. Red light penetrates deeper than blue light, to approximately 2 mm of depth. It effectively reaches the sebaceous glands and activates porphyrins via the Q band at 630 nm. One study evaluated 21 patients treated with 3 h incubation of 16.8 % methylaminolevulinic acid (Metvix®, Photocure) followed by 9 min of 630 nm red light (Aktilite® CL 128, Photocure), for a total dose of 37 J/cm^2 [7]. After two treatments spaced 2 weeks apart, investigators noted a 68 % reduction in inflammatory lesions and no change in the 15 control patients. There was no reduction in noninflammatory lesions in either group. One study found that the combination of blue and red light was superior to either blue light or 5 % benzoyl peroxide alone in reduction of the number of inflammatory acne lesions [8].

Limitations of using an exogenous photosensitizer include intra-procedure pain and post-procedure erythema, edema, and blistering. Of note patients must avoid direct sunlight exposure for 48 h after the procedure, which can be challenging in the teenage acne population.

The pulsed dye laser (PDL, 585–595 nm yellow light), potassium titanyl phosphate (KTP, 532 nm green light), and broadband intense pulsed light (IPL, 500–1,200 nm) with cutoff filters to employ predominately short wavelengths all act on acne by activating endogenous *P. acnes* porphyrins and reducing sebaceous gland function. A 2003 study found a significant reduction of inflammatory acne lesions (49 %) in 31 patients receiving a single PDL treatment versus 10 patients receiving "sham" treatment (10 %) [9]. However, a different, split-face trial of 40 patients receiving 1–2 sub-purpuric PDL treatments found no significant difference in mean papule count versus the untreated control side [10]. A study of the KTP laser found a 35.9 % reduction in inflammatory lesions 1 month after 4 biweekly treatments [11]. Anecdotally the authors find these devices to be more useful for improving the appearance of erythematous "stains" and scars which routinely appear following the resolution of acne lesions.

Mid-infrared light has also been utilized for acne treatment due to its purported ability to shrink sebaceous glands and/or alter their secretion [12]. One study of 32 acne patients treated in a split-face fashion with 3 monthly 1,450 nm diode laser treatments found an equal reduction in inflammatory lesions on both the treatment and control side [13]. The authors state that this may present evidence of a systemic anti-inflammatory effect of the laser, though the mechanism is unclear. Another evaluation of 20 patients treated with a 1,540 nm erbium to glass nonablative fractional laser monthly for 4 months found that acne lesions improved in 85 % of patients and 80 % noted a reduction in sebum production [14].

5.3 Photopneumatic Therapy

Improvement of comedonal acne with lasers and lights has been a challenge to achieve; however the newly developed photopneumatic therapy devices show potential. Photopneumatic therapy combines vacuum suction to mechanically clear pores and concomitant broadband pulsed light. Cutoff filters limit the emission spectrum to 500–1,200 nm, wavelengths that activate endogenous porphyrins to destroy *P. acnes*, as well as short-wavelength visible light that reduces perilesional erythema.

Published data supporting the efficacy of photopneumatic therapy is limited to small, uncontrolled trials. A 2008 study of 11 patients receiving photopneumatic therapy every 3 weeks for four treatments found a statistically significant reduction in both inflammatory (78.8 %) and noninflammatory (57.8 %) lesions at the 3-month follow-up visit post-therapy. Nine of the 11 patients were moderately to very satisfied with their results [15]. Other similar studies corroborate these findings [16, 17]. In the authors' experience, photopneumatic therapy is an effective adjunctive acne treatment.

5.4 Home Devices

Over-the-counter (OTC) handheld laser devices have garnered increasing attention among mass media and consumers. The potential to improve wrinkles, remove or grow hair, and treat acne treatment in the comfort and privacy of one's own home at a cost generally less than in-office procedures has understandably proven attractive. However, in order to ensure safety for self-administration, OTC devices are generally underpowered, require a greater number of treatments, and consequently afford lesser efficacy than their in-office counterparts.

Despite the fact that dozens of devices are available, few have published data supporting their efficacy [18] In a prospective, uncontrolled study of one such device (Omnilux Clear-U®, Photo Therapeutics, Inc, Carlsbad, CA, blue light 415 nm and red light 633 nm), 17 patients with mild to moderate inflammatory acne self-administered a course of eight light treatments, twice daily over 4 weeks.

Each week, the subject administered two alternate exposures: 20 min for blue and 30 min for red light, with 2–3-day intervals between the alternating light treatments. Treatment was associated with statistically significant reduction from baseline in the inflammatory lesion count of 69 % and reduction of 12 % of noninflammatory lesions [19]. It is important to note that treatment time (20 min for blue light and 30 min for red) for the study covered an area of 5 cm × 6 cm. Consequently, a considerably longer time would be required for full-face treatment. Therefore OTC acne devices are best suited for spot treatment and are not routinely recommended by the authors for full-face treatment of acne.

5.5 Future Directions

The future of laser and light therapy for acne is based on the foundation of modern laser therapy—the principle of selective photothermolysis [20]. None of the aforementioned laser and light sources emit wavelengths of light that are preferentially absorbed by the sebaceous gland. One approach recently presented involved the application of gold-coated nanoshells specifically constructed to absorb light at 800 nm. After application to periauricular human skin and subsequent treatment with an 800 nm diode laser, histologic examination showed partial sebaceous gland destruction without damage to the surrounding epidermis or dermis [21]. A recent work investigated the optimal wavelength to target the sebaceous gland found that sebum preferentially absorbs 1,210 and 1,720 nm light [22]. The investigators also estimated that the optimal pulse duration of laser light delivered to confine heat to the target sebaceous gland (thermal relaxation time) to be approximately 100 ms. With these working parameters devices are in development, and perhaps 1 day laser practitioners will be able to satisfyingly specifically target acne the way we currently treat pigmented lesions. Until that day, lasers and lights can provide useful adjuncts to conventional first-line acne therapy.

References

1. Sakomoto FH, Lopes JD, Anderson RR. Photodynamic therapy for acne vulgaris: a critical review from basics to clinical practice. Part I. J Am Acad Dermatol. 2010;63:183–93.
2. Sakomoto FH, Torezan L, Anderson RR. Photodynamic therapy for acne vulgaris: a critical review from basics to clinical practice. Part II. J Am Acad Dermatol. 2010;63:195–211.
3. Hamilton FL, Car J, Lyons M, et al. Laser and other light therapies for the treatment of acne vulgaris: systematic review. Br J Dermatol. 2009;160:1273–85.
4. http://www.clinicaltrials.gov/ct2/show/results/NCT00706433?term=DUSA+Pharmaceuticals&rank=1
5. Shnitkind E, Yaping E, Geen S, et al. Anti-inflammatory properties of narrow-band blue light. J Drugs Dermatol. 2006;5(7):605–10.
6. Fan X, Xing Y-Z, Liu L-H, et al. Effects of 420-nm intense pulsed light in an acne animal model. J Eur Acad Dermatol Venereol. 2012; doi: 10.1111/j.1468-3083.2012.04487.x

7. Wiegell SR, Wulf HC. Photodynamic therapy of acne vulgaris using methyl aminolevulinic acid: a blinded, randomized, controlled trial. Br J Dermatol. 2006;154:969–76.
8. Papageorgiou P, Katsambas A, Chu A. Phototherapy with blue (415 nm) and red (660 nm) light in the treatment of acne vulgaris. Br J Dermatol. 2000;142:973–8.
9. Seaton ED, Charakida A, Mouser PE, et al. Pulsed-dye laser treatment for inflammatory acne vulgaris: randomised controlled trial. Lancet. 2003;362:1347–52.
10. Orringer JS, Kang S, Hamilton T, et al. Treatment of acne vulgaris with a pulsed dye laser: a randomized controlled trial. JAMA. 2004;291:2834–9.
11. Bowes L, Manstein D, Anderson R. Effects of 532 nm KTP laser on acne and sebaceous glands. Laser Med Sci. 2003;18 Suppl 1:S6–7.
12. Perez-Maldonado A, Runger TM, Kreju-Papa N. The 1,450-nm diode laser reduces sebum production in facial skin: a possible mode of action of its effectiveness for the treatment of acne vulgaris. Lasers Surg Med. 2007;39:189–92.
13. Darne S, Hiscutt EL, Seukeran DC. Evaluation of the clinical efficacy of the 1450 nm laser in acne vulgaris: a randomized split-face, investigator-blinded clinical trial. Br J Dermatol. 2011; 165:1256–62.
14. Isarria MJ, Cornejo P, Munos E, et al. Evaluation of clinical improvement in acne scars and active acne in patients treated with the 1540-nm non-ablative fractional laser. J Drugs Dermatol. 2011;10(8):907–12.
15. Gold M, Biron J. Treatment of acne with pneumatic energy and broadband light. J Drugs Dermatol. 2008;7(7):639–42.
16. Shamban AT, Enokibori M, Narurkar V, et al. Photopneumatic technology for the treatment of acne vulgaris. J Drugs Dermatol. 2008;7(2):139–45.
17. Wanitphakdeedcha R, Tanzi E, Alster T. Photopneumatic therapy for the treatment of acne. J Drugs Dermatol. 2009;8(3):239–41.
18. Metelitsa AI, Green JB. Home-use laser and light devices for the skin—an update. Semin Cutan Med Surg. 2011;30:144–7.
19. Sadick NS. Handheld LED, array device in the treatment of acne vulgaris. J Drugs Dermatol. 2008;7:347–50.
20. Anderson RR, Parrish JA. Selective photothermolysis: precise microsurgery by selective absorption of pulsed radiation. Science. 1983;220(4596):524–7.
21. Kauvar A, Lloyd J, Cheung W, et al. Selective photothermolysis of the sebaceous follicle with gold-coated nanoshells for treatment of acne. Presented at 2012 American Society for Laser Medicine and Surgery Annual Meeting, Orlando, Florida.
22. Sakamoto FH, Doukas AG, Farinelli WA, et al. Selective photothermolysis to target sebaceous glands: theoretical estimation of parameters and preliminary results using a free electron laser. Lasers Surg Med. 2012;44:175–83.

Part II
Infectious Diseases Mimicking Acne Vulgaris

Chapter 6
Bacterial Folliculitis

Jessica Gjede and Emmy Graber

6.1 Introduction

Folliculitis is a common disorder characterized by an inflammatory reaction in the superficial aspect of the hair follicle, involving either the follicular opening or the perifollicular area [1]. Folliculitis can be classified based on etiology and is divided into two broad categories: infectious folliculitis and noninfectious folliculitis. Infectious folliculitis is further classified according to the offending organism and may include bacterial folliculitis, fungal folliculitis, viral folliculitis, parasitic folliculitis, and syphilitic folliculitis. Noninfectious etiologies include, but are not limited to, diagnoses such as drug-induced acneiform folliculitis, acne keloidalis nuchae, folliculitis decalvans, and eosinophilic folliculitis. This chapter will focus on bacterial folliculitis.

6.2 Background

Bacterial folliculitis affects both males and females in children and adults [1–3]. An accurate incidence is difficult to determine as many affected patients in the general population do not seek medical attention for this condition. Predisposing factors include occlusion, maceration, hyperhydration, nasal carriage of *Staphylococcus aureus* (*S. aureus*), application of topical steroids, and exposure to oils and certain other chemicals, all of which increase bacterial colonization on the skin [1–3]. Environments that promote occlusion or moisture such as hot or humid weather or prolonged exposure to heated water (i.e., hot tub, heated swimming pool) are predisposing factors as well.

J. Gjede, M.D. (✉) • E. Graber, M.D.
Department of Dermatology, Boston Medical Center, 609 Albany Street, J-203, Boston, MA 02118, USA
e-mail: jessica.luis@gmail.com

J.A. Zeichner (ed.), *Acneiform Eruptions in Dermatology: A Differential Diagnosis*, DOI 10.1007/978-1-4614-8344-1_6, © Springer Science+Business Media New York 2014

Manipulation of the follicular unit by plucking, waxing, or shaving, especially when performed against the normal direction of hair growth, may also be a risk factor. Finally, patients may have other underlying medical conditions that lead to over-colonization of the skin surface with bacteria such as diabetes mellitus and atopic dermatitis.

The most common causative agent in bacterial folliculitis is *S. aureus*; however, species of *Streptococcus*, *Pseudomonas*, *Proteus*, and other Gram-negative bacteria have also been implicated [1]. These other forms of folliculitis will be covered elsewhere in this book.

6.3 Clinical Presentation

The clinical appearance of bacterial folliculitis differs depending on whether infection occurs in the superficial or deep portion of the follicle. Superficial folliculitis, also known as Bockhart impetigo, typically presents with small, folliculocentric pustules with surrounding erythema that evolve into crusted papules with time [1]. If no pustules are present, a clue to the diagnosis of folliculitis may be an erythematous papule with a collarette of scale, especially when the etiologic agent is *S. aureus* (Fig. 6.1) [2, 4]. Associated symptoms include pain, tenderness, and/or pruritus. Cases of methicillin-resistant *S. aureus* (MRSA) often follow a more aggressive course starting with typical erythematous papules and pustules that progress rapidly to painful nodules, often with purulent drainage.

When bacterial infection progresses to involve the deeper portion of the follicle beneath the infundibulum or the tissue adjacent the follicle, a furuncle develops [1]. Furuncles begin as small, folliculocentric, painful, inflammatory nodules, often

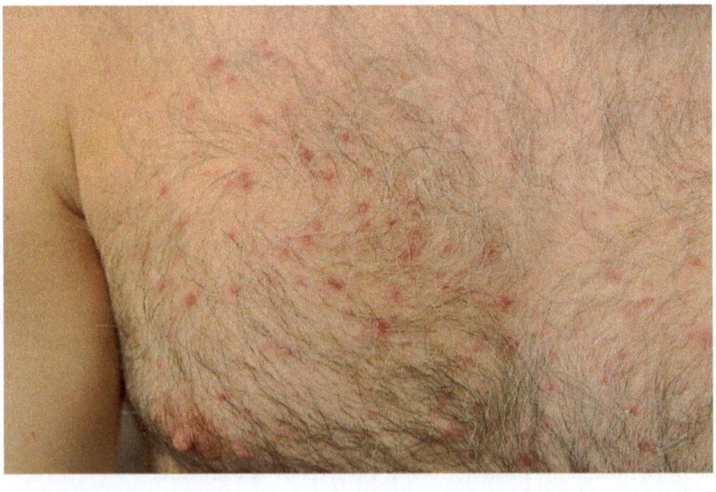

Fig. 6.1 Follicular-based, erythematous papules where pustules had initially existed and subsequently ruptured (Photo credit: Joshua A. Zeichner, M.D.)

with a central pustule that becomes necrotic within a few days [1]. Furuncles are more common in young adult males and favor the face, back of neck, axillae, breast, buttocks, and thighs [1]. Predisposing factors for furunculosis include diabetes mellitus, HIV infection, malnutrition, crowded living conditions such as incarceration, and chronic staphylococcus colonization [1].

Bacterial sycosis is another form of deep folliculitis in which a subacute or chronic staphylococcal infection involves the entire hair follicle [1, 2]. This condition typically occurs in postpubertal males, often in the third to fourth decade, and frequently affects the beard region [1, 2]. Early in the clinical course, the condition presents with an edematous, inflammatory papule or pustule in the beard region with a burning sensation. This is followed by development of numerous papules and pustules involving the surrounding follicles that then coalesce into plaques studded with pustules [1]. In severe or chronic cases persisting for years, the follicles may be destroyed by scarring or a granulomatous appearance may occur. This has been termed lupoid sycosis for its morphologic resemblance to lupus vulgaris [1, 2].

The distribution of folliculitis favors hair-bearing areas, especially the scalp and beard region, but also the upper trunk, buttocks, thighs, axillae, and groin [2]. Areas of involvement vary among different populations. In infants and children, infection favors the face, buttocks, and axillae [1]. Folliculitis in adolescent females is commonly located on the legs, while it affects the flexural areas in adolescent males [1].

6.4 Work-Up

The diagnosis of bacterial folliculitis is typically based on clinical exam. Bacterial culture and Gram stain obtained from swabs of pustular contents help identify the causative organism, especially in cases that are recurrent or resistant to treatment [3]. *S. aureus* is the causative organism in a majority of cases, but bacterial culture and Gram stain are particularly helpful in cases caused by less common bacteria. Correctly identifying the causative pathogen along with culture-directed antibiotic sensitivity enables treatment with appropriate antibiotic therapy. Cultures should be performed prior to initiating antibiotic therapy. In chronic cases, nasal culture may indicate if a patient is a chronic carrier of *S. aureus*.

Other diagnostic tests may be helpful in differentiating bacterial from nonbacterial infectious folliculitis. For example, scraping of pustular contents can be sent for fungal culture, and potassium hydroxide preparations can be performed if a fungal cause is suspected [1]. A Tzanck smear is useful in cases of herpetic folliculitis [1]. Additionally, in some cases of viral folliculitis, polymerase chain reaction (PCR) can be used to identify the causative virus.

A skin biopsy is rarely needed to confirm the diagnosis of folliculitis. However, if performed, salient features include a perifollicular or intrafollicular mixed inflammatory infiltrate composed of lymphocytes, histiocytes, or plasma cells, often progressing to a ruptured follicle surrounded by neutrophils and multinucleated giant cells [5]. Bacteria may be seen within the follicle as well. Older lesions are characterized by perifollicular fibrosis [5]. A furuncle is characterized histopathologically by similar features involving the deeper portions of the follicular unit and occasionally, dermal abscess formation [5].

6.5 Treatment

Treatment in bacterial folliculitis should be targeted at the most common causative organism or the organism identified by bacterial culture. A majority of the evidence-based literature focuses on treatment of other superficial skin and skin structure infections; however, it can be applied to folliculitis because the causative organisms are largely the same. Superficial bacterial folliculitis usually responds to topical antibacterial treatment, specifically agents that cover *S. aureus* with consideration of empiric therapy for MRSA. For culture-negative folliculitis, empiric topical treatments include benzoyl peroxide, topical antibiotics such as clindamycin, and antibacterial washes that contain chlorhexidine or triclosan [2, 3]. In addition to these, mupirocin ointment can be considered for cases of staphylococcal folliculitis, especially those caused by MRSA, although its utility is limited in widespread disease [1, 3]. Other less common options for staphylococcal folliculitis include fusidic acid ointment, which is not available in the United States, and topical retapamulin [1, 6].

When superficial folliculitis becomes widespread or recurrent, oral therapy may be necessary. Oral antibiotics that have been reported to be effective in folliculitis include clindamycin, azithromycin, and tetracycline class antibiotics such as doxycycline and minocycline [2, 6]. Treatment duration of 7–14 days is typically sufficient, although resistant and complicated cases may require several months of therapy. For cases caused by MRSA, systemic therapy may include doxycycline or linezolid in resistant cases, which are both FDA approved for this indication [6]. Additionally, while trimethoprim-sulfamethoxazole is not FDA approved for MRSA-related skin and soft tissue infections, many reports have shown it to be efficacious [6]. The recommended treatment duration for MRSA-folliculitis is 10–14 days, although resistant and complicated cases may necessitate a longer treatment course.

In cases of deep folliculitis or furunculosis, systemic antibiotic therapy is often necessary. A culture should be performed prior to initiating antibiotic therapy to identify the causative organism [1]. Typically, oral antibiotics that cover *S. aureus* are sufficient; however, in some cases, Gram-negative bacteria may be identified, in which culture-directed antibiotics should be considered. Ciprofloxacin is often helpful in these cases [1]. For severe or suppurative folliculitis, intravenous antibiotic therapy with linezolid or daptomycin may be indicated [6].

Treatment failure of bacterial folliculitis is rare, but in cases of recurrent or resistant bacterial folliculitis, eradication of MRSA colonization should be considered [1, 3]. This can be accomplished by applying mupirocin 2 % ointment to the nares twice daily for 5 days [3, 6–8]. Some sources also recommend treating the axillae, groin, anus, and inframammary areas as well [3], while others recommend repeating treatment for 5 days each month to reduce recurrence [8]. Topical fusidic acid and retapamulin can also be used to eradicate MRSA colonization [6, 8].

References

1. Luelmo-Aguilar J, Santandreu MS. Folliculitis: recognition and management. Am J Clin Dermatol. 2004;5(5):301–10.
2. McMichael A, Sanchez DG, Kelly P. Folliculitis and the follicular occlusion tetrad. In: Bolognia JL, Jorizzo JL, Rapini RP, editors. Dermatology. 2nd ed. Mosby: Elsevier; 2008. http://www.expertconsult.com.
3. Halpern AV, Heymann WR. Bacterial diseases. In: Bolognia JL, Jorizzo JL, Rapini RP, editors. Dermatology. 2nd ed. Mosby: Elsevier; 2008. http://www.expertconsult.com.
4. Levy AL, Simpson G, Skinner RB. Medical pearl: circle of desquamation—a clue to the diagnosis of folliculitis and furunculosis caused by Staphylococcus aureus. J Am Acad Dermatol. 2006;55:1079–80.
5. Rapini RP. Practical dermatopathology. Philadelphia, PA: Elsevier; 2005. p. 141.
6. Chon SY, Doan HQ, Mays RM, Singh SM, Gordon RA, Tyring SK. Antibiotic overuse and resistance in dermatology. Dermatol Ther. 2012;25:55–69.
7. Dryden MS, Dailly S, Crouch M. A randomized, controlled trial regimen for the clearance of MRSA colonization. J Hosp Infect. 2004;56:283–6.
8. Bernard P. Management of common bacterial skin infections. Curr Opin Infect Dis. 2008; 21(2):122–8.

Chapter 7
Gram-Negative Folliculitis

Ani L. Tajirian and Leon H. Kircik

7.1 Introduction

Gram-negative folliculitis is a complication of treatment of acne or rosaceas with long-term oral antibiotics, usually tetracyclines. It is caused by the replacement of the gram-positive flora of the mucous membranes of the nose with gram-negative bacteria, which is spread to the face. Common causative organisms include *Escherichia coli*, *Pseudomonas aeruginosa*, *Serratia marcescens*, *Klebsiella*, and *Proteus mirabilis*. Gram-negative folliculitis should be considered in acne patients who have a flare-up of pustular or cystic lesions while on antibiotics and in patients who have no significant improvement of acne lesions after 3–6 months of antibiotic therapy.

7.2 Background

7.2.1 Pathophysiology

Fulton et al. first described gram-negative folliculitis in a group of patients with long-standing treatment-resistant acne in 1968 [1]. Gram-negative folliculitis is characterized by the replacement of gram-positive normal flora of the nares and

A.L. Tajirian, M.D. (✉)
Fletcher Allen Health Care, University of Vermont College of Medicine, Burlington, VT, USA

Webster Management Inc., 3300 Webster Street, Suite 509, Oakland, CA 94609, USA
e-mail: Ani.Tajirian@gmail.com

L.H. Kircik, M.D.
Department of Dermatology, Mt. Sinai School of Medicine, New York, NY, USA

Indiana University School of Medicine, Indianapolis, IN, USA

J.A. Zeichner (ed.), *Acneiform Eruptions in Dermatology: A Differential Diagnosis*,
DOI 10.1007/978-1-4614-8344-1_7, © Springer Science+Business Media New York 2014

adjacent facial skin by gram-negative rods, most commonly Enterobacteriaceae. In patients with acne who are treated with oral antibiotics, the number of *Staphylococcus aureus* and diphtheroids decreases and the number of coagulase-negative staphylococcal and enterobacterial organisms increases in the nares. Gram-negative organisms require a moist environment to survive and proliferate, so they prosper in areas of excessive seborrhea. Sebaceous follicles primarily around the nose and mouth become colonized with these bacteria with subsequent spread to follicles of adjacent skin the development of recalcitrant papules and pustules. Ordinarily, gram-negative bacteria constitute less than 1 % of the total bacterial flora in the nose; however, in patients with gram-negative folliculitis, enterobacteria constitute approximately 4 % of the total bacterial flora. In addition, tetracyclines impair protein synthesis and the function of human lymphocytes as well as the chemotaxis of neutrophils thus increasing the risk of bacterial superinfection [2, 3].

A number of studies have shown changes in the immune defense mechanisms of acne patients with gram-negative folliculitis. In one study by Neubert et al. [2], a subset of patients demonstrated a depressed cell-mediated immunity as shown by weak or absent delayed-type hypersensitivity responses as well as diminished serum concentrations of IgM. A low IgM concentration might lead to a weakened or absent response to the O-antigens of enterobacteria thus increasing the likelihood of a gram-negative rod infection [2]. Alpha-1-antitrypsin deficiency has also been suggested as a cofactor in the development of gram-negative folliculitis through the inactivation of granulocyte neutral protease and the intensification of inflammatory processes [2].

Loofah sponges and exfoliative beauty products might further contribute to the development of gram-negative folliculitis in patients with acne [4].

7.2.2 Epidemiology

Gram-negative folliculitis is a relatively rare complication of prolonged antibiotic therapy, occurring in about 4 % of patients with acne vulgaris on oral antibiotics. It is thought that the frequency of this infection is underreported as it can be mistaken for an acne exacerbation and is infrequently cultured.

There is no racial or sexual predilection for gram-negative folliculitis. A slightly increased age of onset has been observed for gram-negative folliculitis as compared to acne, as most patients who develop gram-negative folliculitis have undergone treatment of acne with a broad-spectrum antibiotic for many years.

7.3 Clinical Presentation

Typical features of acne patients with gram-negative folliculitis include male predominance, severe seborrhea with oily skin, perioral and perinasal papules and pustules, recurrent folliculitis of the scalp, history of prolonged antibacterial

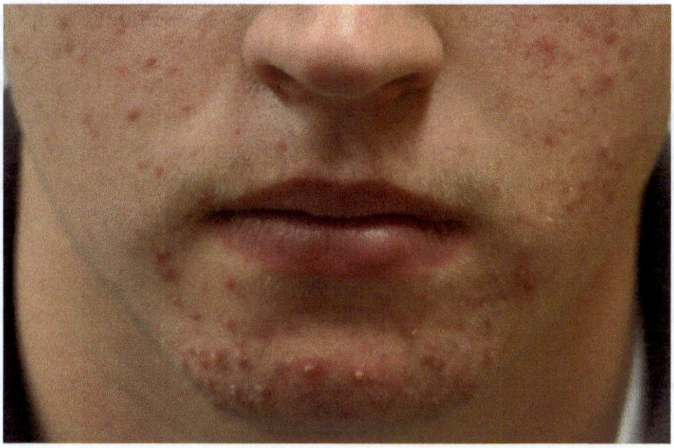

Fig. 7.1 Monomorphic follicular papules in the infranasal area and chin of a teenage boy with acne who developed gram-negative folliculitis after chronic treatment with doxycycline for acne (Photo credit: Joshua A. Zeichner, M.D.)

treatment, and isolation of gram-negative rods from pustules of facial skin and mucous membranes of the nose [2] (Fig. 7.1).

Two main subtypes of gram-negative folliculitis have been described [5]. Type I is much more common and seen in approximately 80 % of patients. These patients develop papules and papulopustules flaring out from the nares and involving the infranasal and perioral skin. In type II, seen in approximately 20 % of patients, deep fluctuant cystic lesions resembling acne conglobata are the key presenting features. The distribution of lesions in both types extends from the infranasal area to the chin and cheeks.

Type I lesions are most commonly associated with a lactose-fermenting, gram-negative rods including *Klebsiella*, *Escherichia*, and *Serratia* species [5]. However, cases associated with Citrobacter, which is another organism of the Enterobacteriaceae family, have been reported [6, 7]. Proteus species is associated with type II lesions; these organisms are motile granting them the ability to invade more deeply, producing large suppurative abscesses resulting in deeper cystic lesions [5].

Gram-negative folliculitis has also been described in patients following recurrent staphylococcal pyoderma [6] as well as after long-term topical antibacterial therapy [8]. Batholow and Maibach described a patient with acne who was treated with topical clindamycin followed by benzoyl peroxide and erythromycin and subsequently developed gram-negative folliculitis secondary to *E. coli* [8].

7.4 Work-Up

Gram-negative folliculitis is most often diagnosed based on history and physical examination alone. However, confirmation with gram stain and culture is recommended. Correct sampling is essential for the proper diagnosis of gram-negative folliculitis. Swabs for bacteriological analysis should be taken from pustules and from the nasal mucosa. The pustule that is sampled should be fresh and preferably on an erythematous base. Gram-negative organisms are sensitive to desiccation and thus samples must be taken rapidly and transported to the laboratory as soon as possible.

It is recommended to culture pustules in any patient with acne who is in their late teens or older and develops a pustular eruption while on antibiotics. It is important to note that gram-negative organisms are not recoverable from every pustule. Selective medium-containing dyes such as methylene blue allow selective growth of gram-negative organisms while inhibiting the growth of gram-positive organisms.

Inadequate sampling, dried-out swabs, and long delay between culturing the pustules/nasal mucosa and the arrival of the specimen in the laboratory may lead to an underestimation of the frequency of gram-negative folliculitis in patients with acne and/or rosacea [9].

7.5 Treatment

Oral isotretinoin is considered to be first-line therapy for gram-negative folliculitis. While culture-directed antibiotics may be tried, they are frequently unsuccessful [9–11]. The effectiveness of isotretinoin has been attributed to its ability to decrease sebaceous gland secretion by 90 % or more [12]. This dries the skin and mucous membranes creating a poor environment for gram-negative bacteria growth. Isotretinoin should be administered at a dose of 0.5–1 mg/kg daily for 4–5 months [5, 9]. Higher doses in excess of 2.0 mg/kg are not superior to lower doses; in fact, the most effective dose with the fewest relapses was shown to be 1 mg/kg [2]. In a subset of patients with recurrent acne lesions and relapses of gram-negative rods, oral antibiotics may be combined with isotretinoin [13].

References

1. Fulton Jr JE, McGinley K, Leyden J, Marples R. Gram-negative folliculitis in acne vulgaris. Arch Dermatol. 1968;98:349–53.
2. Neubert U, Jansen T, Plewig G. Bacteriologic and immunologic aspects of gram-negative folliculitis: a study of 46 patients. Int J Dermatol. 1999;38:270–4.
3. Esterly NB, Koransky JS, Furey NL, Trevisan M. Neutrophil chemotaxis in patients with acne receiving oral tetracycline therapy. Arch Dermatol. 1984;120:1308–13.
4. Bottone EJ, Perez 2nd AA, Oeser JL. Loofah sponges as reservoirs and vehicles in the transmission of potentially pathogenic bacterial species to human skin. J Clin Microbiol. 1994;32:469–72.
5. Leyden JJ, Marples RR, Mills Jr OH, Kligman AM. Gram-negative folliculitis—a complication of antibiotic therapy in acne vulgaris. Br J Dermatol. 1973;88:533–8.
6. Chastain MA. A cycle: recurrent gram-negative folliculitis with Citrobacter diversus (koseri) following eradication of recurrent staphylococcal pyoderma. Arch Dermatol. 2000;136:803.

7. Mostafa WZ. Citrobacter freundii in gram-negative folliculitis. J Am Acad Dermatol. 1989; 20:504–5.
8. Bartholow P, Maibach HI. Gram-negative folliculitis without systemic antibiotics? Arch Dermatol. 1979;115:676.
9. Boni R, Nehrhoff B. Treatment of gram-negative folliculitis in patients with acne. Am J Clin Dermatol. 2003;4:273–6.
10. James WD, Leyden JJ. Treatment of gram-negative folliculitis with isotretinoin: positive clinical and microbiologic response. J Am Acad Dermatol. 1985;12:319–24.
11. Plewig G, Nikolowski J, Wolff HH. Action of isotretinoin in acne rosacea and gram-negative folliculitis. J Am Acad Dermatol. 1982;6:766–85.
12. Landthaler M, Kummermehr J, Wagner A, Plewig G. Inhibitory effects of 13-cis-retinoic acid on human sebaceous glands. Arch Dermatol Res. 1980;269:297–309.
13. Neubert U, Plewig G, Ruhfus A. Treatment of gram-negative folliculitis with isotretinoin. Arch Dermatol Res. 1986;278:307–13.

Chapter 8
Hot-Tub Folliculitis

Paula S. Malhotra and Joseph F. Fowler Jr.

8.1 Introduction

Hot-tub folliculitis is also known as *Pseudomonas aeruginosa* (*P. aeruginosa*) folliculitis. It is characterized by pruritic maculopapular and pustular lesions that have follicular accentuation and can manifest anywhere from 1 to 4 days after bathing in a hot tub, whirlpool, or public swimming pool [1–6]. Hot-tub folliculitis is an infection of the hair follicles that occurs after coming into contact with the bacteria *P. aeruginosa*, which thrives in a warm, wet environment. Diving suits have also been implicated in causing this form of folliculitis as the suits themselves have the potential to become colonized with *P. aeruginosa* [7].

8.2 Background

8.2.1 Pathophysiology

Pseudomonas aeruginosa is a ubiquitous gram-negative bacterial organism found in soil and freshwater that gains its entry through hair follicles or via breaks in the skin. Exposure to water colonized by *P. aeruginosa* leads to a follicular skin infection. Bacterial serotype O:11 is the most commonly reported isolate for water-associated

P.S. Malhotra, B.A., M.D. (✉)
Department of Dermatology, Northwestern University, Chicago, IL, USA
e-mail: paula.malhotra07@gmail.com

J.F. Fowler Jr., M.D.
Division of Dermatology, University of Louisville, 501 S Second Street,
Louisville, KY 40202, USA

J.A. Zeichner (ed.), *Acneiform Eruptions in Dermatology: A Differential Diagnosis*,
DOI 10.1007/978-1-4614-8344-1_8, © Springer Science+Business Media New York 2014

Pseudomonas folliculitis, but other serotypes have also been reported. Serotype O:11 is thought to be more invasive and better adapted to survive in halogenated water than the other serotypes, explaining the prevalence of this serotype in hot-tub folliculitis [8]. As water temperatures rise, free chlorine levels in the water fall, even though the total chlorine levels appear adequate. This provides an ideal environment in which the bacteria can proliferate. Hot water, high pH (>7.8), and low chlorine level (<0.5 mg/L) all predispose to an increased risk for infection.

8.2.2 Epidemiology

The actual incidence of Pseudomonas folliculitis is difficult to assess because of the transient nature of the disease [4]. Most cases of Pseudomonas folliculitis resolve without any adverse reactions or sequelae. There is no known racial or gender predilection.

8.3 Clinical Presentation

The onset of the rash of hot-tub folliculitis is usually 1–4 days after exposure to contaminated water. However, skin lesions can develop as early as 8 h after exposure and as late as 14 days later [9]. Most lesions begin as pruritic, follicular, erythematous macules that progress to papules and pustules. Individual lesions range in size from 2 to 10 mm in diameter and often demonstrate a central pinpoint vesiculopustule. The rash is most prevalent in the intertriginous areas or under bathing suits secondary to compression of contaminated water in those areas. It can also be seen on the trunk and extremities, where the skin is exposed to contaminated water. The face, neck, palms, and soles are usually spared [10]. Other associated complaints are minimal and include earache, sore throat, fever, and malaise. Systemic infections are rare. The rash usually clears spontaneously in 7–14 days without therapy, rarely recurs, and heals without scarring. Sometimes, it may cause desquamation or leave behind post inflammatory hyperpigmented macules which can resolve over time. The rash is not unique in appearance and is most often confused with insect bites.

8.4 Work-Up

The diagnosis of *P. aeruginosa* folliculitis is usually made clinically by obtaining the proper history and physical findings. It can be verified by obtaining bacterial culture results from either a fresh pustule or a sample of contaminated water. Biopsies of active lesions may show a lymphocytic inflammatory response around hair follicles.

8.5 Treatment

The folliculitis usually self-resolves within 7–14 days without therapeutic intervention. However, in patients who present with fever, constitutional symptoms, or prolonged disease, a third-generation cephalosporin or fluoroquinolone like ciprofloxacin or ofloxacin can be useful [11]. Proper maintenance and chlorination of pools, hot tubs, whirlpools, and spas are essential to decrease the population of *Pseudomonas* species. Showering after exposure to contaminated water does not seem to prevent *Pseudomonas* folliculitis.

References

1. Gregory DW, Schaffner W. Pseudomonas infections associated with hot tubs and other environments. Infect Dis Clin North Am. 1987;1(3):635–48.
2. Highsmith AK, Le PN, Khabbaz RF, Munn VP. Characteristics of Pseudomonas aeruginosa isolated from whirlpools and bathers. Infect Control. 1985;6(10):407–12.
3. McCausland WJ. Pseudomonas aeruginosa rash associated with whirlpool. JAMA. 1976; 236(22):2490–1.
4. Price D, Ahearn DG. Incidence and persistence of Pseudomonas aeruginosa in whirlpools. J Clin Microbiol. 1988;26(9):1650–4.
5. Ratnam S, Hogan K, March SB, Butler RW. Whirlpool-associated folliculitis caused by Pseudomonas aeruginosa: report of an outbreak and review. J Clin Microbiol. 1986; 23(3):655–9.
6. Rose HD, Franson TR, Sheth NK, Chusid MJ, Macher AM, Zeirdt CH. Pseudomonas pneumonia associated with use of a home whirlpool spa. JAMA. 1983;250(15):2027–9.
7. Lacour JP, el Baze P, Castanet J, Dubois D, Poudenx M, Ortonne JP. Diving suit dermatitis caused by Pseudomonas aeruginosa: two cases. J Am Acad Dermatol. 1994;31(6):1055–6.
8. Maniatis AN, Karkavitsas C, Maniatis NA, Tsiftsakis E, Genimata V, Legakis NJ. Pseudomonas aeruginosa folliculitis due to non-O:11 serogroups: acquisition through use of contaminated synthetic sponges. Clin Infect Dis. 1995;21(2):437–9.
9. Berger RS, Seifert MR. Whirlpool folliculitis: a review of its cause, treatment, and prevention. Cutis. 1990;45(2):97–8.
10. James W, Berger T, Elston D. Andrews' clinical dermatology. 9th ed. Elsevier, Philadelphia; 2000.
11. Böni R, Nehrhoff B. Treatment of gram-negative folliculitis in patients with acne. Am J Clin Dermatol. 2003;4(4):273–6.

Chapter 9
Malassezia Folliculitis

Patricia K. Farris and Andrea Murina

9.1 Introduction

Malassezia folliculitis, also referred to as Pityrosporum folliculitis, is an underdiagnosed condition that mimics acne vulgaris. This unique type of folliculitis affects the back, chest, and upper arms in healthy teenagers and young adults and can also be seen in patients with underlying immunosuppression. Malassezia folliculitis is caused by an overgrowth of Malassezia yeast that thrives in the sebaceous rich environment of the hair follicle. Direct microscopic examination with potassium hydroxide and skin biopsy can be used to identify the presence of yeast within the follicle thus confirming this often elusive diagnosis.

9.2 Background

The Malassezia genus of yeast is considered to be normal skin flora and is found in the stratum corneum and hair follicles of up to 90 % of individuals [1]. This lipophilic dimorphic yeast can be pathogenic and has been implicated in common skin disorders such as seborrheic dermatitis and pityriasis versicolor [2]. Malassezia folliculitis was first described by Weary et al. in 1969 as an acneiform eruption in the setting of antibiotic therapy with tetracyclines [3]. It is characterized as an invasion of hair follicles by large numbers of Malassezia yeast. Malassezia furfur,

P.K. Farris, M.D. (✉)
Department of Dermatology, Old Metairie Dermatology,
701 Metairie Road, Metairie, LA 70005, USA
e-mail: pkfarmd@gmail.com

A. Murina, M.D.
Department of Dermatology, Tulane University, 1430 Tulane Avenue
New Orleans, LA 70112, USA

J.A. Zeichner (ed.), *Acneiform Eruptions in Dermatology: A Differential Diagnosis*,
DOI 10.1007/978-1-4614-8344-1_9, © Springer Science+Business Media New York 2014

M. pachydermatis, and M. globosa are the predominant causative organisms [4]. This disease is often seen in healthy teens and young adults and is thought to be the result of follicular occlusion creating the sebaceous rich environment in which Malassezia thrives [5]. In this regard, the pathogenesis is similar to that of acne vulgaris. Staphylococcus and Propionibacteria can also be present in the follicles.

Although they are distinct clinical entities, acne vulgaris can occur concomitantly with Malassezia folliculitis. Sweeney et al. reported a series of adolescent girls who had traditional papules, pustules, and comedones of acne but also displayed monomorphic papules and pustules that were pruritic and flared during hot humid weather [6]. Potassium hydroxide examination of the latter showed Malassezia yeast and all patients responded to topical and systemic antifungal treatment.

Steroid acne seen after topical or systemic corticosteroid therapy has been associated with an overgrowth of Malassezia. A study looking at direct microscopic examination of material gathered using a comedo extractor from lesions of 34 patients with steroid acne demonstrated that 76 % were positive for Malassezia spores [7]. Treatment with itraconazole resulted in clinical improvement and reduced spore loads in these patients. The authors suggest that in view of these results, all patients with steroid acne should have a direct microscopic examination and/or biopsy to rule out colonization with Malassezia.

Likewise, Malassezia spores have been noted on biopsies of patients with clinical presentation consistent with eosinophilic pustular folliculitis [8, 9]. Similar to Malassezia folliculitis, eosinophilic pustular folliculitis (EPF) or Ofuji's disease is characterized by an intensely pruritic eruption of erythematous follicular papules. Histopathology of classic EPF shows a predominance of eosinophils and lack of organisms [9]. In contrast, biopsy specimens on patients with HIV-associated EPF may show both eosinophils and Malassezia indicating that Malassezia may play a role [8].

Malassezia yeasts have also been found in the acneiform eruption that occurs as a side effect of Cetuximab [10]. Acneiform folliculitis is a class effect of EGFR inhibitors [11]. It is believed that EGFR inhibition in the skin results in follicular occlusion by keratinocytes resulting in acneiform folliculitis. Both Staphylococcus and Malassezia have been reported in patients with this acneiform cutaneous reaction [10].

Finally, Malassezia folliculitis has a higher incidence in patients who are immunosuppressed [12, 13] as a result of conditions such as HIV [14], Hodgkin's disease [15], diabetes [13], and solid organ and bone marrow transplant recipients [16–18]. Patients on broad-spectrum antibiotics may also be more prone to the disease [3]. It is unknown exactly what immune mechanisms lead to the overgrowth of Malassezia yeast within the follicles. It has been hypothesized that the overgrowth of Malassezia in the follicles is favored by the lipophilic nature of the yeasts, diminished T cell function, and the decreased number of Langerhans cells that are present in the skin in immunocompromised patients [19]. There should be a low threshold to KOH or biopsy patients with acneiform eruptions and immunosuppression to evaluate for the presence of Malassezia yeast.

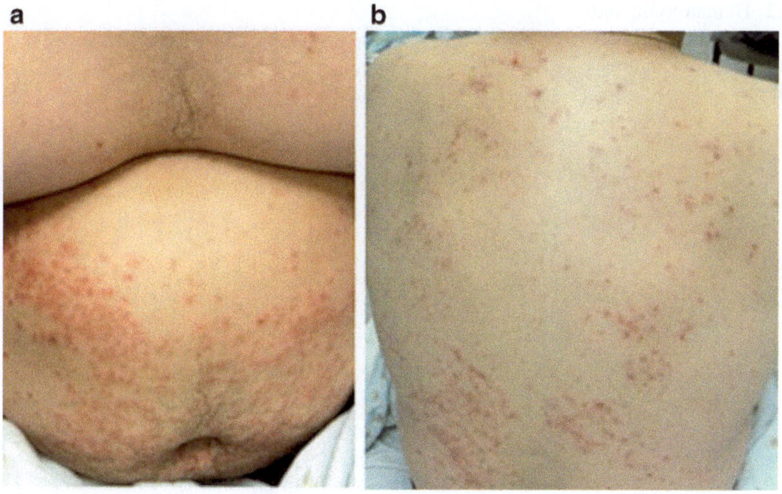

Fig. 9.1 (**a**, **b**) Malassezia folliculitis in a patient following broad-spectrum antibiotics

9.3 Clinical Presentation

Malassezia folliculitis is common in young to middle-age adults. Lesions can be asymptomatic or pruritic and are distributed on the back, chest, and upper arms [20, 21]. The most common presentation is monomorphic dome-shaped follicular papules with a central dell although in severe cases pustules, nodules and cysts may be present (Fig. 9.1). There are no comedones in Malassezia folliculitis which is an important differentiating point between this condition and chest and back acne. When the conditions coexist, the acne will usually be present on the face while the folliculitis occurs on the trunk and upper arms.

Malassezia folliculitis is more frequent in tropical climates due to effects of heat and humidity with a prevalence reported in the Philippines at 16.5 % [22]. In these environments, an atypical distribution can occur including spread to the face and cheeks.

9.4 Work-Up

Malassezia folliculitis should be suspected in patients who have papular lesions on the trunk and upper arms unresponsive to acne treatments, in those who have taken broad-spectrum antibiotics, or who are immunocompromised. Direct microscopic examination is preferable to culture since Malassezia is normal skin flora. The organisms can be seen on direct microscopic examination at high power (40×) when mounted with 10–15 % potassium hydroxide [23]. Examination of the follicular contents after

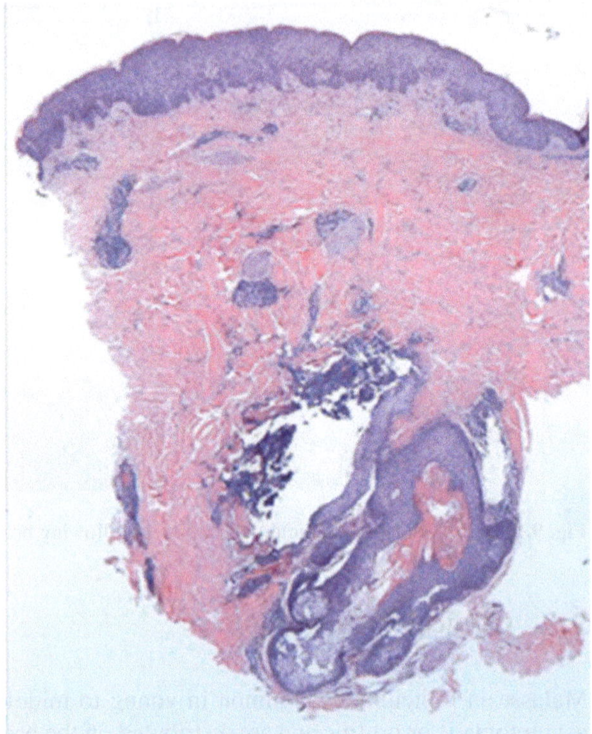

Fig. 9.2 Hematoxylin and Eosin stain showing focal inflammation surrounding the follicle

extraction with a comedo extractor may provide superior results to simple skin scrapings [7]. Biopsy specimens will show abundant round budding yeasts with occasional hyphae (Fig. 9.2). PAS stain can further highlight the organisms (Fig. 9.3). An inflammatory infiltrate surrounding the hair follicle consisting of lymphocytes, histiocytes, and neutrophils is seen on histology [24, 25]. This inflammatory response may be due in part to the fact that Malassezia yeasts have been shown to hydrolyze triglycerides into free fatty acids [21, 23, 24]. Hair follicles tend to be dilated, full of keratinous material, and may have focal rupture. The diagnosis can be made from clinical presentation, a positive direct microscopic examination, histopathology demonstrating yeast engorged hair follicles, and a positive response to antifungal treatment.

9.5 Treatment

Treatment of Malassezia folliculitis can be difficult due to the propensity for recurrence. Topical medications such as 2 % selenium sulfide lotion, 50 % propylene glycol in water, and 20 % sodium thiosulfate lotion are effective [20]. In a study of 26 cases, the cure rate with topical ketoconazole cream alone, oral ketoconazole

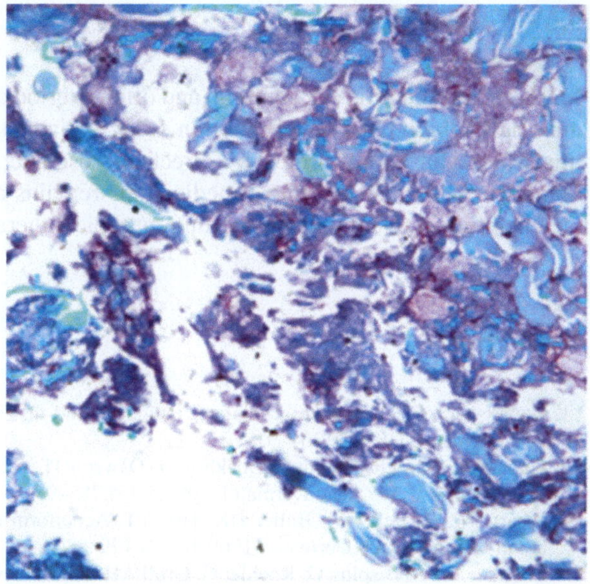

Fig. 9.3 PAS stain at 40× showing multiple spores within the follicle

alone, or topical plus oral ketoconazole was 12 %, 75 %, and 75 %, respectively, indicating the superior efficacy of systemic therapy [26]. Additionally, there was high rate of recurrence 3–4 months after therapy was discontinued even in those who received systemic therapy. Thus, it may be prudent to recommend the use of topical antifungal preparations periodically to prevent recurrences. Itraconazole, which is both lipophilic and keratophilic, is also effective in treating Malassezia folliculitis. In a double-blind placebo-controlled study, short-term itraconazole therapy (200 mg daily for 7 days) resulted in a negative direct microscopic KOH examination at 5 weeks in 84.6 % of patients compared to 8.3 % who received placebo [27]. Fluconazole has also been found to be effective [28].

Isotretinoin has been proposed as a treatment for Malassezia folliculitis in view of the fact that it reduces sebum secretion [29]. In a case report, 40 mg isotretinoin daily for 20 weeks (0.65 mg/kg/day) resulted in dramatic improvement of biopsy-proven Malassezia folliculitis. The authors note that condition reoccurred 10 months after discontinuation of the isotretinoin. In view of the temporary benefit and potential for adverse events, isotretinoin is not a favored treatment option in this condition.

For patients who are not candidates for oral antifungal medications or who have failed treatment, photodynamic therapy may be an option [30]. In a small study, six patients with recalcitrant Malassezia folliculitis were pretreated with methyl-5-aminolevulinic acid cream for 3 h followed by noncoherent red light using light-emitting diodes for 7.5 min. The patients received three treatments at 2-week intervals. Investigators note that four patients responded well to treatment, one patient responding slightly, while the other was considered a nonresponder. Although these results are preliminary, further studies are indicated to determine if photodynamic therapy might be beneficial for treating Malassezia folliculitis.

9.6 Conclusion

Malassezia folliculitis is a common and often overlooked condition. Dermatologists must have a high level of suspicion in order to diagnose this unique type of folliculitis which can be confirmed by direct microscopic examination or skin biopsy. Treatment with oral antifungal medications remains a mainstay of therapy, and it may be prudent to administer intermittent topical therapy to prevent recurrences.

References

1. Roberts SO. Pityrosporum orbiculare: incidence and distribution on clinically normal skin. Br J Dermatol. 1969;81:264–9.
2. Gupta AK, Batra R, Bluhm R, Boekhout T, Dawson TL. Skin diseases associated with malassezia species. J Am Acad Dermatol. 2004;51(5):785–98.
3. Weary PE, Russell CM, Butler HK, Hsu YT. Acneiform eruption resulting from antibiotic administration. Arch Dermatol. 1969;100(2):179–83.
4. Tragiannidis A, Bisping G, Koehler G, Groll AH. Minireview: Malassezia infections in immunocompromised patients. Mycoses. 2009;53:187–95.
5. Hill MK, Goodfield MJ, Rodgers FG, Crowley JL, Saihan EM. Skin surface electron microscopy in Pityrosporum folliculitis: the role of follicular occlusion in disease and the response to oral ketoconazole. Arch Dermatol. 1990;126:1071–4.
6. Sweeney K. Pityrosporum folliculitis: diagnosis and management in 6 female adolescents with acne vulgaris. Arch Pediatr Adolesc Med. 2005;159(1):64–7.
7. Yu H, Lee S, Son SJ, Kim YS, Yang HY, Kim JH. Steroid acne vs. pityrosporum folliculitis: the incidence of Pityrosporum ovale and the effect of antifungal drugs in steroid acne. Int J Dermatol. 1998;37(10):772–7.
8. Ferrandiz C, Ribera M, Barranco JC, Clotet B, Lorenzo JC. Eosinophilic pustular folliculitis in patients with acquired immunodeficiency syndrome. Int J Dermatol. 1992;31(3):193–5.
9. Nervi SJ, Schwartz RA, Dmochowski M. Eosinophilic pustular folliculitis: a 40 year retrospect. J Am Acad Dermatol. 2006;855(2):285–9.
10. Cholongitas E, Pipili C, Ioannidou D. Malassezia folliculitis presented as acneiform eruption after cetuximab administration. J Drugs Dermatol. 2009;8(3):274–5.
11. Duvic M. EGFR inhibitor-associated acneiform folliculitis. Am J Clin Dermatol. 2008; 9(5):285–94.
12. Archer-Dubon C, Icaza-Chivez M, Orozco-Topete R, Reyes E, Baez-Martinez R, de León SP. An epidemic outbreak of malassezia folliculitis in three adult patients in an intensive care unit: a previously unrecognized nosocomial infection. Int J Dermatol. 1999;38(6):453–6.
13. Yohn JJ, Lucas J, Camisa C. Malassezia folliculitis in immunocompromised patients. Cutis. 1985;35(6):536–8.
14. Fearfield LA, Rowe A, Francis N, Bunker CB, Staughton RC. Itchy folliculitis and human immunodeficiency virus infection: clinicopathological and immunological features, pathogenesis and treatment. Br J Dermatol. 1999;141(1):3–11.
15. Helm KF, Lookingbill DP. Pityrosporum folliculitis and severe pruritus in two patients with Hodgkin's disease. Arch Dermatol. 1993;129(3):380–1.
16. Rhie S, Turcios R, Buckley H, Suh B. Clinical features and treatment of malassezia folliculitis with fluconazole in orthotopic heart transplant recipients. J Heart Lung Transplant. 2000; 19(2):215–9.
17. Koranda FC, Dehmel EM, Kahn G, Penn I. Cutaneous complications in immunosuppressed renal homograft recipients. JAMA. 1974;229(4):419–24.

18. Bufill JA, Lum LG, Caya JG, Chitambar CR, Ritch PS, Anderson T, et al. Pityrosporum folliculitis after bone marrow transplantation. Ann Intern Med. 1988;108(4):560.
19. Gueho EF, Faegemann J, Lyman C, Anaissie EJ. Malassezia and Trichosporin: two emerging pathogenic basidiomycetous yeast-like fungi. J Med Vet Mycol. 1994;32:367–78.
20. Bäck O, Faergemann J, Hörnqvist R. Pityrosporum folliculitis: a common disease of the young and middle-aged. J Am Acad Dermatol. 1985;12(1, Part 1):56–61.
21. Faergemann J, Johansson S, Back O, Scheynius A. An immunologic and cultural study of pityrosporum folliculitis. J Am Acad Dermatol. 1986;14(3):429–33.
22. Jacinto-Jamora S, Tamesis J, Katigbak ML. Pityrosporum folliculitis in the philippines: diagnosis, prevalence, and management. J Am Acad Dermatol. 1991;24(5 Pt 1):693–6.
23. Potter BS, Burgoon Jr CF, Johnson WC. Pityrosporum folliculitis: report of seven cases and review of the pityrosporum organism relative to cutaneous disease. Arch Dermatol. 1973; 107(3):388–91.
24. Faergemann J, Bergbrant I, Dohsé M, Scott A, Westgate G. Seborrhoeic dermatitis and pityrosporum (malassezia) folliculitis: characterization of inflammatory cells and mediators in the skin by immunohistochemistry. Br J Dermatol. 2001;144(3):549–56.
25. Sina B, Kauffman CL, Samorodin CS. Intrafollicular mucin deposits in pityrosporum folliculitis. J Am Acad Dermatol. 1995;32(5 Pt 1):807–9.
26. Levy A, Feuilhade de Chauvin M, Dubertret L, Morel P, Flageul B. Malassezia folliculitis: characteristics and therapeutic response in 26 patients. Ann Dermatol Venereol. 2007; 134:823–8.
27. Parsad D, Saini R, Negi KS. Short-term treatment of pityrosporum folliculitis: a double blind placebo-controlled study. J Eur Acad Dermatol Venereol. 1998;11(2):188–90.
28. Faergemann J. Treatment of pityriasis versicolor with a single dose of fluconazole. Acta Derm Venereol. 1992;72(1):74–5.
29. Friedman SJ. Pityrosporum folliculitis: treatment with isotretinoin. J Am Acad Dermatol. 1987;16:632–3.
30. Lee J, Kim B, Kim M. Photodynamic therapy: new treatment for recalcitrant malassezia folliculitis. Lasers Surg Med. 2010;42(2):192–6.

Chapter 10
Tinea Barbae

Lauren Kole and Boni Elewski

10.1 Introduction

Tinea barbae is an uncommon dermatophytosis of the beard and moustache areas with invasion of coarse hairs; thus, it is a condition almost exclusively found in adult males [1]. Historically, tinea barbae was frequently transmitted by barbers using contaminated razors before single-use razors became readily available. Currently, in most cases, the causative organisms are zoophilic ectothrix, namely, *Trichophyton mentagrophytes* and *Trichophyton verrucosum*, acquired from animals. The clinical presentation is variable and may be severe with intense inflammation or superficial and less inflammatory, similar to tinea corporis [2]. Diagnosis typically relies on clinical presentation with confirmatory mycological culture [3]. The treatment of tinea barbae requires oral antifungal therapy [2].

10.2 Background

Tinea barbae is most frequently seen in tropical countries with high temperatures and high humidity. The incidence has decreased in recent years due to the increased availability of disposal razors, as the infection was regularly transmitted by barbers using unsanitary razors. Today, tinea barbae is more often found among rural inhabitants exposed to zoophilic dermatophytes from sources such as cattle, horses, cats, and dogs (Table 10.1). The species commonly isolated include *T. mentagrophytes* and *T. verrucosum*. *Microsporum canis* and *T. mentagrophytes* var. *erinacei* are less common. In certain geographic regions, other anthropophilic dermatophytes,

L. Kole, M.D. (✉) • B. Elewski, M.D.
Department of Dermatology, University of Alabama, Birmingham, 414 CEFH, 1720 2nd Avenue South, Birmingham, AL 35294, USA
e-mail: kole.lauren@gmail.com; beelewski@gmail.com

J.A. Zeichner (ed.), *Acneiform Eruptions in Dermatology: A Differential Diagnosis*, DOI 10.1007/978-1-4614-8344-1_10, © Springer Science+Business Media New York 2014

Table 10.1 Zoophilic etiologies of tinea barbae and their animal sources

Zoophilic dermatophytes	Animal sources
Trichophyton mentagrophytes	Rodents
Trichophyton verrucosum	Cattle and horses
Microsporum canis	Dogs and cats
Trichophyton mentagrophytes var. *erinacei*	Hedgehogs

Trichophyton schoenleinii, *Trichophyton violaceum*, and *Trichophyton megninii*, are endemic and can cause tinea barbae [2]. Recently, there have been several case reports of *Trichophyton rubrum* infections caused by autoinoculation from onychomycosis and tinea pedis [4, 5].

10.3 Clinical Presentation

Tinea barbae, as the name suggests, is a dermatophyte infection of the bearded areas of the face and neck of adult males [1]. The clinical presentation maybe either one of two types: inflammatory or noninflammatory, depending on the infecting fungus and the patient's immune response. The zoophilic dermatophyte infections typically cause severe, deep inflammation, characterized commonly by inflammatory nodules and multiple follicular pustules [4]. Abscesses, sinus tracts, kerion-like plaques, and bacterial superinfections may also occur. Furthermore, patients may have constitutional symptoms such as malaise and lymphadenopathy. The involved hairs can become loose or broken, and this variety of tinea barbae may lead to permanent, scarring alopecia [2].

The second type of tinea barbae is clinically similar to tinea corporis, as it is superficial and less inflammatory and is usually caused by *T. rubrum*. The characteristic lesion is an annular, erythematous plaque with an active, papular border (Fig. 10.1). Vesicles and overlying crust are other features that are not uncommon. Reversible alopecia in the center of the lesion may also be present [5].

A third variant of chronic tinea barbae may present similar to sycosis (inflammation of the hair follicles), with papules and pustules in a follicular distribution [4]. The differential diagnosis of tinea barbae includes bacterial folliculitis, pseudofolliculitis barbae, atypical rosacea, periorbital dermatitis, acne vulgaris, cervicofacial actinomycosis, and viral infections such as herpes simplex or herpes zoster [6].

10.4 Work-up

Tinea barbae is typically diagnosed by a combination of clinical presentation and confirmatory laboratory tests. In the clinic, a quick potassium hydroxide test may be performed with direct microscopic fungal element visualization sampled

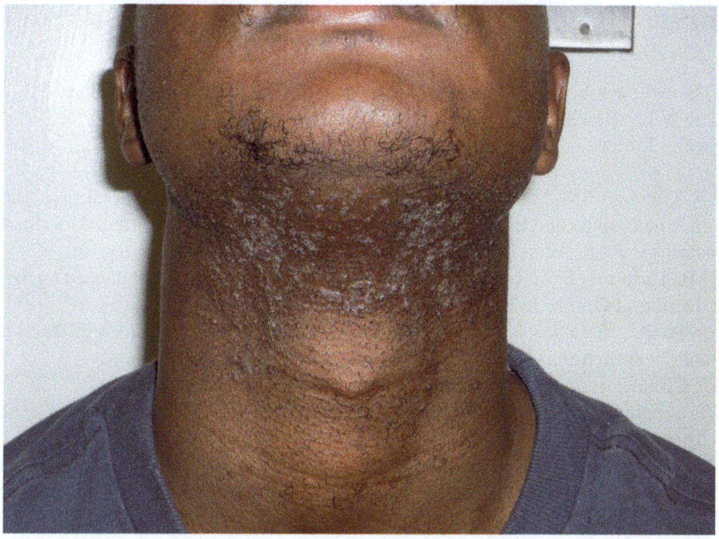

Fig. 10.1 Scaly papules affecting the skin within the beard of the anterior neck of a young man. Fungal culture revealed *Trichophyton* species (Photo credit: Joshua A. Zeichner, M.D.)

from infected hair and pustules. The dermatophyte Microsporum canis may also be visualized with Wood's light, and a biopsy can be diagnostic as well. Fungal culture is performed on agar with cycloheximide to identify the causative organism [7].

10.5 Treatment

Tinea barbae should be treated with systemic antifungal therapy, as these drugs are able to penetrate the infected hair shaft, whereas topical therapies cannot. Debridement and shaving of the affected hairs is also recommended [2]. Griseofulvin up to 1 g daily, FDA approved for the treatment of tinea capitis, is dosed daily for 6–12 weeks [8]. However, some authors advocate a 4-week course of terbinafine 250 mg daily [7]. Terbinafine should not be the first line of therapy if the causative organism is unknown, as *M. canis* is resistant to terbinafine. Treatment with itraconazole 200 mg or fluconazole 200 mg daily for 4–6 weeks is also effective [2]. Adjuvant therapy with antifungal shampoos, such as ketoconazole 2 % shampoo and selenium sulfide 2.5 % shampoo, used at least three times weekly, will decrease shedding of the infectious fungal elements [9]. Furthermore, elimination of the source of the infection, whether by treatment of infected animals or treatment of onychomycosis, is very important [4].

References

1. Burns T, Breathnach S, Cox N, Griffiths C, editors. Rook's textbook of dermatology. 8th ed. San Francisco: Wiley-Blackwell; 2010.
2. Bolognia JL, Jorizzo JL, Rapini RP, editors. Dermatology. 2nd ed. St. Louis: Mosby Elsevier; 2008.
3. Drake LA, Dinehart SM, Farmer ER, et al. Guidelines of care for superficial mycotic infections of the skin: tinea capitis and tinea barbae. Guidelines/Outcomes Committee. American Academy of Dermatology. J Am Acad Dermatol. 1996;34:290–4.
4. Xavier MH, Torturella DM, Rehfeldt FVS, et al. Sycosiform tinea barbae caused by *Trichophyton rubrum*. Dermatol Online J. 2008;14:10.
5. Szepietowski JC, Matusiak L. *Trichophyton rubrum* autoinoculation from infected nails is not such a rare phenomenon. Mycoses. 2008;51:345–6.
6. Habif TP. Clinical dermatology. 5th ed. St. Louis: Mosby Elsevier; 2010.
7. Baran W, Szepietowski JC, Schwartz RA. Tinea barbae. Acta Dermatovenerol Alp Panonica Adriat. 2004;13:91–4.
8. Gupta AK, Dlova N, Taborda P, et al. Once weekly fluconazole is effective in children in the treatment of tinea capitis: a prospective, multicenter study. Br J Dermatol. 2000;142:965–8.
9. Elewski BE. Treatment of tinea capitis: beyond griseofulvin. J Am Acad Dermatol. 1999; 40:S27–30.

Chapter 11
Flat Warts

Ted Rosen and Sara Risner-Rumohr

11.1 Introduction

Verruca plana, or flat warts, are virally induced papules caused by the human papillomavirus (HPV) that can mimic a closed comedone or an acneiform papule. This chapter will discuss the etiology, risk factors, diagnosis, and treatment of flat warts. Table 11.1 summarizes the similarities and differences between flat warts and acne.

11.2 Background

HPV includes greater than 100 genotypes of a double-stranded DNA virus [1]. Cutaneous HPV types comprise a group of viruses that infect the skin and induce common warts, palmar and plantar warts, flat warts, and butcher's warts. Classification of warts is based upon morphology, anatomic localization, and HPV typing.

Common warts are hyperkeratotic, exophytic papules, or nodules typically associated with HPV-1, HPV-2, or HPV-4 [2]. They are most commonly located on fingers, the dorsal surfaces of hands, and other sites prone to trauma. They typically spare the face but can occur at any anatomical location. HPV types 2, 27, and 57 caused the majority of palmoplantar warts [2]. Myrmecia are large, deep burrowing warts on the plantar surface caused by HPV-1. Most commonly, flat warts that have been analyzed by polymerase chain reaction (PCR) studies contain HPV-3 and, less often, types 10, 28, 29, and 41 [2–6].

T. Rosen, M.D. (✉) • S. Risner-Rumohr, M.D.
Department of Dermatology, Baylor College of Medicine,
1977 Butler Blvd, Suite E6.200, Houston, TX 77030, USA
e-mail: vampireted@aol.com; risner.rumohr@gmail.com

J.A. Zeichner (ed.), *Acneiform Eruptions in Dermatology: A Differential Diagnosis*,
DOI 10.1007/978-1-4614-8344-1_11, © Springer Science+Business Media New York 2014

Table 11.1 Similarities and differences between acne and flat warts

Features	Flat warts	Acne
Affected age group—childhood and young adult	Yes	Yes
Koebner phenomenon	Yes	Occasionally[a]
Follicular-based papules	No	Yes
Flat-topped papules	Yes	No
Virally induced	Yes	No
Ultraviolet light influenced	Yes—worsened	Yes—most often improved
Can heal with a scar	Occasionally[b]	Yes
Hormonally influenced	No	Yes
Cellular immunity related	Yes	No
Spontaneously resolve	Yes	Yes
Response to retinoid therapy	Yes	Yes

[a]Acne can be triggered by minor trauma/friction (e.g., acne mechanica)
[b]Treatments can lead to permanent scarring

The papillomavirus species-specific life cycle is completed only in fully differentiated human squamous epithelia. The infection and induction of hyperproliferation are initiated when the virus enters the basal layer [2]. Unlike other viruses, such as herpes simplex or molluscum contagiosum, HPV does not encode the enzymes required for the replication of viral DNA. HPV is dependent on the host's cellular machinery for replication. HPV proteins can amplify cell replication acting as viral oncoproteins. However, unlike the high-risk HPV infections located on mucosal surfaces, flat warts have not been linked to dysplasia and cancer [4].

Nongenital warts occur in 7–10 % of the general population, flat warts being the least common variant [6]. Children and young adults are primarily affected by flat warts [5–7]. Sun exposure appears to be a risk factor for flat warts, as the latent virus has the ability to induce lesions following after ultraviolet exposure [8]. Flat warts may also develop at sites of trauma (the Koebner phenomenon) as a result of autoinoculation. This may be clinically manifest as linear configurations. For example, men who shave their beards and women who shave their legs often exhibit this pattern [9]. The development of multiple warts has also been reported after tattooing [8, 10].

11.3 Clinical Presentation

Flat warts are 2–4 mm in diameter, slightly elevated, flat-topped, smooth papules (Fig. 11.1). They can be skin colored or slightly erythematous on pale skin and hyperpigmented on darker skin. They are generally multiple and grouped. The forehead, cheeks, and nose, perioral region, and dorsal hands are classic locations [9]. Hyperpigmented lesions may be confused with lentigines or ephelides. Skin-colored to erythematous lesions located on the central face may be confused with closed

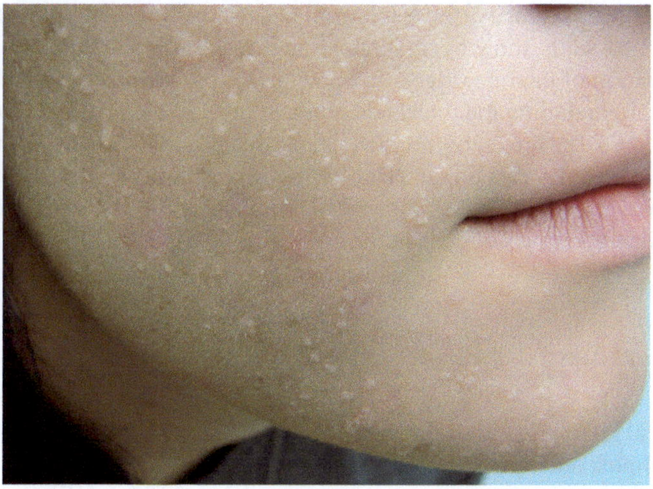

Fig. 11.1 Adolescent woman who presented for treatment of "acne" with typical facial flat warts

comedones or acneiform papules [9]. Filiform warts, a variant of common warts with characteristic frond-like projections, are often seen on the face but rarely cause diagnostic confusion [8].

11.4 Work-up

Multiple flat warts are commonly seen in healthy individuals but may also be a sign of a compromised immune system. When there is extensive involvement in an adult with no obvious risk factors, or in a treatment-refractory case, the patient's cellular immune function should be evaluated. Extensive flat warts have been reported in patients with human immunodeficiency virus infection (HIV) [11]. Widespread flat warts have also been reported in immune-reconstitution syndrome in HIV patients on HAART (Highly Active Anti-Retroviral Treatment) [12]. Similarly, the transplant population and primary immunodeficiency diseases, such as common variable immunodeficiency, severe combined immunodeficiency, Hyper-IgM, Hyper-immunoglobulin E syndrome, idiopathic CD4+ T-cell lymphocytopenia [13], and WHIM (warts, hypogammaglobulinemia, infections, and myelokathexis) [14] have a higher incidence of viral warts.

Epidermodysplasia verruciformis (EDV) is a rare, autosomal recessive disorder with widespread skin colonization by HPV. The clinical presentation is of disseminated flat warts or large pityriasis versicolor-like patches induced most commonly by HPV-3 and HPV-10 [15]. One-third to one-half of patients will develop squamous cell carcinoma, associated most frequently with HPV subtypes 5, 8, and 47 [2, 15].

A flat wart can be easily discerned from an acneiform lesion with a histological evaluation. Flat warts show hyperkeratosis and acanthosis, no papillomatosis, only slight elongation of the rete ridges, and no areas of parakeratosis. In the upper stratum malpighii, including the thickened granular layer, there is diffuse vacuolization of the cells [16]. The nuclei of the vacuolated cells lie at the centers of the cells, and some appear deeply basophilic. The dermis appears normal. In spontaneously regressing warts, there is often a superficial lymphocytic infiltrate in the dermis with exocytosis and apoptosis of cells in the epidermis [16].

11.5 Treatment

Of all clinical HPV infections, flat warts have the highest rate of spontaneous remission; they almost universally resolve without treatment over several months to years [9]. This makes evaluation of any treatment modality difficult [17]. Among immunosuppressed patients, the warts typically persist longer and are more resistant to treatment [11, 14].

Wart regression is probably the result of cell-mediated immune mechanisms, although the process is not completely understood [18]. Considerations related to treatment of flat warts include the patient's age, immune status, skin integrity, and potential cosmetic outcome. Despite the fact that a wide range of local treatments for nongenital cutaneous warts exists, there is only limited reliable evidence regarding the efficacy of various potential interventions [17]. Viral wart survival is based on evading the immune detection apparatus within the epidermis. Inflammation of the skin may stimulate a concurrent immunologic response against HPV. Keratolytics, such as many over-the-counter products containing with salicylic acid or prescription strength retinoids, are frequently used for flat warts. These cause chemical irritation and debridement of the wart's keratotic surface. In reality, topical salicylic acid products have the highest grade clinical evidence regarding their superiority to placebo [17]. Topical retinoids are potent keratolytics but also assist in the treatment of warts by the disruption of epidermal growth and differentiation, as well as via modest immunomodulatory effects. One study investigating tretinoin 0.05 % cream resulted in an 85 % clearance in a series of children with flat warts compared to 32 % spontaneous clearance in the controls [19]. Astringent chemicals such as trichloroacetic acid and cantharidin are also frequently used in the office setting. Cantharidin is a chemical derived from the blister beetle, *Cantharis vesicatoria*. When applied it causes dermal blistering and local necrosis. Responses are variable, and this material can cause scarring or spread of warts around the index, treated lesion. Podophyllin, topical 5 % 5-fluorouracil, and intralesional bleomycin are other topical therapies that have varying degrees of antimitotic effect; however, they tend to be more beneficial for mucosal lesions and exophytic warts.

Destructive techniques, such as curettage, electrodesiccation, laser therapy, photodynamic therapy, or cryotherapy using liquid nitrogen, have all been utilized with good results. Nonetheless, destructive techniques are considered second-line therapy as they carry the risk of scar formation and recurrence in or around the treatment site. This is especially true for smaller, less exophytic warts, such as verruca plana. Prolonged occlusive duct tape treatment followed by periodic manual debridement has been shown to be superior or at least comparable to cryotherapy for common warts but has not been reported for flat warts [20].

Many laser therapies have been employed. The carbon dioxide (CO_2) laser emits an infrared light emission (10,600 nm) that causes a nonselective thermal tissue destruction; the lost skin then heals by secondary intent [21]. The erbium:yttrium/aluminum/garnet (Er:YAG) emits an infrared light emission (2,940 nm) which is absorbed more efficiently by epidermal water, thus allowing for a more precise ablation and a smaller zone of thermal damage than the CO_2 laser [22]. No randomized studies on the efficacy of laser therapy for flat warts have been published. Infectious hazards have also been demonstrated for both laser and electrocoagulation, as HPV DNA has been identified in the vaporized laser plume [23]. Other laser therapies such as pulse dye laser have been used to selectively destroy the dilated capillaries within the warts, producing less pain and scarring than CO_2 laser. This technique has been utilized more for flat warts in children and for facial lesions in all ages due to a preferable safety profile [24].

Contact immunotherapy can be an effective treatment. Dinitrochlorobenzene diphenylcyclopropenone or squaric acid have been used as non-mutagenic sensitizers eliciting a contact allergy that theoretically concomitantly heightens the immune response against the virus. Intralesional immunotherapy has little role in flat warts due to their thin nature. A topical immune response modifier, imiquimod, has been FDA approved for external anogenital warts. Imiquimod has been shown to interact with Toll-like receptors 7 and 8, resulting in activation of cytokine secretion from monocytes/macrophages (including α-interferon, interleukin-12, and TNF-α), as well as stimulation of antigen-presenting dendritic cells [2, 25]. No randomized controlled studies have been performed with imiquimod cream at any of the available concentrations (5, 3.75, and 2.5 %) for the management of flat warts. Nonetheless, imiquimod has been widely utilized in children and for facial flat warts in all ages as it generally elicits less discomfort compared to many of the other available treatments. In 2006, the FDA approved an ointment extract of green tea (*Camellia sinensis*) containing 15 % sinecatechins for treatment of genital warts. No studies have been published to date regarding efficacy in flat warts, but it may well represent a novel topical approach for recalcitrant lesions [26].

Systemic therapies including garlic supplements (*Allium sativum*) have been shown to inhibit cellular proliferation of virally infected cells [27]. Oral cimetidine (20–40 mg/kg/day) and oral zinc sulfate supplementation (10 mg/kg/day) have been used in an attempt to enhance cell-mediated immunity [28, 29]. Systemic retinoids, both isotretinoin and acitretin, have been used for extensive flat warts. In immunocompromised patients (both EDV and HIV populations), systemic and 1–3 % topical cidofovir, an antiviral that inhibits DNA synthesis, has been used effectively [30].

A combination of therapies is often pursued due to the frequent resilience of warts. There is no single gold standard wart treatment. The specific treatment regimen should be individualized to the needs and desires of the patient and subsequently altered or modified based upon the clinical response obtained. With the exception of topical tretinoin, none of the typical repertoire of topical or systemic acne interventions would benefit flat warts.

References

1. de Villiers EM, Fauquet C, Broker TR, et al. Classification of papillomaviruses. Virology. 2004;324:17–27.
2. Kirnbauer R, Lenz P, Okun M. Human papillomavirus, Chapter 78. In: Bolognia JL, Jorizzo JL, Rapini RP, editors. Dermatology. 2nd ed. Philadelphia: Mosby-Elsevier; 2008. p. 1183–98.
3. Harwood CA, Spink PJ, Surentheran T, et al. Degenerate and nested PCR: a highly sensitive and specific method for detection of human papillomavirus infection in cutaneous warts. J Clin Microbiol. 1999;37:3545–55.
4. Pfister H. Chapter 8: Human papillomavirus and skin cancer. J Natl Cancer Inst Monogr. 2003;31:52–6.
5. Plasencia JM. Cutaneous warts: diagnosis and treatment. Prim Care. 2000;27:423–34.
6. Brentjens M, Yeung-Yue KA, Lee P, Tyring SK. Human papillomaviruses and warts, Chapter 142. In: Gorbach S, Bartlett J, Blacklow N, editors. Infectious diseases. 3rd ed. Philadelphia: Lippincott Williams & Wilkins; 2004. p. 1215–20.
7. Lebwohl MG, Rosen T, Stockfleth E. The role of human papillomavirus in common skin conditions: current viewpoints and therapeutic options. Cutis. 2010;86(5):Suppl 1–11.
8. Brajac I, Loncarek K, Stojnić-Sosa L, Gruber FJ. Delayed onset of warts over tattoo mark provoked by sunburn. J Eur Acad Dermatol Venereol. 2005;19:247–8.
9. James WD, Elston DM, Berger TG. Viral diseases, Chapter 19. In: Andrews GC, Domonkos AN, Arnold HL, Odom RB, editors. Andrews' diseases of the skin: clinical dermatology. 11th ed. Philadelphia: Saunders-Elsevier; 2011. p. 397–406.
10. Baxter SY, Deck DH. Tattoo-acquired verruca plana. Am Fam Physician. 1993;47:732.
11. Berger TG, Obuch ML, Goldschmidt RH. Dermatologic manifestations of HIV infection. Am Fam Physician. 1990;41:1729–42.
12. Iarikov D, Duke W, Skiest D. Extensive development of flat warts as cutaneous manifestation of immune reconstitution syndrome. AIDS Read. 2008;18:524–7.
13. Fischer LA, Norgaard A, Permin H, et al. Multiple flat warts associated with idiopathic CD4-positive T lymphocytopenia. J Am Acad Dermatol. 2008;58:S37–8.
14. Dotta L, Tassone L, Badolato R. Clinical and genetic features of warts, hypogammaglobulinemia, infections and myelokathexis (WHIM) syndrome. Curr Mol Med. 2011;11:317–25.
15. Patel T, Morrison LK, Rady P, Tyring S. Epidermodysplasia verruciformis and susceptibility to HPV. Dis Markers. 2010;29:199–206.
16. Xu X, Erickson L, Chen L, Elder DE. Diseases caused by viruses, Chapter 25. In: Elder DE, Elenitsas R, Johnson BL, Murphy GF, editors. Lever's histopathology of the skin. 10th ed. Philadelphia: Lippincott Williams & Wilkins; 2004. p. 637–66.
17. Gibbs S, Harvey I. Topical treatments for cutaneous warts. Cochrane Database Syst Rev. 2006;3, CD001781.
18. Aiba S, Rokugo M, Tagami H. Immunohistologic analysis of the phenomenon of spontaneous regression of numerous flat warts. Cancer. 1986;58:1246–51.
19. Kubeyunje EP. Evaluation of the efficacy and safety of 0.05% tretinoin cream in the treatment of plane warts in Arab children. J Dermatolog Treat. 1996;7:21–2.
20. Focht III DR, Spicer C, Fairchok MP. The efficacy of duct tape vs. cryotherapy in the treatment of verruca vulgaris. Arch Pediatr Adolesc Med. 2002;156:971–4.
21. Lauchli S, Kempf W, Dragieva G, et al. CO_2 laser treatment of warts in immunosuppressed patients. Dermatology. 2003;206:148–52.

22. Park JH, Hwang ES, Kim SN, Kye YC. Er:YAG laser treatment of verrucous epidermal nevi. Dermatol Surg. 2004;30:378–81.
23. Sawchuk WS, Weber PJ, Lowy DR, Dzubow LM. Infectious papillomavirus in the vapor of warts treated with carbon dioxide laser or electrocoagulation: detection and protection. J Am Acad Dermatol. 1989;21:41–9.
24. Vargas H, Hove CR, Dupree ML, Milliams EF. The treatment of facial verrucae with pulsed dye laser. Laryngoscope. 2002;112:1573–6.
25. Gaspari A, Tyring SK, Rosen T. Beyond a decade of 5% imiquimod topical therapy. J Drugs Dermatol. 2009;8:467–74.
26. Viera MH, Amini S, Huo R, et al. Herpes simplex virus and human papillomavirus genital infections: new and investigational therapeutic options. Int J Dermatol. 2010;49:733–49.
27. Seki R, Tsuji K, Hayato Y, et al. Garlic and onion oils inhibit proliferation and induce differentiation of HL-60 cells. Cancer Lett. 2000;160:29–35.
28. Al-Gurairi FT, Al-Waiz M, Sharquie KE. Oral zinc sulphate in the treatment of recalcitrant viral warts: randomized placebo-controlled clinical trial. Br J Dermatol. 2002;146:423–31.
29. Rogers CJ, Gibney MD, Siegfried EC, et al. Cimetidine therapy for recalcitrant warts in adults: is it any better than placebo? J Am Acad Dermatol. 1999;41:123–7.
30. Grone D, Treudler R, de Villiers EM, et al. Intravenous cidofovir treatment for recalcitrant warts in the setting of a patient with myelodysplastic syndrome. J Eur Acad Dermatol Venereol. 2006;20:202–5.

Chapter 12
Molluscum Contagiosum

Yvonne Clark and Lawrence F. Eichenfield

12.1 Introduction

Molluscum contagiosum is a benign cutaneous and mucosal viral infection manifested by dome-shaped flat-topped papules with occasional nodules. Molluscum contagiosum can be seen at any age but predominantly affects children. Molluscum lesions are spread by direct skin to skin contact with fomites, and fomite facilitators can include shaving, tattoos, electrolysis, and bath towels. The incubation period is quite variable, most commonly ranging from 2 to 7 weeks, while in some cases, the latency period can be as long as 6 months after exposure. The process of identifying initial infection can be difficult. Molluscum may be spread through sexual contact as in more commonly seen in young adults and individuals with decreased immunity, including human immunodeficiency virus (HIV) or acquired immune deficiency syndrome (AIDS), or those receiving immunosuppressive therapy. Molluscum contagiosum in neonates and infants is rare, presumably as a result of maternal antibodies [1, 2].

Y. Clark, MPAS-C
Department of Dermatology, Sharp Rees-Stealy, La Mesa, CA, USA
e-mail: Yvonne.clark@sharp.com

L.F. Eichenfield, M.D. (✉)
Division of Pediatric and Adolescent Dermatology, Rady Children's Hospital, San Diego, 8010 Frost Street, Suite 620, San Diego, CA 92123, USA
e-mail: leichenfield@ucsd.edu

J.A. Zeichner (ed.), *Acneiform Eruptions in Dermatology: A Differential Diagnosis*,
DOI 10.1007/978-1-4614-8344-1_12, © Springer Science+Business Media New York 2014

12.2 Background

Molluscum contagiosum is caused by the molluscum contagiosum virus, the sole member of the genus Molluscipoxvirus. It is a large double-stranded deoxyribonucleic acid virus constructed of a 190-kbp genome that encodes 163 proteins. Most of the proteins encoded by the molluscum genome do not illicit a virus–host interaction, differentiating it from another virus in the poxvirus family, variola, the causative agent of smallpox. Research in molluscum–host interactions is needed but has been hindered by the inability to grow molluscum contagiosum virus in tissue culture cells or animal models [3, 4].

The transmission through water and swimming pools remains controversial. It is unclear if transmission is due to swimming in contaminated water versus fomites used during swimming activities, including toys, kickboards, or towels [1]. The Center for Disease Control and Prevention recommends children with molluscum to cover all visible lesions with watertight bandages and to dispose of all bandages at home. The Center for Disease Control and Prevention also recommends "no sharing of toys, equipment or kickboards during swimming activities. Individuals with open sores should not go into swimming pools [5]." The American Academy of Pediatrics does not restrict children with molluscum contagiosum from attending day care, school, or swimming in public pools [6].

12.3 Clinical Presentation

Characteristic molluscoid lesions are pearly, flesh- to pink-colored dome-shaped papules that can be translucent ranging in size from 2 to 8 mm usually with a distinct white annular area in the center. Lesions can be umbilicated but this finding is not necessary for diagnosis (Fig. 12.1). Occasionally lesions may be much larger, up to several centimeters termed "giant molluscum." Significant erythema is common as a reactive eczematous dermatitis that is usually local but may generalize similar to a dermatophytid eruption. Rarely bacterial superinfection can occur with abscess formation. Most individuals present with more than 15 lesions in common areas like axilla, groin, popliteal fossa, genitals, and perianal due to rubbing, friction, and moisture. It is not uncommon to see ill-defined areas of erythematous patches and plaques surrounding molluscoid lesions known as "molluscum dermatitis." Autoinoculation from scratching pruritic skin spreads the virus to other areas of the body. Lesions can be seen in linear distribution (koebnerization) due to scratching and trauma [2].

Spontaneous resolution usually occurs but timing can vary. Significant erythema can be an indication of host immune response. The majority of infections clear within 6–12 months, but some cases can take years for complete clearance. Children with atopic dermatitis and those who are immunosuppressed have more widespread disease and a prolonged course [7].

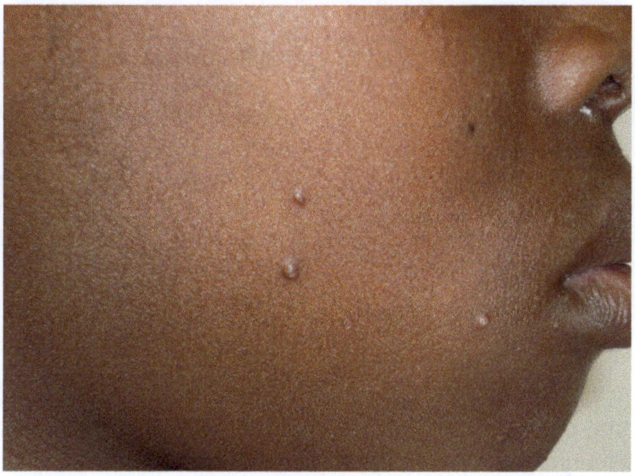

Fig. 12.1 Umbilicated, flesh-colored papules on the cheek of an adolescent boy. He presented to the office with a complaint of acne (Photo credit: Joshua A. Zeichner, M.D.)

12.4 Work-Up

Molluscum contagiosum is a clinical diagnosis requiring little to no work-up. Differential diagnosis includes warts (both flat and common), keratosis pilaris, xanthomas, and adnexal tumors [8]. Wright and Giemsa stains of cells from the core show intracytoplasmic basophilic bodies. Electron microscopy reveals typical poxvirus particles. Dermoscopy can visualize specific characteristic vascular patterns [9]. Biopsy may be necessary when the diagnosis is unclear, revealing large intracytoplasmic basophilic bodies that push the host nucleus to the periphery, giving a signet ring appearance to the superficial epidermal cells. Real-time polymerase chain reaction is available for homologous p43k and MC080R genes but rarely used [10]. Bacterial cultures may be considered for lesions with signs and symptoms of secondary bacterial infections.

12.5 Treatment

Treatment options include observation, destructive methods, and immune modulating modalities. Observation is a reasonable option since spontaneous resolution is common but due to cosmetic impact, pruritus, and concerns of others, teachers, school nurses, and other parents, treatment is often requested [1, 2].

Destructive methods include cantharidin, curettage, cryotherapy, tape stripping, topical tretinoin cream, 5–10 % potassium hydroxide and keratolytics such as salicylic acid and alpha hydroxyl acid, and pulse dye laser. Immune modulating therapies include oral cimetidine, intralesional candida antigen, topical imiquimod 5 % cream, and topical cidofovir [11, 12]. With a variety of therapy options

Table 12.1 Clinical pearls

Facial lesions	Topical tretinoin 0.025 % cream, caution with irritation and sun sensitivity
Body lesions	Cantharidin with 4 h wash off. Do not occlude lesions
Extensive facial and/or body lesions >50	Oral cimetidine 35–40 mg/kg/day for 6–12 weeks. Side effects: headaches, diarrhea, nausea, inhibitor of cytochrome P450, intolerable taste (solution formulation)
Adults, older children or teenagers	Cryotherapy (caution post inflammatory pigment changes and scarring) or
	Intralesional candida antigen (localized erythema and pain)

available, patient's age, pain tolerance, and accessibility to clinic should be taken into consideration when choosing a remedy. Destructive methods can be painful to younger children but well tolerated in older children and adults. To date there are no standard treatment protocols or reliable evidence-based recommendations for treating molluscum contagiosum [13].

The most commonly utilized treatment amongst pediatric dermatologist is cantharidin [14]. Cantharidin has been available and used to treat molluscum since 1950. Cantharidin is derived from the blistering beetle, *Cantharis vesicatoria*, and causes vesiculation of the epidermis. Application in office by a physician or other qualified and well-trained professional is recommended. Side effects include blistering, temporary burning, localized pain, erythema, and pruritus. Occlusion of treated areas is not recommended and a typical wash-off period can range from 2 to 6 h or sooner if blistering or discomfort is noted. Cantharidin is a powerful toxin that should not be ingested or absorbed; therefore application to mucosal areas is not recommended. Cantharidin generally is not used on the face or on occluded areas such as under a diaper [15]. Facial lesions may be treated with topical tretinoin cream. Systemic therapy with oral cimetidine has been advocated by some as monotherapy or in conjunction with cantharidin for extensive lesions or recalcitrant lesions to cantharidin, though there is a minimal evidence to support its utility (Table 12.1).

References

1. Braue A, Ross G, Varigos G, Kelly H. Epidemiology and impact of childhood molluscum contagiosum: a case series and critical review of the literature. Pediatr Dermatol. 2005;22:287–94. doi:10.1111/j.1525-1470.2005.22401.x.
2. Paller A, Mancini AJ. Molluscum contagiosum. Hurwitz clinical pediatric dermatology: a textbook of skin disorders of childhood and adolescence. Philadelphia, PA: Elsevier Saunders; 2006. p. 412–5.
3. Senkevich TG, Bugert JJ, Sisler JR, Koonin EV, Darai G, Moss B. Genome sequence of a human tumorigenic poxvirus: prediction of specific host response-evasion genes. Science. 1996;273(5276):813–6.
4. King AMQ, Adams MJ, Carstens EB, Lefkowitz EJ, editors. Virus taxonomy: classification and nomenclature of viruses: Ninth Report of the International Committee on Taxonomy of Viruses. San Diego: Elsevier Academic; 2011.

5. Homepage | CDC Molluscum Contagiosum. Centers for Disease Control and Prevention. 2011. Web 11 Dec 2011. http://www.cdc.gov/ncidod/dvrd/molluscum/.
6. American Academy of Pediatrics. Summaries of infectious disease. In: Pickering LK, Baker CJ, Kimberlin DW, Long SS, editors. Red Book: 2009 Report of the committee on infectious diseases. 28th ed. Elk Grove Village, IL: American Academy of Pediatrics; 2009. p. 466.
7. Dohil M, Lin P, Lee J, Lucky A, Paller A, Eichenfield L. The epidemiology of molluscum contagiosum in children. J Am Acad Dermatol. 2006;54(1):47–54.
8. Krishnamurthy J, Nagappa DK. The cytology of molluscum contagiosum mimicking skin adnexal tumor. J Cytol. 2010;27(2):74.
9. Ianhez M, Sda Cestari C, Enokihara MY, Seize MB. Dermoscopic patterns of molluscum contagiosum: a study of 211 lesions confirmed by histopathology. An Bras Dermatol. 2011;86(1):74–9.
10. Trama JP, Adelson ME, Mordechai E. Identification and genotyping of molluscum contagiosum from genital swab samples by real-time PCR and pyrosequencing. J Clin Virol. 2007; 40(4):325–9.
11. Maronn M, Salm C, Lyon V, Galbraith S. One-year experience with Candida antigen immunotherapy for warts and molluscum. Pediatr Dermatol. 2008;25:189–92. doi:10.1111/j.1525-1470.2008.00630.x.
12. Enns LL, Evans MS. Intralesional immunotherapy with *Candida* antigen for the treatment of molluscum contagiosum in children. Pediatr Dermatol. 2011;28:254–8. doi:10.1111/j.1525-1470.2011.01492.x.
13. van der Wouden JC, van der Sande R, van Suijlekom-Smit LWA, Berger M, Butler CC, Koning S. Interventions for cutaneous molluscum contagiosum. Cochrane Database Syst Rev. 2009;4, CD004767. doi:10.1002/14651858.CD004767.pub3.
14. Coloe J, Morrell DS. Cantharidin use among pediatric dermatologists in the treatment of molluscum contagiosum. Pediatr Dermatol. 2009;26:405–8. doi:10.1111/j.1525-1470.2008.00860.x.
15. Silverberg N, Sidbury R, Mancini AJ. Childhood molluscum contagiosum: experience with cantharidin therapy in 300 patients. J Am Acad Dermatol. 2000;43(3):503–7.

Chapter 13
Herpes Simplex Virus

Rachel Gordon and Stephen Tyring

13.1 Introduction

Our understanding of human herpes simplex virus (HSV) has increased tremendously since the early descriptions of disease provided by Hippocrates [1, 2]. Notable advances include the correlation of herpetic lesions with genital infections in the eighteenth century [3] and Vidal's recognition of human-to-human transmission in 1893 [2]. Antigenic differences between HSV subtypes, suspected on clinical observations by Lipschitz [4], were confirmed in 1968 [5]. In modern day, there is successful antiviral treatment available for most HSV infections [6]. Insight into the viral life cycle and gene expression has been a driving force behind the development of antiviral treatment, including new vaccines and gene therapy [4].

13.2 Background

Transmission of HSV occurs when a mucosal surface or abraded skin in a seronegative individual comes into contact with virus. Viral replication at the site of primary infection is followed by retrograde axonal transportation of a virion to the dorsal ganglion cells where latency is established by another episode of viral replication [12]. Recurrent infections occur randomly, but there is a positive correlation with

R. Gordon, M.D. (✉)
Department of Dermatology, The University of Texas Medical School at Houston,
6655 Travis Street, Suite 600, Houston, TX 77030, USA
e-mail: Rachel.gordon@gmail.com

S. Tyring, M.D., Ph.D., M.B.A.
Department of Dermatology, The University of Texas at Houston, Houston, TX, USA
e-mail: styring@ccstexas.com

J.A. Zeichner (ed.), *Acneiform Eruptions in Dermatology: A Differential Diagnosis*,
DOI 10.1007/978-1-4614-8344-1_13, © Springer Science+Business Media New York 2014

stress, immunosuppression, UV light, fever, and tissue damage [4, 7]. The severity of the initial infection correlates with the chance of recurrence. Rarely, life-threatening infections occur in cases of severe immune compromise, pregnancy, and neonatal disseminated HSV. "Primary infections" are considered first-time events, but their occurrence in seropositive individuals indicates that latent infection can be established without prior symptoms [6].

HSV infections are ubiquitous, even in remote areas [8]. More than 57 % of the US population between the ages of 14 and 49 are seropositive for HSV1 [9]. Incidence correlates with age in a linear fashion, globally reaching 60–90 % in older adults [10]. HSV1 is most commonly transmitted in childhood and adolescence. The overall incidence of HSV1 is significantly higher than that of HSV2 [10], which occurs more commonly in women and in subpopulations with high-risk sexual behavior [4, 10]. Humans are the only reservoir for HSV infection, and there have been no reported animal vectors [4].

13.3 Clinical Presentation

13.3.1 Oropharyngeal and Orolabial HSV

Infections around the mouth are the most common sites and reservoirs of HSV. Primary infection is usually asymptomatic [11]. Symptomatic cases may include extensive orolabial vesiculo-ulcerative lesions, gingivostomatitis, fever, and localized lymphadenopathy [4]. Adolescents can present with acute pharyngitis and mononucleosis-like symptoms [12, 13]. Dehydration from poor oral intake is the most frequent reason for hospitalization [6].

The incubation period for HSV infections is 4 days on average, and clinical symptoms may persist for 2–3 weeks [4, 14]. Vesicles form within 1–2 days of prodromal symptoms, progress to ulcers in another 1–2 days, and heal within 8–10 days. Pain is most severe with the appearance of lesions [15]. The frequency of recurrences varies among individuals [4], but is estimated to occur in 20–40 % of adults [6], most commonly on the vermillion border. Viral shedding increases with active lesions [16], during episodes of the common cold, oral trauma, and false prodromes [17]. Shedding persists in the absence of symptoms in an estimated 7 % of the healthy population [18] (Figs. 13.1 and 13.2).

13.3.2 HSV Keratoconjunctivitis

Keratoconjunctivitis acquired during birth is usually caused by HSV2. Outside the neonatal period, it is usually caused by HSV1 [4]. These infections result in corneal scarring and vision loss [19] and are the second most common cause of corneal blindness in America [4]. Primary infections can be unilateral or bilateral. Presenting symptoms of pain, tearing, chemosis, and photophobia [6] are associated with

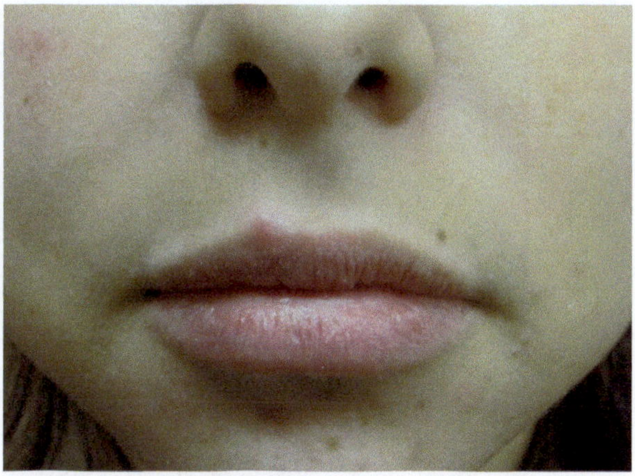

Fig. 13.1 Herpes labialis in early stage on the upper vermillion border

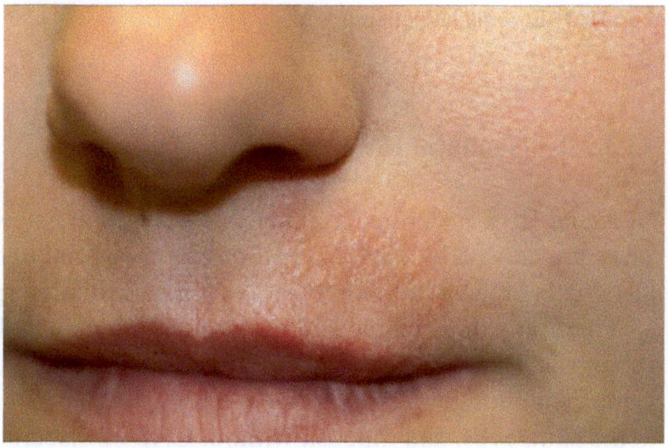

Fig. 13.2 Recurrent herpes labialis with nearby cutaneous involvement

periorbital edema and preauricular lymphadenopathy [1]. Corneal lesions with a branching dendritic pattern are pathognomonic [4]. Even with antiviral therapy, healing of the cornea can take up to a month [4, 6]. Approximately one-third of individuals experience a recurrence [1]; when they do occur, they are typically unilateral [4] and resolve over a period of weeks [4].

13.3.2.1 HSV in Immunocompromised Individuals

The degree of immune suppression correlates with the risk of developing HSV outbreaks. Organ transplant recipients and individuals with HIV/AIDS are at high risk for severe infections and frequent recurrences [4, 20]. The most frequent complication is progressive, chronic mucocutaneous infection with subsequent tissue necrosis [6]. Progressive disease involving the esophagus, respiratory, and gastrointestinal tract has been reported [4].

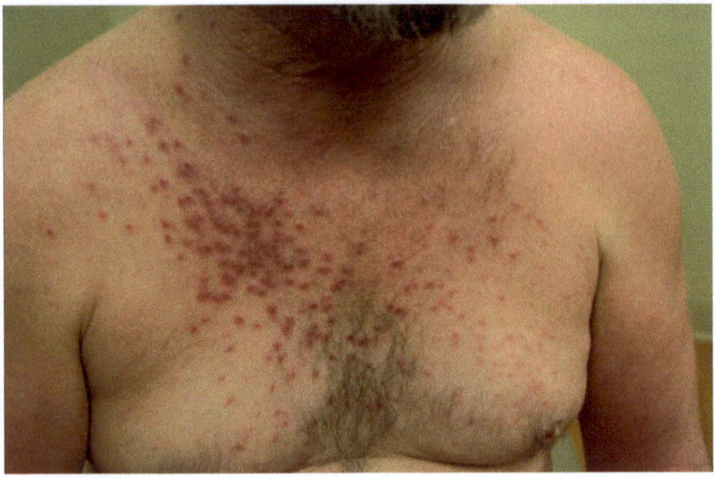

Fig. 13.3 Eczema herpeticum

13.3.2.2 Neonatal HSV

Neonatal HSV is defined as an HSV infection in a newborn within 28 days of birth. They are caused by viral exposure during vaginal delivery [21]. The risk of transmission is highest in mothers who acquire genital herpes near term [22].

There are three clinical presentations of neonatal HSV, each with a different prognosis. Because a rash is absent in 50 % of cases, all infants with CNS or sepsis symptoms should be evaluated for HSV. First, in 45 % of cases, infection is limited to the skin, eyes, and mucosa without CNS or visceral organ involvement. The vesicles that appear in these areas commonly recur in early childhood. Second, CNS involvement occurs in 30 % of cases; cutaneous signs are variable. Complications of CNS involvement include developmental delay, cognitive disabilities, blindness, and epilepsy. More than 50 % of children with HSV2 CNS infection have neurologic abnormalities. Finally, disseminated HSV occurs in 25 % of cases. It is indistinguishable from sepsis and has a 30 % mortality rate [21].

13.3.2.3 Miscellaneous HSV Infections

Individuals with a damaged epithelial barrier, most commonly from atopic dermatitis [23], are susceptible to eczema herpeticum. This presents as a vesiculopustular eruption in areas of underlying skin disease; lesions may erode and become secondarily infected. Recurrent episodes are generally less severe [24]. In wrestlers, herpes gladiatorum occurs in areas of close contact, usually the face and neck [25]. Facial HSV folliculitis presents as folliculocentric vesiculopapules and is confirmed histopathologically by HSV changes limited to the pilosebaceous unit [26] (Fig. 13.3).

13.4 Work-Up

Classically, detection is performed by viral culture in media that will show the HSV cytopathic effect, followed by typing with monoclonal antibodies [27, 28]. Viral swabs may be obtained from vesicles or other involved sites: oral mucosa, cerebrospinal fluid, or conjunctiva [4]. Polymerase chain reaction (PCR) has been the gold standard for diagnosing CNS infections and may become the standard test to diagnose HSV infections in other sites [29]. It has shown greater sensitivity than culture in detecting virus from oral [30] and genital lesions [31]. Serologic assays using enzyme-linked immunosorbent assay (ELISA) distinguish between HSV1 and HSV2 infections and detect infection in the absence of symptoms. Utilization of Western blot is restricted to research labs [4].

While not as sensitive as PCR [32], Tzanck smears allow for the cytopathologic detection of HSV. They are prepared by scraping the periphery of an ulcer, smearing the material on a glass slide, fixing immediately in cold ethanol, and then staining with Giemsa, Papanicolaou, or Wright stain [4]. Herpetic giant cells have multiple nuclei with molding and a ground-glass appearance, and intranuclear inclusion bodies [33]. Intranuclear inclusion bodies are not specific and may be seen in VZV infections as well [4]. Biopsy samples may show intraepidermal vesicles containing acantholytic keratinocytes with these cytologic changes [34] (Fig. 13.4).

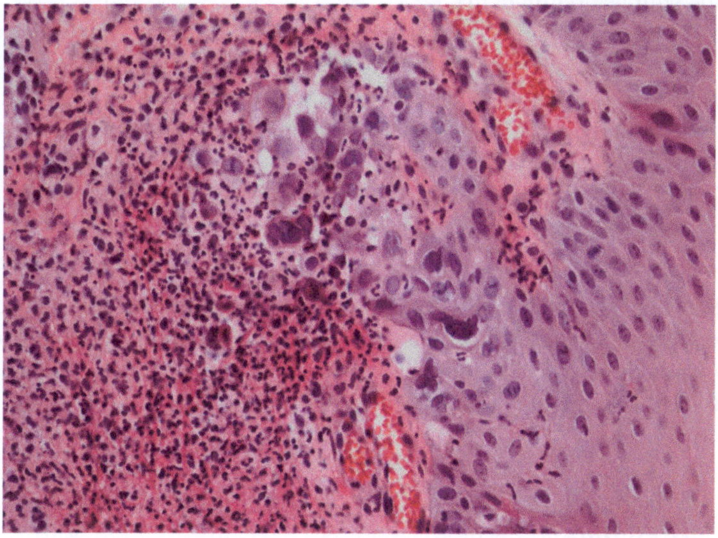

Fig. 13.4 HSV-infected cells with ground-glass nuclei, marginated peripheral chromatin, and a multinucleated giant cell with molding

13.5 Treatment

Most HSV infections are treated with acyclovir, its prodrug valacyclovir, and famciclovir (prodrug of penciclovir). These nucleoside analogues are activated by viral thymidine kinase and selectively inhibit viral DNA production by competing as substrate for DNA polymerase [6, 35].

13.5.1 Oropharyngeal and Orolabial HSV Infections

In moderate to severe primary disease in children, acyclovir 15 mg/kg five times per day for 7 days has been shown to decrease the duration of lesions from 10 to 4 days [11, 36]. Appropriate regimens for treatment of primary infections in adults include acyclovir 400 mg TID for 7–10 days, valacyclovir 1 g BID for 7–10 days, famciclovir 500 mg BID for 7 days, or 250 mg TID for 7–10 days [11, 37].

The ability to change the course of recurrent disease by administering antiviral therapy at the onset of symptoms has long been recognized [4, 15, 38]. Beginning treatment in this narrow therapeutic window is possible with patient-initiated episodic therapy, which reduces healing time to a greater extent than physician-initiated therapy [39]. First-line therapy in recurrent herpes labialis consists of famciclovir 1,500 mg once a day or valacyclovir 2 g twice daily for 1 day initiated at the first prodromal symptom [40, 41]. Suppressive treatment is not frequently practiced [40], but is effective at reducing recurrences [41, 42]. Valacyclovir 500 mg once daily is the simplest regimen [4].

Topical therapy includes docosanol 10 % cream (Abreva®) which demonstrated an 18-h reduced median time to healing in treated patients compared to placebo [43]. Penciclovir 1 % cream (Denavir®) and acyclovir 5 % cream (Zovirax®) both demonstrate therapeutic efficacy in early- and late-stage lesions [44].

13.5.2 HSV Keratoconjunctivitis

Trifluridine 1 % ophthalmic solution (Viroptic®) is the treatment of choice for primary and recurrent disease. Dosing is one drop every 2 h while awake (not to exceed nine drops per day). Once reepithelialization of the ulcer occurs, dosing continues at one drop every 4 h while awake for 7 days [4].

13.5.3 Mucocutaneous HSV in Immunocompromised Individuals

Acyclovir is effective in the prevention and treatment of HSV infections [4, 45]. For adults intravenous dosing is 5 mg/kg over 1 h, every 8 h for 7 days. In children, the dose is 250 mg/m^2 with the same schedule. For limited disease, topical 5 % acyclovir ointment can be used every 3 h for 7 days [4]. One recent review found no evidence that valacyclovir is more efficacious than acyclovir [45]. In patients with HIV, episodic treatment with famciclovir 500 mg BID for 7 days or valacyclovir 500 mg to 1 g BID for 7 days is appropriate. The same regimen can be used off-label for chronic suppressive therapy [4].

Antiviral-resistant herpes virus, usually secondary to mutations in viral thymidine kinase, is a special concern in this population as suppressive therapy has become standard. In such cases, treatment with the pyrophosphate analogue foscarnet and the nucleotide analogue cidofovir are appropriate [46]. Standard drug-sensitivity tests take more than 10 days for a result, but newer, faster methods are being developed [47].

13.5.4 Neonatal HSV

Intravenous acyclovir 20 mg/kg every 8 h for 14 days is recommended for disease restricted to the skin and mucosa. The same regimen is extended to 21 days for disseminated and CNS disease. The 14-day regimen is considered appropriate therapy for asymptomatic infants born to mothers who acquired HSV infection near term [21].

13.5.5 Miscellaneous HSV Infections

Without controlled studies, it is intuitive that primary and recurrent cutaneous infections may be treated with valacyclovir or famciclovir at doses used to treat primary and recurrent herpes genitalis [4]. Prophylactic use of valacyclovir (500 mg or 1 g once or twice daily) is effective at preventing recurrences of herpes gladiatorum during the wrestling season [48].

References

1. Beswick TS. The origin and the use of the word herpes. Med Hist. 1962;6:214–32.
2. Roizman B, Whitley RJ. The nine ages of herpes simplex virus. Herpes. 2001;8:23–7.
3. Hutfield DC. History of herpes genitalis. Br J Vener Dis. 1966;42:263–8.
4. Tyring SK, Yen-Moore A, Lupi O. Mucocutaneous manifestations of viral diseases. London: Informa Healthcare; 2010. p. 65–97.
5. Nahmias AJ, Dowdle WR. Antigenic and biologic differences in herpesvirus hominis. Prog Med Virol. 1968;10:110–59.
6. Arvin A, Roizman B, Whitley R, Mocarski E, Campadelli-Fiume G, Yamanishi K, editors. Human herpes-virus: biology, therapy & immunoprophylaxis. Cambridge: Cambridge University Press; 2007.

7. El Hayderi L, Raty L, Failla V, Caucanas M, Paurobally D, Nikkels AF. Severe herpes simplex virus type-I infections after dental procedures. Med Oral Patol Oral Cir Bucal. 2011; 16(1):e15–8.
8. Lin H, He N, Su M, Feng J, Chen L, Gao M. Herpes simplex virus infections among rural residents in eastern China. BMC Infect Dis. 2011;11:69.
9. Xu F, Sternberg MR, Kottiri BJ, McQuillan GM, Lee FK, Nahmias AJ, Berman SM, Markowitz LE. Trends in herpes simplex virus type 1 and type 2 seroprevalence in the United States. JAMA. 2006;296(8):964–73.
10. Smith JS, Robinson NJ. Age-specific prevalence of infection with herpes simplex virus types 2 and 1: a global review. J Infect Dis. 2002;186 Suppl 1:S3–28.
11. Wheeler Jr CE. The herpes simplex problem. J Am Acad Dermatol. 1988;18:163–8.
12. Glezen WP, Fernald GW, Lohr JA. Acute respiratory disease of university students with special reference to the etiologic role of Herpesvirus hominis. Am J Epidemiol. 1975;101(2):111–21.
13. McMillan JA, Weiner LB, Higgins AM, Lamparella VJ. Pharyngitis associated with herpes simplex virus in college students. Pediatr Infect Dis J. 1993;12(4):280–4.
14. Young SK, Rowe NH, Buchanan RA. A clinical study for the control of facial mucocutaneous herpes virus infections. I. Characterization of natural history in a professional school population. Oral Surg Oral Med Oral Pathol. 1976;41:498–507.
15. Spruance SL, Overall Jr JC, Kern ER, Krueger GG, Pliam V, Miller W. The natural history of recurrent herpes simplex labialis: implications for antiviral therapy. N Engl J Med. 1977; 297:69–75.
16. Daniels CA, LeGoff SG. Shedding of infectious virus/antibody complexes from vesicular lesions of patients with recurrent herpes labialis. Lancet. 1975;2:524–8.
17. Spruance SL. Pathogenesis of herpes simplex labialis: excretion of virus in the oral cavity. J Clin Microbiol. 1984;19(5):675–9.
18. Buddingh GJ, Schrum DI, Lanier JC, Guidry DJ. Studies of the natural history of herpes simplex infections. Pediatrics. 1953;11:595–610.
19. Simmons A. Clinical manifestations and treatment considerations of herpes simplex virus infection. J Infect Dis. 2002;186 Suppl 1:S71–7.
20. Shiley K, Blumberg E. Herpes viruses in transplant recipients: HSV, VZV, human herpes viruses, and EBV. Infect Dis Clin North Am. 2010;24:373–93.
21. Corey L, Wald A. Maternal and neonatal herpes simplex virus infections. N Engl J Med. 2009;361:1376–85.
22. Brown ZA, Selke S, Zeh J, Kopelman J, Maslow A, Ashley RL, et al. The acquisition of herpes simplex virus during pregnancy. N Engl J Med. 1997;337:509–15.
23. Mooney MA, Janniger CK, Schwartz RA. Kaposi's varicelliform eruption. Cutis. 1994;53: 243–5.
24. Kramer SC, Thomas CJ, Tyler WB, Elston DM. Kaposi's varicelliform eruption: a case report and review of the literature. Cutis. 2004;73:115–22.
25. Anderson BJ. The epidemiology and clinical analysis of several outbreaks of herpes gladiatorum. Med Sci Sports Exerc. 2003;35:1809–14.
26. Al-Dhafiri SA, Molinari R. Herpetic folliculitis. J Cutan Med Surg. 2002;6:19–22.
27. Scott DA, Coulter WA, Lamey PJ. Oral shedding of herpes simplex virus type 1: a review. J Oral Pathol Med. 1997;26:441–7.
28. Aarnaes SL, Peterson EM, de la Maza LM. Evaluation of a new herpes simplex virus typing reagent for tissue culture confirmation. Diagn Microbiol Infect Dis. 1989;12(3):269–70.
29. Strick LB, Wald A. Diagnostics for herpes simplex virus: is PCR the new gold standard? Mol Diagn Ther. 2006;10:17–28.
30. Tateishi K, Toh Y, Minagawa H, Tashiro H. Detection of herpes simplex virus (HSV) in the saliva from 1,000 oral surgery outpatients by the polymerase chain reaction (PCR) and virus isolation. J Oral Pathol Med. 1994;23:80–4.
31. Cone RW, Hobson AC, Palmer J, Remington M, Corey L. Extended duration of herpes simplex virus DNA in genital lesions detected by the polymerase chain reaction. J Infect Dis. 1991; 164:757–60.

32. Nahass GT, Goldstein BA, Zhu WY, Serfling U, Penneys NS, Leonardi CL. Comparison of Tzanck smear, viral culture, and DNA diagnostic methods in detection of herpes simplex and varicella-zoster infection. JAMA. 1992;268:2541–4.
33. Douglas D, Richman RJW, Hayden FG, editors. Clinical virology. Washington, DC: ASM Press; 2002.
34. Weedon D. Skin pathology. Edinburgh: Churchill Livingstone; 2002.
35. Derse D, Cheng YC, Furman PA, St Clair MH, Elion GB. Inhibition of purified human and herpes simplex virus-induced DNA polymerases by 9-(2-hydroxyethoxymethyl)guanine triphosphate. Effects on primer-template function. J Biol Chem. 1981;256:11447–51.
36. Amir J, Harel L, Smetana Z, Varsano I. Treatment of herpes simplex gingivostomatitis with aciclovir in children: a randomised double blind placebo controlled study. BMJ. 1997; 314(7097):1800–3.
37. Thomas Kreig DRB, Miyachi Y, editors. Therapy of skin diseases: a worldwide perspective on therapeutic approaches and their molecular basis. London: Springer; 2010.
38. Spruance SL, Schnipper LE, Overall Jr JC, Kern ER, Wester B, Modlin J, et al. Treatment of herpes simplex labialis with topical acyclovir in polyethylene glycol. J Infect Dis. 1982;146:85–90.
39. Reichman RC, Badger GJ, Mertz GJ, Corey L, Richman DD, Connor JD, Redfield D, Savoia MC, Oxman MN, Bryson Y, et al. Treatment of recurrent genital herpes simplex infections with oral acyclovir. A controlled trial. Treatment of recurrent genital herpes simplex infections with oral acyclovir. JAMA. 1984;251(16):2103–7.
40. Modi S, Van L, Gewirtzman A, Mendoza N, Bartlett B, Tremaine AM, Tyring S. Single-day treatment for orolabial and genital herpes: a brief review of pathogenesis and pharmacology. Ther Clin Risk Manag. 2008;4(2):409–17.
41. Rooney JF, Straus S, Mannix ML, Wohlenberg CR, Alling DW, Dumois JA, Notkins AL. Oral acyclovir to suppress frequently recurrent herpes labialis. A double-blind, placebo-controlled trial. Ann Intern Med. 1993;118(4):268–72.
42. Baker D, Eisen D. Valacyclovir for prevention of recurrent herpes labialis: 2 double-blind, placebo-controlled studies. Cutis. 2003;71(3):239–42.
43. Sacks SL, Thisted RA, Jones TM, Barbarash RA, Mikolich DJ, Ruoff GE, Jorizzo JL, Gunnill LB, Katz DH, Khalil MH, Morrow PR, Yakatan GJ, Pope LE, Berg JE, Docosanol 10% Cream Study Group. Clinical efficacy of topical docosanol 10% cream for herpes simplex labialis: a multicenter, randomized, placebo-controlled trial. J Am Acad Dermatol. 2001;45(2):222–30.
44. Spruance SL, Nett R, Marbury T, Wolff R, Johnson J, Spaulding T. Acyclovir cream for treatment of herpes simplex labialis: results of two randomized, double-blind, vehicle-controlled, multicenter clinical trials. Antimicrob Agents Chemother. 2002;46(7):2238–43.
45. Glenny AM, Fernandez Mauleffinch LM, Pavitt S, Walsh T. Interventions for the prevention and treatment of herpes simplex virus in patients being treated for cancer. Cochrane Database Syst Rev. 2009;1, CD006706.
46. Piret J, Boivin G. Resistance of herpes simplex viruses to nucleoside analogues: mechanisms, prevalence, and management. Antimicrob Agents Chemother. 2011;55:459–72.
47. Shiota T, Lixin W, Takayama-Ito M, Iizuka I, Ogata M, Tsuji M, et al. Expression of herpes simplex virus type 1 recombinant thymidine kinase and its application to a rapid antiviral sensitivity assay. Antiviral Res. 2011;91:142–9.
48. Anderson BJ. The effectiveness of valacyclovir in preventing reactivation of herpes gladiatorum in wrestlers. Clin J Sport Med. 1999;9:86–90.

Chapter 14
Varicella Zoster Virus

Rachel Gordon, Stephen Tyring, Whitney Lapolla, and Rana Mays

14.1 Introduction

Varicella zoster virus causes two clinical syndromes. Chicken pox, or varicella, is a self-limiting disease of childhood characterized by a highly pruritic rash. Shingles, or herpes zoster, is a reactivation of the virus typically seen in adults. Heberden first distinguished these illness as separate entities in 1767 [1], and Osler emphasized the distinction in his book on clinical medicine [2]. Their relation was suggested by von Bokay in 1892 when he noted that children developed varicella after coming into contact with herpes zoster patients [3]. Weller et al. proved a common etiological agent [3–5], and Garland and Hope-Simpson were the first to propose a reactivation of latent varicella as the cause of herpes zoster [3]. In 1995, the FDA approved the first vaccine for the prevention of varicella, significantly changing the epidemiology of this disease [6].

R. Gordon, M.D. (✉)
Department of Dermatology, The University of Texas Medical School at Houston, 6655 Travis Street, Suite 600, Houston, TX 77030, USA
e-mail: Rachel.gordon@gmail.com

S. Tyring, M.D., Ph.D., M.B.A. • W. Lapolla, M.D.
Department of Dermatology, The University of Texas at Houston, Houston, TX, USA

R. Mays, M.D.
Department of Dermatology, Baylor College of Medicine, Houston, TX, USA

J.A. Zeichner (ed.), *Acneiform Eruptions in Dermatology: A Differential Diagnosis*,
DOI 10.1007/978-1-4614-8344-1_14, © Springer Science+Business Media New York 2014

14.2 Background

Varicella virus is transmitted both by direct contact and through airborne spread when a patient breathes or sneezes. Transmission may occur more easily in temperate environments as compared to tropical climates, though seasonal peaks are seen in both climates [2]. In the United States, April has the highest incidence of VZV infection [7]. Before the advent of vaccination, primary varicella was commonplace and approximately 11,000 hospitalizations per year in the United States resulted from complications of the illness in otherwise healthy children [2]. Vaccination decreased the incidence of disease in all age groups with the greatest decline in children aged 12 months to 4 years [8]. By 2004, mortality associated with varicella had decreased 82 % from the pre-vaccine era [9].

While the incidence of varicella has decreased by 76–90 % as a result of vaccination [10, 11], roughly 90–95 % of adults in the United States are seropositive for varicella [12, 13]. Therefore, most people are susceptible to herpes zoster, the lifetime risk of which has been estimated to be 10–30 % [10, 14]. Age is a major risk factor for herpes zoster, and its prevalence increases dramatically every 5 years; the sharpest spike is between 50 and 60 years of age [15]. Other risk factors include HIV [16], malignancy (especially lymphoproliferative cancers), immunosuppressive therapy, history of organ transplant [17], and possibly trauma [18]. Genetics may also be a risk factor as 39 % of herpes zoster patients recall a blood relative with a history of shingles compared to 11 % of control patients without herpes zoster who report shingles in a blood relative [19]. Recurrent zoster is rare, but may occur in 1.7–6 % of patients [15, 20].

VZV is a DNA alpha-herpesvirus that adheres to respiratory mucosa with the glycoproteins on its outer lipid-containing envelope. Viral replication occurs in regional lymph nodes and the reticuloendothelial system, followed respectively by viremia at 4–6 and again at 14 days [21]. Involvement of the skin is due to transmission of the virus from infected CD4+ T cells expressing skin-homing factors to dermal fibroblasts and keratinocytes [22]. During primary infection, the virus spreads to the cranial or dorsal root ganglia, possibly by retrograde transport, infects ganglia tissue, and then enters a latent state [23]. VZV resides in both neurons and satellite cells, unlike herpes simplex virus, which is restricted to neurons [24].

Primary infection occurs typically in childhood when susceptible individuals inhale airborne virus or directly contact the rash of primary varicella or herpes zoster. VZV is highly contagious and 61–100 % of contacts develop clinical infection after exposure. Transmission by airborne respiratory droplets occurs 1–2 days before the development of lesions. Virus can be transmitted from the rash up to a week after lesions appear [2]. Once lesions are crusted, they are no longer contagious [21].

Herpes zoster results from VZV reactivation following an unknown trigger, possibly when cell-mediated immunity decreases below a crucial level [15]. Replication in affected ganglia and anterograde spread via secondary afferent sensory neurons are associated with inflammation and necrosis of neuronal and non-neuronal cells [2, 3]. The neuropathic pain associated with shingles is caused by damage to neurons and altered central nervous system (CNS) signal processing [2, 25].

14.3 Clinical Presentation

14.3.1 Primary Varicella (Chicken Pox)

Primary varicella infection presents with fever and a rash starting on the head and extending to the trunk and extremities. Adults and adolescents may have a prodrome of fever, malaise, and headache 1–2 days before the rash, while in children the fever and rash develop at the same time. The rash begins as macules and then evolves through stages of papules, vesicles, and pustules before forming scabs [2]. Pruritus is universal [26]. A unique characteristic is that new lesions appear as older ones crust; thus lesions will be at different stages [27]. Lesions may involve mucosal surfaces [28], and scarring is unusual [2].

Varicella is usually a self-limiting disease, but complications exist and morbidity and mortality are significantly higher in adults. In 1990–1994, adults had a risk of dying from varicella 25 times greater than children 1–4 years old, and most people who died were previously healthy [29]. One severe complication, varicella pneumonia, develops within 6 days of rash onset [2]. In a study of adult men, the mortality rate was 10 % or 30 % in immunocompetent and immunocompromised people, respectively [30]. The most common complication is bacterial superinfection (usually with staphylococcus or streptococcus), which frequently scars, but rarely leads to septicemia. CNS complications occur in less than 1 out of 1,000 cases and include encephalitis, meningoencephalitis, acute cerebellar ataxia, and Guillain-Barre syndrome [2]. Since introduction of the vaccine, the most common neurological complication is meningitis [31].

If primary varicella is acquired during pregnancy, there is a 10 % risk of developing pneumonia [32]. Risk to the fetus is highest in the first trimester with a 2.2 % chance of embryopathy [33]. Defects include hypoplastic limbs, cortical atrophy, ocular abnormalities, psychomotor retardation, and low birth weight (37). It is recommended that susceptible women be vaccinated before pregnancy [32] (Figs. 14.1 and 14.2).

14.3.2 Herpes Zoster (Shingles)

Herpes zoster is characterized by a prodrome with acute stinging, itching, tingling, burning, paresthesias, and hyperesthesia in a single dermatome 1–5 days before the rash [2]. Patients may also have constitutional symptoms of headache, malaise, and fever and present with dependent lymphadenopathy [15]. Pain in a dermatome preceding cutaneous manifestations can cause misdiagnoses such as myocardial infarction, peptic ulcer, and appendicitis [28]. A unilateral rash of erythematous macules and papules evolves into vesicles, with new vesicles forming up to 7 days. Vesicles evolve into pustules and ultimately scabs which fall off within 4 weeks. Most commonly, the midthoracic to upper lumbar (T3-L2) and ophthalmic (V1) regions are involved [34]. Classically, the rash is unilateral and does not cross the

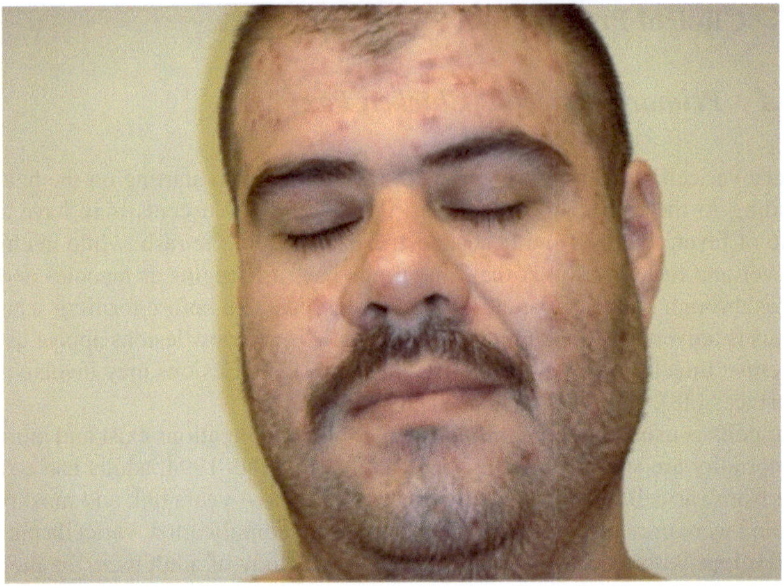

Fig. 14.1 Primary varicella (chickenpox) in an adult

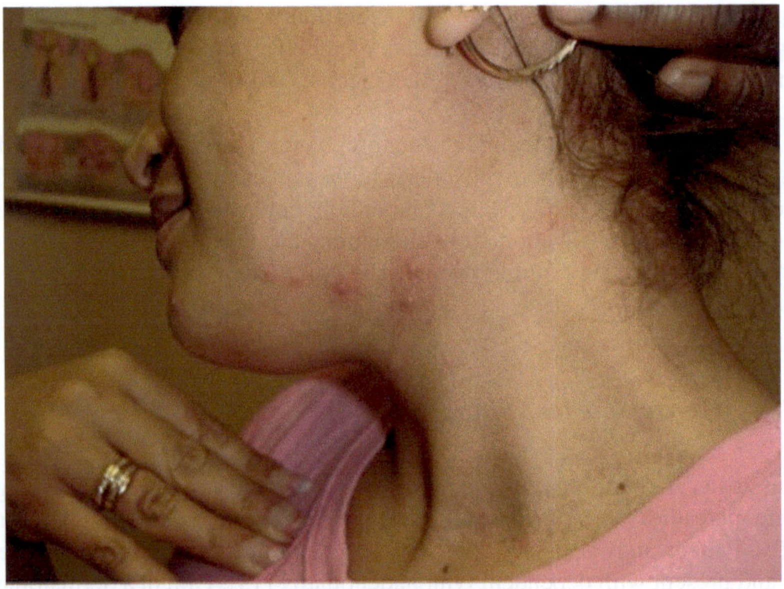

Fig. 14.2 Primary varicella (chickenpox) in an adult

midline, but bilateral zoster has been reported in both immunocompromised and immunosuppressed patients [2]. Symptoms of zoster along with its serologic or virologic evidence presenting without cutaneous signs are called zoster sine herpete; it rarely occurs.

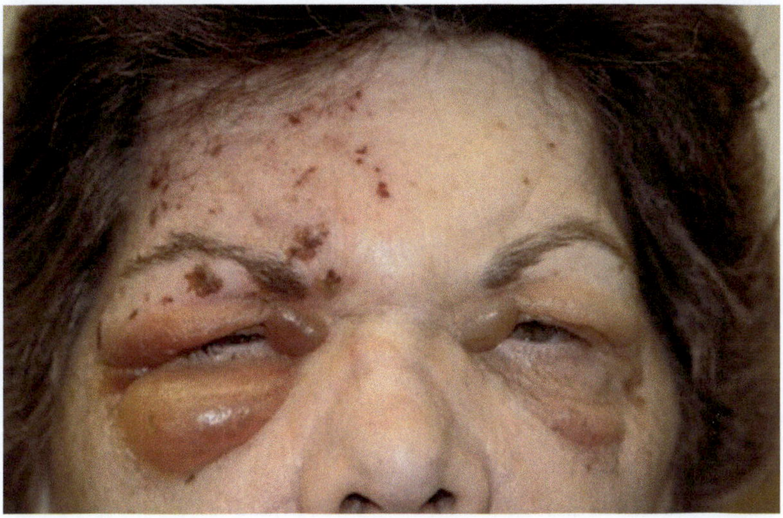

Fig. 14.3 Herpes zoster in V1 distribution of the trigeminal nerve with contralateral edema

The neuralgia of herpes zoster usually resolves as the lesion crusts fall off [2]. However, 20 % of all patients will experience the most common complication of herpes zoster post-herpetic neuralgia (PHN) [15]. Under the age of 40, PHN is uncommon [2], but more than one third of patients over 60 years [2, 34], and 75 % of those over 75 years will develop PHN [35]. In addition to age, risk factors include female sex, immunosuppression, and severity of rash and acute pain [36]. The intensity of PHN typically lessens in 1–6 months, but the duration varies [2] (Fig. 14.3).

Reactivation in the ophthalmic division of the trigeminal nerve (V1) occurs in 10–20 % of zoster cases and is known as herpes zoster ophthalmicus (HZO) [37]. The development of ocular disease occurs in 20–70 % of these cases [2], validating referral to an ophthalmologist [15]. Ocular complications include scleritis, acute epithelial keratitis, uveitis, chorioretinitis, oculomotor palsies, optic neuritis, and panophthalmitis secondary to bacterial infection [2, 38]. Impaired corneal sensation may result in ulceration. Involvement of the second or third divisions of the trigeminal nerve may result in lesions in the mouth, pharynx, larynx, or ears. In Ramsay-Hunt syndrome, involvement of the facial or auditory nerves may cause symptoms of vertigo, loss of taste, tinnitus, and otalgia [2]. Cutaneous and visceral dissemination is rare in immunocompetent individuals (Figs. 14.4, 14.5, and 14.6).

14.4 Work-Up

Most cases of varicella and herpes zoster can be diagnosed on the basis of clinical history and exam. However, herpes simplex virus (HSV) can be a very good imitator of VZV, especially when it occurs outside of its typical distribution. Differentiation

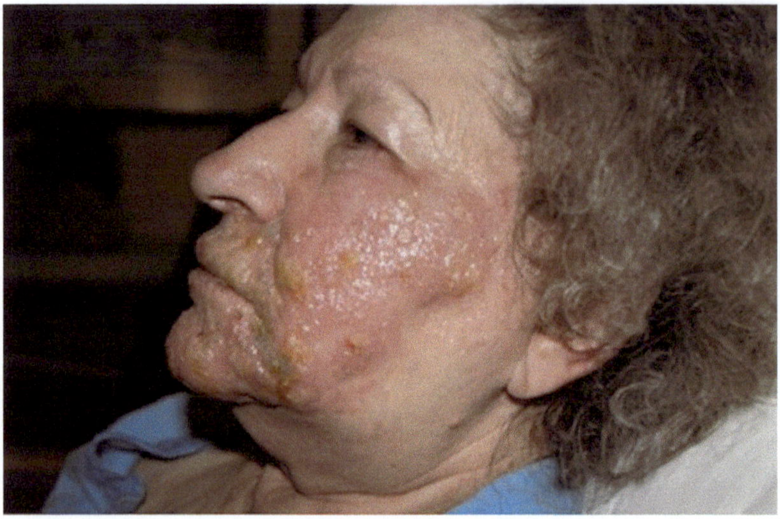

Fig. 14.4 Herpes zoster in V2 distribution of the trigeminal nerve

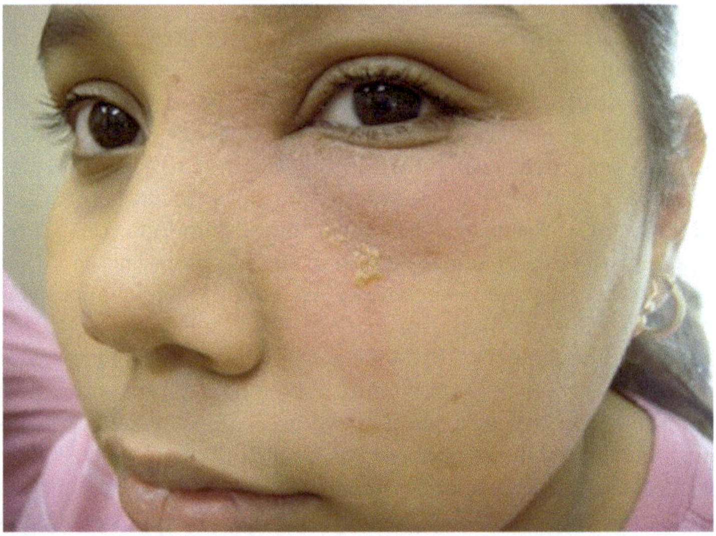

Fig. 14.5 Herpes zoster in V2 distribution of the trigeminal nerve in a child

of VZV from HSV with viral culture is most specific, but it takes 1–2 weeks for results and the sensitivity is 60–75 % [2, 15]. Serologic testing is limited by possible preexistence of antibodies to VZV as well as to HSV 1 or 2. In addition, commercial ELISA tests are usually not sufficiently sensitive to identify the level of immunity that develops in vaccines [10]. PCR is the most sensitive and specific test [15] and has been used to detect VZV from skin lesions, peripheral blood, CSF, and other

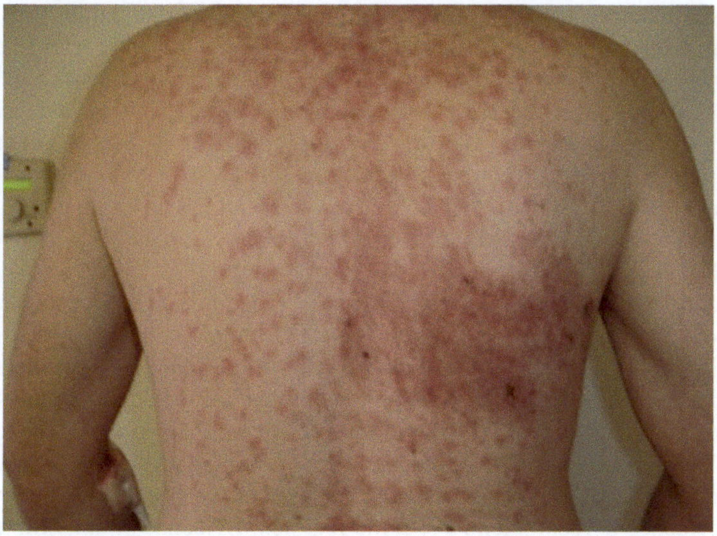

Fig. 14.6 Disseminated herpes zoster on the back

tissues from infected patients. Because of their rapid results and high sensitivity, direct immunofluorescence and PCR are currently the preferred methods of diagnosis. Histopathology and cytopathology are not clinically useful in the differentiation of varicella from herpes zoster or VZV [2].

14.5 Treatment

Primary prevention is preferred over treatment of an outbreak. For the prevention of varicella in infants and children, two vaccines are available: a monovalent varicella vaccine and a quadrivalent (measles, mumps, rubella, and varicella – MMRV) vaccine. MMRV is associated with a twofold increase in febrile seizures when compared with MMR and varicella given separately. A two-dose schedule is currently recommended to reduce breakthrough varicella [39]. Some pregnant women have received the vaccine inadvertently, and there have been no reported varicella syndromes from these instances [2]. Zostavax® was developed to boost VZV-specific cell-mediated immunity and has been approved for use in adults older than 50 years. It has greater efficacy in preventing zoster in the age group 60–69, and it prevents PHN to a greater extent in those over 70 [40].

Treatment for primary varicella often uses antiviral therapy. Oral acyclovir has been shown to significantly reduce the severity and duration of illness and is approved for the treatment of primary varicella after the age of 2. The dose is 20 mg/kg QID for 5 days, or 800 mg five times a day for 7 days in children over 40 kg and adults. The same regimens of valacyclovir and famciclovir used in treating zoster are also commonly used to treat primary varicella, though it is not specifically FDA approved [2].

In cases of herpes zoster, treatment within 72 h of vesicle formation with antiviral medications has been found to reduce the duration of the rash and zoster-related pain by nearly half. If patients present outside 72 h, they still may benefit from antiviral therapy [15]. First-line treatment in immunocompetent patients is valacyclovir 1 g every 8 h or famciclovir 500 mg every 8 h for 7 days [2, 15, 41]. Novel anti-VZV drugs, including the bicyclic nucleoside analog FV-100, the helicase-primase inhibitor ASP2151, and valomaciclovir, have recently been evaluated in clinical trials. To date, it seems these drugs should be as safe as, and possibly more effective than, valacyclovir [42].

Immunocompromised patients with primary varicella or herpes zoster are at high risk for disseminated VZV. Hospitalization for treatment with IV acyclovir 10 mg/kg Q8H for 7 days, or until the infection is controlled, should be considered. After this point, oral medication may be used to complete a course of 7–10 days [2, 15]. Acyclovir resistance is rare, but should be considered if there is vesicle formation beyond 7 days. In such cases, IV foscarnet and cidofovir are appropriate [15].

Controlling acute pain and PHN is a challenge in zoster patients; however there is poor evidence to recommend a specific regimen. Evidence of antiviral treatment reducing the incidence and duration of PHN is conflicting [41], but early, concomitant use of valacyclovir and gabapentin has been effective at reducing the incidence of PHN [43]. Management of PHN is palliative, and topical lidocaine 5 % plus gabapentin or pregabalin is first-line treatment [15]. Pregabalin offers a more rapid clinical effect than gabapentin [41]. Alternative agents include opioid analgesics, NSAIDS, tricyclic antidepressants (amitriptyline), and capsaicin cream [15, 41]. Systemic corticosteroids administered within 72 h of rash onset have a clinically significant benefit on acute pain, but no demonstrable effect on PHN [41].

14.6 Conclusion

In an age of vaccinations, primary prevention of both varicella and zoster is increasing. While not as rampant an infection as it was several decades ago, correct diagnosis and treatment is extremely important when cases arrive. An acute onset of herpes zoster on the face is clinically distinguishable from acne, but such a diagnosis may not be clear to patients. Prompt antiviral therapy for these patients can clear the infection while minimizing any cutaneous or neurological sequelae.

References

1. Gordon JE. Chickenpox: an epidemiological review. Am J Med Sci. 1962;244:362–89.
2. Tyring SK, Moore AY, Lupi O, editors. Mucocutaneous manifestations of viral diseases. London: Informa Healthcare; 2010.
3. Arvin AM. Varicella-zoster virus. Clin Microbiol Rev. 1996;9:361–81.
4. Weller TH, Witton HM. The etiologic agents of varicella and herpes zoster; serologic studies with the viruses as propagated in vitro. J Exp Med. 1958;108:869–90.

5. Weller TH, Witton HM, Bell EJ. The etiologic agents of varicella and herpes zoster; isolation, propagation, and cultural characteristics in vitro. J Exp Med. 1958;108:843–68.
6. Creed R, Satyaprakash A, Ravanfar P. Varicella zoster vaccines. Dermatol Ther. 2009;22:143–9.
7. Shah AP, Smolensky MH, Burau KD, Cech IM, Lai D. Seasonality of primarily childhood and young adult infectious diseases in the United States. Chronobiol Int. 2006;23:1065–82.
8. Seward JF, Watson BM, Peterson CL, Mascola L, Pelosi JW, Zhang JX, et al. Varicella disease after introduction of varicella vaccine in the United States, 1995–2000. JAMA. 2002;287:606–11.
9. Roush SW, Murphy TV. Vaccine-preventable disease table working G. Historical comparisons of morbidity and mortality for vaccine-preventable diseases in the United States. JAMA. 2007;298:2155–63.
10. Gershon AA. Varicella-zoster virus infections. Pediatr Rev. 2008;29:5–10. quiz 1.
11. Guris D, Jumaan AO, Mascola L, Watson BM, Zhang JX, Chaves SS, et al. Changing varicella epidemiology in active surveillance sites–United States, 1995–2005. J Infect Dis. 2008;197 Suppl 2:S71–5.
12. Choo PW, Donahue JG, Manson JE, Platt R. The epidemiology of varicella and its complications. J Infect Dis. 1995;172:706–12.
13. Johnson RW. Herpes zoster and postherpetic neuralgia. Expert Rev Vaccines. 2010;9:21–6.
14. Ragozzino MW, Melton 3rd LJ, Kurland LT, Chu CP, Perry HO. Population-based study of herpes zoster and its sequelae. Medicine (Baltimore). 1982;61:310–6.
15. Lapolla W TS. Clinical decision support in dermatology: herpes zoster. Heyman et al., Elsevier 2011.
16. Buchbinder SP, Katz MH, Hessol NA, Liu JY, O'Malley PM, Underwood R, et al. Herpes zoster and human immunodeficiency virus infection. J Infect Dis. 1992;166:1153–6.
17. Gnann Jr JW, Whitley RJ. Clinical practice. Herpes zoster. N Engl J Med. 2002;347:340–6.
18. Lee MR, Ryman W. Herpes zoster following cryosurgery. Australas J Dermatol. 2005;46:42–3.
19. Hicks LD, Cook-Norris RH, Mendoza N, Madkan V, Arora A, Tyring SK. Family history as a risk factor for herpes zoster: a case–control study. Arch Dermatol. 2008;144:603–8.
20. Yawn BP, Wollan PC, Kurland MJ, St Sauver JL, Saddier P. Herpes zoster recurrences more frequent than previously reported. Mayo Clin Proc. 2011;86:88–93.
21. Heininger U, Seward JF. Varicella. Lancet. 2006;368:1365–76.
22. Taylor SL, Moffat JF. Replication of varicella-zoster virus in human skin organ culture. J Virol. 2005;79:11501–6.
23. Eshleman E, Shahzad A, Cohrs RJ. Varicella zoster virus latency. Future Virol. 2011;6:341–55.
24. Abendroth A, Arvin A. Varicella-zoster virus immune evasion. Immunol Rev. 1999;168: 143–56.
25. Kost RG, Straus SE. Postherpetic neuralgia–pathogenesis, treatment, and prevention. N Engl J Med. 1996;335:32–42.
26. McCrary ML, Severson J, Tyring SK. Varicella zoster virus. J Am Acad Dermatol. 1999;41:1–14. quiz 5–6.
27. Cohen JI, Brunell PA, Straus SE, Krause PR. Recent advances in varicella-zoster virus infection. Ann Intern Med. 1999;130:922–32.
28. Chen TM, George S, Woodruff CA, Hsu S. Clinical manifestations of varicella-zoster virus infection. Dermatol Clin. 2002;20:267–82.
29. Meyer PA, Seward JF, Jumaan AO, Wharton M. Varicella mortality: trends before vaccine licensure in the United States, 1970–1994. J Infect Dis. 2000;182:383–90.
30. Weber DM, Pellecchia JA. Varicella pneumonia: study of prevalence in adult men. JAMA. 1965;192:572–3.
31. Pahud BA, Glaser CA, Dekker CL, Arvin AM, Schmid DS. Varicella zoster disease of the central nervous system: epidemiological, clinical, and laboratory features 10 years after the introduction of the varicella vaccine. J Infect Dis. 2011;203:316–23.
32. Gnann Jr JW. Varicella-zoster virus: atypical presentations and unusual complications. J Infect Dis. 2002;186 Suppl 1:S91–8.
33. Pastuszak AL, Levy M, Schick B, Zuber C, Feldkamp M, Gladstone J, et al. Outcome after maternal varicella infection in the first 20 weeks of pregnancy. N Engl J Med. 1994;330:901–5.

34. Burgoon Jr CF, Burgoon JS, Baldridge GD. The natural history of herpes zoster. J Am Med Assoc. 1957;164:265–9.
35. Vander Straten M, Carrasco D, Lee P, Tyring SK. Reduction of postherpetic neuralgia in herpes zoster. J Cutan Med Surg. 2001;5:409–16.
36. Jung BF, Johnson RW, Griffin DR, Dworkin RH. Risk factors for postherpetic neuralgia in patients with herpes zoster. Neurology. 2004;62:1545–51.
37. Liesegang TJ. Herpes zoster ophthalmicus natural history, risk factors, clinical presentation, and morbidity. Ophthalmology. 2008;115:S3–12.
38. Liesegang TJ. The varicella-zoster virus: systemic and ocular features. J Am Acad Dermatol. 1984;11:165–91.
39. Lai J, Fay KE, Bocchini JA. Update on childhood and adolescent immunizations: selected review of US recommendations and literature: part 2. Curr Opin Pediatr. 2011;23:470–81.
40. Kimberlin DW, Whitley RJ. Varicella-zoster vaccine for the prevention of herpes zoster. N Engl J Med. 2007;356:1338–43.
41. Whitley RJ, Volpi A, McKendrick M, Wijck A, Oaklander AL. Management of herpes zoster and post-herpetic neuralgia now and in the future. J Clin Virol. 2010;48 Suppl 1:S20–8.
42. Andrei G, Snoeck R. Emerging drugs for varicella-zoster virus infections. Expert Opin Emerg Drugs. 2011;16(3):507–35.
43. Lapolla W, Digiorgio C, Haitz K, Magel G, Mendoza N, Grady J, et al. Incidence of postherpetic neuralgia after combination treatment with gabapentin and valacyclovir in patients with acute herpes zoster: open-label study. Arch Dermatol. 2011;147(8):901–7.

Part III
Variants of Acne Vulgaris

Chapter 15
Acne Conglobata

Jonathan S. Weiss and Elijah Wilder

15.1 Introduction

The term acne conglobata is reserved for the most severe form of inflammatory acne. While uncommon, the condition presents as a highly inflammatory, extensive nodulocystic eruption. Acne conglobata is differentiated from acne fulminans by the former's lack of systemic symptoms, including fever [1]. Severe disfigurement and scarring are a common result leading to potential psychological impairment, including anxiety and depression. Acne conglobata comprises one part of the follicular occlusion triad, along with perifolliculitis capitis abscedens et suffodiens (dissecting cellulitis of the scalp) and hidradenitis suppurativa [2].

15.2 Background

The primary cause of acne conglobata remains unknown. Distinctly uncommon, it has a predilection for males over females with an age of onset most often between 18 and 30 years. The condition is seen rarely, if ever, in infants and children [3]. Certainly the pathophysiologic factors of acne vulgaris play a role, including Propionibacterium acnes (P. acnes), release of inflammatory mediators, and hormonal influences. Anabolic/androgenic steroid use, androgen-producing tumors, and testosterone therapy have all been associated with the development of acne conglobata [4]. Environmental factors that lead to acne vulgaris have been present

J.S. Weiss, M.D., F.A.A.D. (✉)
Department of Dermatology, Emory University, Atlanta, GA 30322, USA
e-mail: jonweissmd@gmail.com

E. Wilder, D.O.
Philadelphia College of Osteopathic Medicine, Georgia, Atlanta, GA USA

J.A. Zeichner (ed.), *Acneiform Eruptions in Dermatology: A Differential Diagnosis*,
DOI 10.1007/978-1-4614-8344-1_15, © Springer Science+Business Media New York 2014

in some patients with this most severe form of inflammatory acne, including exposure to halogenated hydrocarbons or ingestion of halogens [3]. Chromosomal defects have been found in some patients with acne conglobata, namely, an XXY karyotype in individuals that do not exhibit Klinefelter's syndrome [5]. PAPA syndrome, consisting of pyoderma gangrenosum, acne conglobata, and pyogenic aseptic arthritis, has been mapped to a locus on the long arm of chromosome 15 and may be associated with mutations CD 2 binding protein 1 (CD2BP1) [6, 7].

15.3 Clinical Presentation

Acne conglobata may arise in preexisting acne vulgaris or as an acute onset eruption. Areas of involvement include the chest, shoulders, back, buttocks, and face [8, 9]. Lesion types include extensive nodules, cysts, sinus tracts, along with papules, pustules, and severe double comedones. As inflammation progresses, interconnecting/communicating abscesses form and foul-smelling purulent drainage ensues. Crusts may form over healing erosions and ulcers. Active lesions are often tender. Atrophic and hypertrophic scars are common following resolution of the inflammation (Fig. 15.1). Patients who exhibit acne conglobata along with sacroiliitis have also been found to have anterior uveitis [10]. Renal amyloidosis and musculoskeletal syndrome have also been associated [11]. Cutaneous associations include hidradenitis suppurativa, dissecting cellulitis of the scalp and

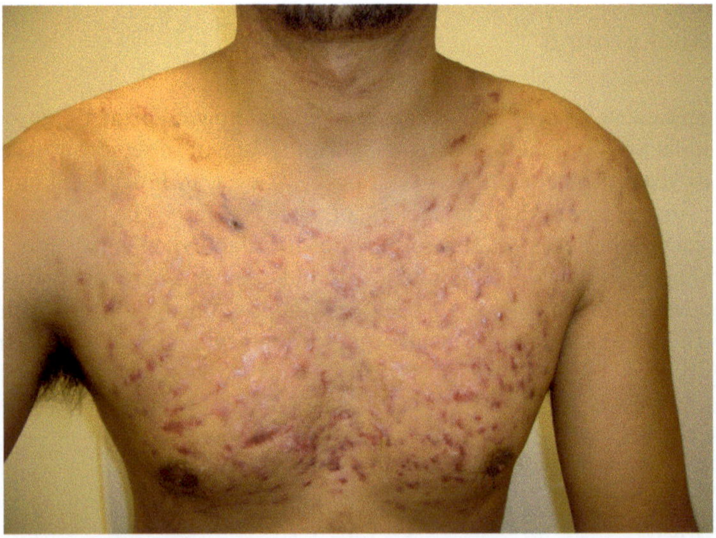

Fig. 15.1 Hypertrophic scars on the chest of a young man with acne conglobata (Photo credit: Joshua A. Zeichner, M.D.)

pyoderma gangrenosum [12]. The differential diagnosis of acne conglobata includes acne fulminans, severe acne vulgaris, other acneiform eruptions/drug-induced acne, and sporotrichosis [3].

15.4 Work-Up

Acne conglobata is generally a clinical diagnosis. A good history and physical to rule out acne fulminans is indicated. While uncommon in women, the presence of acne conglobata may indicate the need for an endocrinologic work-up to include total and free testosterone, DHEAS, prolactin, LH, and FSH [2]. Concerns of abnormalities should prompt referral to an endocrinologist or general internist, either of whom might feel it prudent to perform a glucose tolerance test and/or lipid profile. Depending on therapeutic considerations, such as isotretinoin, a CBC, liver function studies, and lipid profile may be indicated, along with serum or urine pregnancy tests in women. Draining cysts and sinus tracts should be cultured to ensure they are not superinfected with gram-negative bacteria or coagulase-positive Staphylococcus.

15.5 Treatment

Isotretinoin in a dosage of 0.5–1 mg/kg per day is the treatment of choice for fully developed acne conglobata [3]. Its effects on remission of nodulocystic lesions are unparalleled in acne therapeutics. Because isotretinoin can increase inflammation early in the course of therapy, in the absence of contraindications, the prudent practitioner may also add systemic corticosteroids (prednisone/prednisolone) 40–60 mg daily with taper over the first 2–4 weeks of therapy. By reducing the overall inflammation and severity of nodules and cysts, corticosteroids may alleviate discomfort and reduce ultimate scarring. If cultures are positive for pathogenic organisms, antibiotics are also indicated, the choice being guided by sensitivity testing. During isotretinoin therapy, tetracycline antibiotics are relatively contraindicated due to risks of pseudotumor cerebri. If isotretinoin is contraindicated or refused by the patient, less optimal therapeutic options include oral antibiotics. Tetracycline, doxycycline, minocycline, clarithromycin, and sulfamethoxazole/trimethoprim would be good initial choices. Dapsone in dosages of 50–150 mg daily can be used as adjuvant therapy in patients showing suboptimal responses to either isotretinoin or antibiotics [13]. For patients on antibiotic therapy, topical retinoid treatment may help with comedonal and microinflammatory lesions.

Procedures that may be indicated to assist with resolution of acne conglobata include aspiration of cysts/sinuses and injection of intralesional corticosteroids. Both may be performed in association with either isotretinoin or systemic antibiotic therapy, either alone or together. Triamcinolone 2.5–3 mg/ml is the authors' agent of choice for intralesional injection. Incision and drainage of cysts or excision of nodules have been previously advocated but should be avoided during isotretinoin treatment due to poor healing tendencies under the influence of systemic retinoids [14]. Cryotherapy of nodules has also been advocated by some authors [15]. After resolution, fractional laser resurfacing, CO_2 laser, dermabrasion, and chemical peeling have been utilized to reduce the appearance of scarring [16].

Psychological implications of acne conglobata cannot be overlooked. Depression, feelings of shame, and anxiety over one's appearance all contribute to a decreased quality of life. Depression can also be a rare but highly publicized side effect of isotretinoin therapy. At the very least, the treating practitioner should question patients and/or their family members regarding their psychological state and the effects that the condition and therapies are having on their lives. Referral to appropriate mental health professionals should always be considered.

References

1. Bolognia J, Jorizzo J, Rapini R, editors. Dermatology. 2nd ed. Philadelphia: Mosby-Elsevier; 2008.
2. Habif T. Clinical dermatology. 5th ed. Philadelphia: Mosby-Elsevier; 2010.
3. Schwartz R. Acne conglobata. Medscape Reference. http://emedicine.medscape.com/article/1072716-overview. Accessed 12 Dec 2011.
4. Melnik B, Jansen T, Grabbe S. Abuse of anabolic-androgenic steroids and bodybuilding acne: an underestimated health problem. J Dtsch Dermatol Ges. 2007;5(2):110–7.
5. Wollenberg A, Wolff H, Jansen T, Schmid MH, Rocken M, Plewig G. Acne conglobata and Klinefelter's syndrome. Br J Dermatol. 1997;136(3):421–3.
6. Ziff M, Maliakkal J. Acne conglobata and arthritis. Ann Intern Med. 1983;98(3):417.
7. Yeon HB, Lindor NM, Seidman JG, Seidman CE. Pyogenic arthritis, pyoderma gangrenosum, and acne syndrome maps to chromosome 15q. Am J Hum Genet. 2000;66(4):1443–8.
8. Patterson WM, Stibich AS, Dobke M, Schwartz RA. Mutilating facial acne conglobata. Cutis. 2000;66(2):139–40.
9. Shimomura Y, Nomoto S, Yamada S, Ito A, Ito K, Ito M. Chronic glomerulonephritis remarkably improved after surgery for acne conglobata of the buttocks. Br J Dermatol. 2001; 145(2):363–4.
10. Leybishkis B, Fasseas P, Ryan KF, Roy R. Hidradenitis suppurativa and acne conglobata associated with spondyloarthropathy. Am J Med Sci. 2001;321(3):195–7.
11. Perez-Villa F, Campistol JM, Ferrando J, Botey A. Renal amyloidosis secondary to acne conglobata. Int J Dermatol. 1989;28(2):132–3.
12. Velez A, Alcala J, Fernandez-Roldan JC. Pyoderma gangrenosum associated with acne conglobata. Clin Exp Dermatol. 1995;20(6):496–8.
13. Tan BB, Lear JT, Smith AG. Acne fulminans and erythema nodosum during isotretinoin therapy responding to dapsone. Clin Exp Dermatol. 1997;22(1):26–7.
14. Weinrauch L, Peled I, Hacham-Zadeh S, Wexler MR. Surgical treatment of severe acne conglobata. J Dermatol Surg Oncol. 1981;7(6):492–4.
15. Leyden JJ, Mills OH, Kligman AM. Cryoprobe treatment of acne conglobata. Br J Dermatol. 1974;90(3):335–41.
16. Hasegawa T, Matsukura T, Suga Y, et al. Case of acne conglobata successfully treated by CO(2) laser combined with topical tretinoin therapy. J Dermatol. 2007;34(8):583–5.

Chapter 16
Acne Excoriée

Jillian Wong Millsop and John Y.M. Koo

16.1 Introduction

There are a variety of psychiatric problems that relate to dermatological conditions. Psychiatric and psychosocial factors are reportedly significant in at least 25–33 % of dermatology patients [1]. Acne can have a negative impact physically and psychologically, resulting in social isolation and even more severe secondary consequences on the psyche. Moreover, acne itself can be aggravated by underlying psychopathology. Acne excoriée is one such condition, resulting from the relationship between acne and a psychiatric disorder.

16.2 Background

Acne excoriée is a psychodermatological condition that refers to the behavior of picking acne lesions (Fig. 16.1) [2]. The primary pathophysiologic source is in the psyche and not in the skin [3]. Acne excoriée is characterized by picking or scratching at acne or skin with minor epidermal abnormalities [4]. This subtype of excoriating behavior in acne patients is also referred to by various other names, including neurotic excoriation, psychogenic excoriation, pathological or compulsive skin picking, and dermatillomania.

Though the patient has a skin condition, there is a primary psychiatric disturbance that focuses on acne. The disturbance can simply be the habit of picking; however, there can also be a more serious source for the behavior. Patients with acne

J.W. Millsop, M.D., M.S. (✉) • J.Y.M. Koo, M.D.
Department of Dermatology, University of California San Francisco, Psoriasis and Skin Treatment Center, 515 Spruce Street, San Francisco, CA 94118, USA
e-mail: jillianwwong@gmail.com

J.A. Zeichner (ed.), *Acneiform Eruptions in Dermatology: A Differential Diagnosis*,
DOI 10.1007/978-1-4614-8344-1_16,

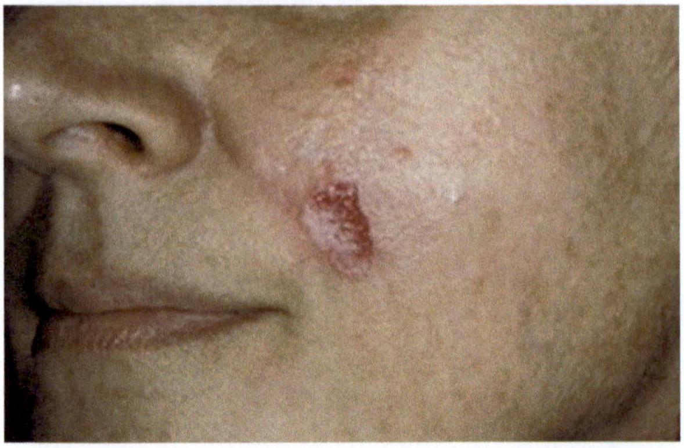

Fig. 16.1 Facial acne excoriation

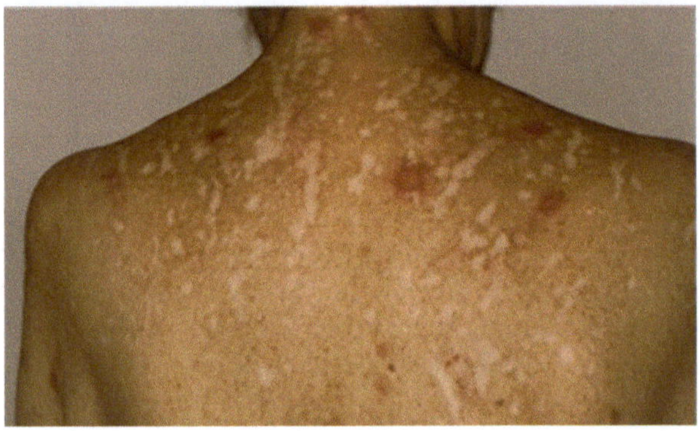

Fig. 16.2 Acne excoriation over the back with scarring

excoriée can have a variety of underlying psychopathology, but depression and anxiety appear to be the two most common underlying psychiatric conditions [3]. Many patients also report the compulsion for picking the skin associated with poor self-image [5]. Scar formation as a result of excoriation (Fig. 16.2) has a further negative psychosocial impact, exacerbating the patient's social isolation, depression, and anxiety. This continues in a vicious cycle.

Approximately 2 % of all dermatology clinic patients are found to have some form of psychogenic excoriation [4]. The age of onset of the condition typically ranges from 15 to 45 years, and the duration of symptoms has a range of 5 and 21 years [4]. Though onset of this condition generally occurs in adulthood, acne excoriée is one of the most common presentations of psychodermatology in the pediatric age group [5]. More females than males are affected with acne excoriée, while the female to male ratio for all psychogenic excoriations is 8:1 [4, 6]. Case studies reporting Caucasian patients with acne excoriée are more common than those of African Americans or other racial groups, but no confirmatory studies of racial distribution in the general population exist. In addition, the lifetime prevalence of the condition is unknown.

16.3 Clinical Presentation

A patient with acne excoriée most commonly presents as a young, Caucasian female with excoriated acne and scars. As a result of the self-inflicting nature of the condition, patients tend to pick at skin regions most easily accessible. Therefore, the distribution of scars or excoriations over the body can provide a useful clue to clinicians. The patient with acne excoriée can have a distribution of lesions resembling the shape of butterfly wings on the back, referred to as the "butterfly sign" [3]. In the butterfly sign, there is sparing of the upper, lateral sides of the back bilaterally resulting from the fact that the patient cannot reach these areas. Similarly, there tends to be more involvement of the extensor arm as compared to the medial arm and more involvement of the anterior thigh as compared to the posterior thigh. Often, patients report a sense of tension immediately prior to picking at their skin and a sense of relief after the behavior is complete [6].

Patients can present with severe psychosocial impairment. Comorbidities of acne excoriée include mood and anxiety disorders. Mood disorders are found in 48–68 % of patients, which include major depression, dysthymia, and bipolar disorders [7, 8]. Anxiety disorders are found in 41–65 % of patients and include generalized anxiety disorder, agoraphobia, panic disorder, social and more specific phobia, obsessive-compulsive disorder, and post-traumatic stress disorder [7, 8]. Additionally, if a patient has a mood or anxiety disorder, he or she frequently has comorbid psychiatric disorders related to the mood or anxiety disorder, particularly a compulsive-impulsive spectrum disorder [9], including body dysmorphic disorder, eating disorder, substance use disorder, or an impulse control disorder, which includes kleptomania, compulsive buying, and trichotillomania [7, 8, 10]. For very rare patients, acne excoriée may even present as a manifestation of a delusional disorder [2].

Significant functional impairment is a common occurrence. Patients are often embarrassed to admit their behavior to a physician. Many report impairment in social functioning including avoidance of activities that expose their skin to the public, such as sexual activity, going to the beach, and attending sports and community events [4, 11]. Patients often use cosmetics, bandages, and clothing to hide their excoriations.

16.4 Work-Up

As a result of the psychiatric nature of the condition, there are no laboratory measures to make the diagnosis of acne excoriée. Instead, diagnosis is based on clinical presentation.

The approach that the authors recommend includes taking a thorough history, conducting a detailed physical examination, and assessing the patient for an underlying psychiatric disorder that may be related to the condition. In particular, evaluating the patient for the exact nature of the underlying psychopathology such as depression, anxiety, and obsessive-compulsive disorder (OCD) is key.

In order to evaluate the patient for major depression or depression-related disorder, one should ask the patient about subjective and physiological symptoms of depression. Subjective symptoms include depressed mood, excessive guilt, anhedonia, feelings of worthlessness, hopelessness, helplessness, and crying spells. Physiological symptoms of depression include loss of appetite, hyperphagia, insomnia, hypersomnia, fatigue, memory loss, poor concentration, and psychomotor agitation or retardation [3]. In order to assess the patient for anxiety, ask the patient about feeling tense or restless, becoming easily fatigued, difficulty concentrating, irritability, significant muscle tension, and difficulty sleeping [12]. In order to evaluate the patient for OCD, inquire about repugnant thoughts and compulsive behaviors. OCD patients can be distinguished from delusional patients by retention of insight that their behavior is destructive. OCD patients believe their behavior is damaging in contrast to delusional patients who have no insight and believe that what they are doing to the skin is justified no matter how destructive the behavior [2].

16.5 Treatment

Due to the nature of the disorder, therapy targeting the psyche can help decrease destructive behavior involved in acne excoriée. For a patient with depression as the underlying cause of the acne excoriée, an antidepressant with psychotherapy can be provided [1, 13, 14]. A patient with anxiety as the underlying source for acne excoriée can use an anti-anxiolytic medication combined with psychotherapy. Patients with obsessive thoughts and compulsive urges to damage the skin may find relief through an anti-OCD medication such as paroxetine (Paxil®) and fluoxetine (Prozac®) along with behavioral therapy to reduce the obsessions and compulsions [4, 15]. Behavioral therapy is generally thought to be more efficacious for the treatment of OCD than insight-oriented psychotherapy [16]. For mixed depression-OCD patients, selective serotonin reuptake inhibitors (SSRIs) are the preferred choice of therapy because of their dual antidepressant and anti-OCD properties [2]. In general, SSRIs are commonly used to treat patients in dermatology with psychiatric comorbidity, especially major depressive disorder [1, 11]. It is important to understand that pharmacologic therapy alone may not be effective if the patient is not motivated to control the compulsive urges such as a case in which a teenager is brought in by his/her parents. If the clinician perceives a "power struggle" between the teenager and the parent over the issue of excoriation, it is often helpful to see the teenager alone and first try to build therapeutic rapport with the teenage patient. In this situation, it is important to establish rapport so that the dermatologist is not seen as another "authority figure" to rebel against.

Case reports have also documented efficacy of pulsed dye laser irradiation along with cognitive psychotherapy. Treatment of hypertrophic scars and acne lesions with laser was first introduced with argon laser [17]. In a case series, 585-nm flashlamp-pumped pulsed dye with concomitant cognitive psychodynamic therapy was used to stop skin picking and scar formation in two OCD patients with acne excoriée [18]. In the cases, practical behavior modification techniques, including removal of mirrors in the home and avoidance of situations that would induce stress or conflict, were helpful.

Finally, biofeedback techniques and hypnosis have also been documented to improve acne excoriée and other dermatoses with a psychological component [19]. Posthypnotic suggestion has also been used to treat the condition. In two case reports, patients were instructed to remember the word "scar" when they felt the urge to pick at the face and to say "scar" to refrain from picking. In both cases, acne excoriée resolved [19]. Aversion therapy techniques and habit reversal have been noted in case reports as successful strategies for cognitive-behavioral therapy [20–22]. Aversion therapy occurs when self-destructive behavior is linked to an aversive stimulus. Habit reversal treatment involves making the patient aware of the scratching behavior, teaching the patient about the negative social impact of the habit, and developing competing response of isometric exercise using fist clenching to prevent scratching.

It is important to recognize the clinical presentation and work-up of acne excoriée, as the underlying source of the condition can be found in the psychopathology rather than in the skin itself. Working closely with the patient to serve his or her specific needs and establishing a solid therapeutic alliance can significantly improve outcomes with all treatments.

Acknowledgements Figures 16.1 and 16.2 are courtesy of Joseph Bikowski, M.D.

References

1. Gupta MA, Gupta AK. The use of antidepressant drugs in dermatology. J Eur Acad Dermatol Venereol. 2001;15:512–8.
2. Koo JYM, Lee CS, editors. Psychocutaneous medicine. New York: Marcel Dekker; 2003.
3. Koo J. Psychodermatology: a practical manual for clinicians. Current problems in dermatology 1995; Nov/Dec: 204–32.
4. Arnold LM, Auchenbach MB, McElroy SL. Psychogenic excoriation: clinical features, proposed diagnostic criteria, epidemiology and approaches to treatment. CNS Drugs. 2001;15:351–9.
5. Shah KN, Fried RG. Factitial dermatosis in children. Curr Opin Pediatr. 2006;18:403–9.
6. Bach M, Bach D. Psychiatric and psychometric issues in acne excoriée. Psychother Psychosom. 1993;60:207–10.
7. Arnold LM, McElroy SL, Mutasim DF, Dwight MM, Lamerson CL, Morris EM. Characteristics of 34 adults with psychogenic excoriation. J Clin Psychiatry. 1998;59:509–14.
8. Wilhelm S, Keuthen NJ, Deckersbach T, Engelhard IM, Forker AE, Baer L, O'Sullivan RL, Jenike MA. Self-injurious skin picking: clinical characteristics and comorbidity. J Clin Psychiatry. 1999;60:454–9.
9. McElroy SL, Phillips KA, Keck PE. Obsessive compulsive spectrum disorder. J Clin Psychiatry. 1994;55(10 Suppl):33–53.
10. Oldham JM, Hollander E, Skodol AE. Impulsivity and compulsivity. Washington, DC: American Psychiatric Press; 1996.
11. Simeon D, Stein DJ, Gross S, Islam N, Schmeidler J, Hollander E. A double-blind trial of fluoxetine in pathologic skin picking. J Clin Psychiatry. 1997;58:509–14.

12. American Psychiatric Association. Diagnostic and statistical manual of mental disorders. 4th ed. Washington, DC: American Psychiatric Association; 2000.
13. Kalivas J, Kalivas L, Gilman D, Hayden CT. Sertraline in the treatment of neurotic excoriations and related disorders. Arch Dermatol. 1996;132:589–90.
14. Klobenzer CS. Psychocutaneous disease. New York, NY: Grune and Stratton; 1987.
15. Kearney CA, Silverman WK. Treatment of an adolescent with obsessive-compulsive disorder by alternating response prevention and cognitive therapy: an empirical analysis. J Behav Ther Exp Psychiatry. 1990;21:39–47.
16. Mancebo MC, Elsen JL, Sibrava NJ, Dyck IR, Rasmussen SA. Patient utilization of cognitive-behavioral therapy for OCD. Behav Ther. 2011;42:399–412.
17. Alster TS, Kurban AK, Grove GL, Grove MJ, Tan OT. Alteration of argon laser-induced scars by the pulsed dye laser. Lasers Surg Med. 1993;13:368–73.
18. Bowes LE, Alster TS. Treatment of facial scarring and ulceration resulting from acne excoriée with 585-nm pulsed dye laser irradiation and cognitive psychotherapy. Dermatol Surg. 2004; 30:934–8.
19. Shenefelt PD. Biofeedback, cognitive-behavioral methods, and hypnosis in dermatology: is it all in your mind? Dermatol Ther. 2003;16:114–22.
20. Ratliffe R, Stein N. Treatment of neurodermatitis by behavior therapy: a case study. Behav Res Ther. 1968;6:397–9.
21. Rosenbaum MS, Ayllon T. The behavioral treatment of neurodermatitis through habit reversal. Behav Res Ther. 1981;19:313–8.
22. Kent A, Drummond LM. Acne excoriée- a case report of treatment using habit reversal. Clin Exp Dermatol. 1989;14:163–4.

Chapter 17
Acne Fulminans

Alison Schram and Misha Rosenbach

17.1 Introduction

Acne fulminans is a rare, severe form of acne vulgaris associated with the acute onset of systemic symptoms. This entity was first described in 1959 when Burns and Colville reported a case of acne conglobata with septicemia in a 16-year-old boy with an acute febrile illness [1]. In 1971, Kelly and Burns described two patients with a syndrome they termed "acute febrile ulcerative conglobate acne with polyarthralgia." The features of this syndrome included the sudden onset of severe ulcerative acne conglobata without cyst formation, fever, polyarthralgia, failure to respond to usual antibiotic therapy, and a favorable response to debridement in combination with steroid therapy [2]. In 1975, Plewig and Kligman named this disease *acne fulminans* [3]. This rare entity may occur in isolation or as part of the SAPHO syndrome (synovitis, acne, pustulosis, hyperostosis, and osteitis).

17.2 Background

The etiology of acne fulminans remains unclear, although infection, exogenous drug reaction, immunologic abnormalities, and genetic causes have all been proposed. Bacterial cultures reveal no unusual organisms and systemic antibiotics are ineffective when used as monotherapy, suggesting bacterial infection in isolation is

A. Schram, B.S.
School of Medicine, University of Pennsylvania, Philadelphia, PA, USA

M. Rosenbach, M.D. (✉)
Department of Dermatology, University of Pennsylvania, 3600 Spruce Street, 2nd Floor, Maloney Building, Philadelphia, PA 19014, USA
e-mail: misha.rosenbach@uphs.upenn.edu

J.A. Zeichner (ed.), *Acneiform Eruptions in Dermatology: A Differential Diagnosis*,
DOI 10.1007/978-1-4614-8344-1_17,

unlikely to be the causative mechanism. One theory suggests that acne fulminans is the manifestation of a severe immunologically mediated hypersensitivity reaction to *Propionibacterium acnes* (*P. acnes*) antigens. Cases of acne fulminans precipitated by isotretinoin therapy have been described, leading some to postulate that isotretinoin-induced fragility of the pilosebaceous unit increases the immune system's contact with *P. acnes* antigens [4, 5]. This theory is consistent with data suggesting that isotretinoin may initially increase superoxide ion and myeloperoxidase release from neutrophils in the early stages of acne treatment [6]. Genetically determined changes in neutrophil activity may put some individuals at increased risk for this aberrant immune response. Interestingly, a pair of siblings has been reported in whom one developed isotretinoin-induced eruptive pyogenic granulomas and the other isotretinoin-induced acne fulminans [5]. There have been reports of monozygotic twins and HLA-matched siblings who presented at the same age with similar clinical features, lending support to the role of hereditary factors in the pathogenesis of this entity [7–9].

Circulating immune complexes have been documented in patients with acne fulminans, causing some to postulate that the mechanism is that of an autoimmune disease. Other factors that favor the autoimmune hypothesis include the increase in γ-globulins and decrease in complement (C3) levels seen in some patients [10–12]. Additionally, patients often respond rapidly to systemic steroids.

Acne fulminans develops almost exclusively in adolescent boys, raising the question of whether hormonal factors are relevant in the pathogenesis of this condition. One report describes acne fulminans in three boys treated with testosterone for excessively tall stature [13]. Additionally, a 21-year-old body builder developed acne fulminans after taking 4 weeks of testosterone and anabolic steroids; however, on measurement his serum testosterone levels were found to be within normal limits [14]. Androgenic steroids augment sebum excretion in postpubertal men, leading to an increase in *P. acnes*. In some individuals, this may lead to an immunological reaction that manifests as acne fulminans.

The precise etiopathogenesis of this rare entity is uncertain and may involve a combination of factors including genetic susceptibility (potentially with abnormal hormone levels or immune response) and a vigorous reaction to bacterial antigens.

Acne fulminans occurs primarily in adolescent, Caucasian males, aged 13–19 years old. While it may occur in women, it is exceptionally rare. The disease usually begins as mild cystic acne that becomes fulminant after 1–2 years on average, although de novo presentations with acne fulminans as the initial presentation of acne have been reported [15].

17.3 Clinical Presentation

Patients usually present with a history of mild to moderate acne that suddenly erupts into spreading, ulcerative acne lesions with intense inflammation and necrosis. The lesions most often occur on the chest, and back, or face, and rarely the

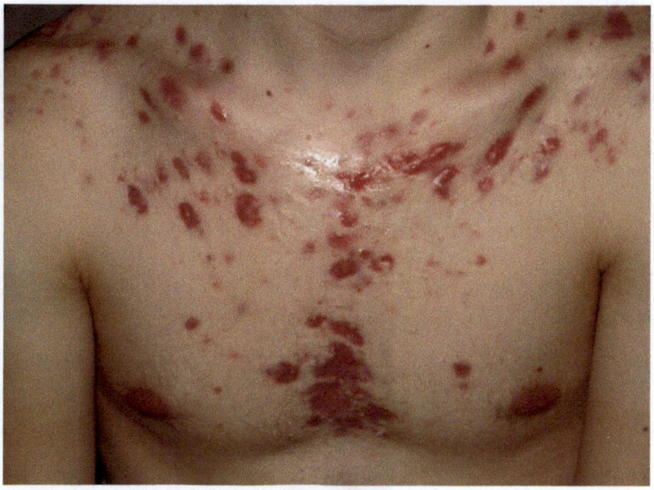

Fig. 17.1 Severe depressed scarring and post-inflammatory erythema in a patient with resolving acne fulminans

scalp and thighs [15]. The face is usually less severely affected than the trunk, and isolated lesions on the face are uncommon [4]. The highly inflammatory lesions initially resemble acne conglobata; however, they quickly form hemorrhagic nodules and plaques that undergo suppurative degeneration. The resultant lesions appear as ragged ulcerations with gelatinous, necrotic debris at their bases [10] (Figs. 17.1, 17.2, and 17.3). In contrast to acne vulgaris, open and closed comedones are uncommon. These fulminant eruptions are extremely tender and painful.

A broad spectrum of systemic reactions can be seen in patients with acne fulminans. The majority of cases are accompanied by systemic signs and symptoms, such as fever, fatigue, malaise, arthralgias, and myalgias. Other systemic findings of arthritis, myositis, erythema nodosum, hepatosplenomegaly, and aseptic bone lesions are less common [11, 15–17]. Musculoskeletal pain is often located in the chest, shoulder girdle, lower back, and large joints [15]. Patients may experience painful joint swelling in the iliosacral, iliac, and knee joints, resulting in a bent-over posture when walking. If present, erythema nodosum usually occurs on the shins [11, 16, 17]. Additionally, a patient has been reported with concurrent posterior scleritis and pyoderma gangrenosum-like eruptions on the lower legs [18].

17.4 Work-Up

Laboratory findings in acne fulminans are not consistent and may include leukocytosis, thrombocytosis, anemia, proteinuria, microscopic hematuria, and elevated erythrocyte sedimentation rate (ESR), C-reactive protein (CRP), and liver enzymes. Occasionally, a leukemoid reaction is present with an increased percentage of

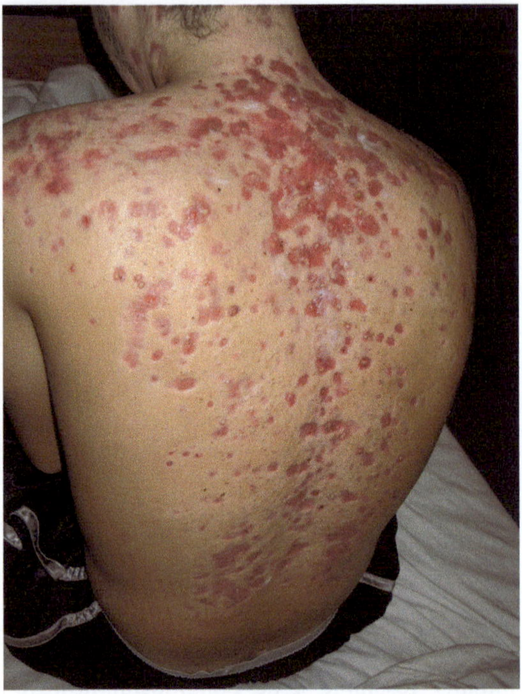

Fig. 17.2 Extensive areas of broad erosion with granulation and scattered inflammatory pustules and comedones

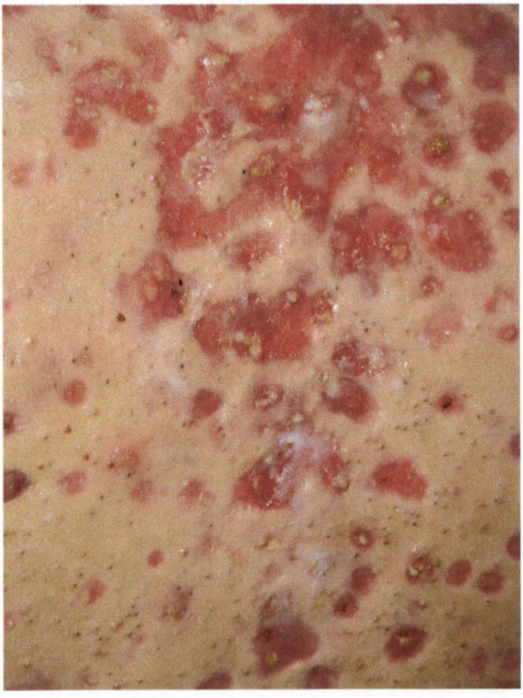

Fig. 17.3 Close up view of comedones, inflammatory pustules, and broad areas of erosion with scattered resolving lesions leaving depressed atrophic scars

myeloblasts, promyelocytes, and myelocytes in the peripheral blood [19]. Serum proteins may show decreased albumin or increased α-globulin and γ-globulin. Circulating immune complexes have been reported, as well as low C3 levels [10–12]. Rheumatoid factor and antinuclear antibody (ANA) tests have been negative, and there is no known association with HLA-B27 [4]. In contrast to patients with acne vulgaris, those with acne fulminans have shown depressed delayed hypersensitivity to various antigens on skin testing [20].

Bone involvement in acne fulminans is rare but well described. Lesions are initially osteolytic but become sclerotic with periosteal formation of new bone. Radiographs may demonstrate lytic bone lesions, and bone scans often show increased uptake of technetium "hot spots" [4, 21].

Histologically, early pustules show an intense dermal infiltrate of granulocytes with the destruction of follicles and sebaceous glands. The epidermis necroses secondary to hyalinized thrombotic vessels and profuses bleeding into the skin. The hemorrhagic skin becomes surrounded by a mixed granulocytic and lymphocytic infiltrate [10]. Some follicles distend with accumulating keratinized cells but do not form comedones. Late nodules show a regenerating acanthotic epidermis with a dense dermal mixed cellular infiltrate, vascular hyperplasia, and numerous stellate fibroblastic cells [4]. Direct immunofluorescence testing can rarely reveal a linear immunoglobulin M and fibrin band at the dermo-epidermal junction, in addition to fibrin deposition around the sebaceous glands [10].

Bone lesions in acne fulminans have historically been biopsied to rule out malignancy or infection. These specimens show benign, reactive changes. The inflammatory infiltrate and granulation tissue observed can mimic osteomyelitis; however, there is no evidence of microorganisms [22, 23].

Bacterial cultures from blood, joint fluid, skin, and bone lesions are usually negative. In addition to the usual organisms cultured from skin, *Staphylococcus aureus* can occasionally be seen. Antistaphylococcal and antistreptococcal antibody levels are usually normal [10]. *P. acnes* has been isolated from bone lesions of patients with acne fulminans, although the clinical significance of this finding is unclear, and contamination from the skin puncture site was not ruled out [22].

17.5 Treatment

The mainstay of treatment in patients with acne fulminans includes local wound care, supportive systemic care, and systemic corticosteroids. Patients often feel sick and require bed rest or hospitalization. The first step in management is gentle surgical debridement and frequent application of warm compresses with 20–40 % urea solutions to prevent the accumulation of crusts. Urea is also beneficial for its deodorant and antiseptic properties. Other topical treatments, including local antimicrobial agents, may be used as well. High-potency topical corticosteroids can effectively decrease inflammation when applied to the ulcerated nodules twice daily for 7–10 days [10]. Pulsed laser has also been reported to improve local control [24].

Systemic corticosteroids (0.5–1.0 mg/kg prednisolone) are indicated in patients with acne fulminans to manage the skin lesions, reduce fever, and improve musculoskeletal symptoms. Oral therapy should be gradually reduced to avoid the adverse effects of prolonged treatment with systemic steroids; however, relapse can occur 2–8 weeks after the acute attack when corticosteroid therapy is decreased [15]. The required duration of treatment seems to be 2–5 months to avoid relapse. Patients should be counseled about the anticipated long course of steroids and monitored closely for steroid-related side effects.

The use of isotretinoin in combination with oral corticosteroids is controversial. Systemic isotretinoin has been used in the successful treatment of acne fulminans; however, it has also been reported to precipitate the condition [4, 5, 15]. Isotretinoin should be started 2–4 weeks after corticosteroid therapy. It is recommended that physicians initiate isotretinoin at low doses (e.g., 0.1 mg/kg/day) initially to avoid exacerbation of lesions in patients with crusting. The final recommended dosage is 0.5–2.0 mg/kg/day, treated to a minimum total dose of 120 mg/kg. Occasionally, a repeat course of isotretinoin may be required. Although the utility of dapsone is unclear in acne fulminans, it may be used if isotretinoin is contraindicated [4].

Additional treatment may be useful in controlling the symptoms of acne fulminans. The myalgia, arthritis, and fever often respond to nonsteroidal anti-inflammatory drugs. Antibiotic therapy is indicated if there are signs of secondary bacterial infection. Other therapies have been tried with variable results, including intra-articular corticosteroids, methotrexate, sulfasalazine, cyclosporine A, bisphosphonates, and infliximab [4]. Regular measurement of ESR and white blood cell count provide an objective measure of treatment response and may correlate with the clinical course [10].

The long-term prognosis for patients with acne fulminans is good. Although relapse can occur when steroid treatment is reduced quickly, the risk of relapse is small after 1 year. The cutaneous lesions may result in significant scarring. Residual bone changes, including sclerosis and hyperostosis, remain visible radiographically [4].

References

1. Burns RE, Colville JM. Acne conglobata with septicemia. Arch Dermatol. 1959;79:361–3.
2. Kelly AP, Burns RE. Acute febrile ulcerative conglobate acne with polyarthralgia. Arch Dermatol. 1971;104:182–7.
3. Plewig G, Kligman AM. Acne: morphogenesis and treatment. Berlin: Springer; 1975. p. 196.
4. Zaba R, Schwartz RA, Jarmuda S, Czarnecka-Operacz M, Silny W. Acne fulminans: explosive systemic form of acne. J Eur Acad Dermatol Venereol. 2011;25(5):501–7.
5. Blanc D, Zultak M, Wendling D, et al. Eruptive pyogenic granulomas and acne fulminans in two siblings treated with isotretinoin: a possible common pathogenesis. Dermatologica. 1988;177(1):16–8.
6. Perkins W, Crocket KV, Hodgins MB, Mackie RM, Lackie JM. The effect of treatment with 13-*cis*-retinoic acid on the metabolic burst of peripheral blood neutrophils from patients with acne. Br J Dermatol. 1991;124:429–32.
7. Darley CR, Currey HL, Baker H. Acne fulminans with arthritis in identical twins treated with isotretinoin. J R Soc Med. 1984;77:328–30.

8. Gonzales T, Gantes M, Bustabad S, et al. Acne fulminans associated with arthritis in monozygotic twins. J Rheumatol. 1985;12:389–90.
9. Wong SS, Pritchard MH, Holt PJA. Familial acne fulminans. Clin Exp Dermatol. 1992; 17:351–3.
10. Jansen T, Plewig G. Acne fulminans: review. Int J Dermatol. 1998;37:254–7.
11. Kellett J, Beck MH, Chalmers RJG. Erythema nodosum and circulating immune complexes in acne fulminans after treatment with isotretinoin. Br Med J. 1985;290:820.
12. Woolfson H. Acne fulminans with circulating immune complexes and leukaemoid reaction treated with steroids and azathioprine. Clin Exp Dermatol. 1986;12:463–6.
13. Traupe H, von Muhlendahl KE, Bramswig J, et al. Acne of the fulminans type following testosterone therapy in three excessively tall boys. Arch Dermatol. 1988;124:414–7.
14. Heydenreich G. Testosterone and anabolic steroids and acne fulminans. Arch Dermatol. 1989;125:571–2.
15. Karvonen SL. Acne fulminans: report of clinical findings and treatment of twenty-four patients. J Am Acad Dermatol. 1993;28:572–9.
16. Reizis Z, Trattner A, Hodak E, et al. Acne fulminans with hepatosplenomegaly and erythema nodosum migrans. J Am Acad Dermatol. 1991;24:886–8.
17. Williamson DM, Cunliffe WJ, Gatecliff M, Scott FG. Acute ulcerate acne conglobata (acne fulminans) with erythema nodosum. Clin Exp Dermatol. 1977;2:351–4.
18. Kurokawa S, Tokura Y, Nham NX, et al. Acne fulminans coexisting with pyoderma gangrenosum-like eruptions and posterior scleritis. J Dermatol. 1996;23:37–41.
19. Strom S, Thyresson N, Bostrom H. Acute febrile ulcerative conglobate acne with leukemoid reaction. Acta Derm Venereol. 1973;53:306–12.
20. Palatsi R. Delayed hypersensitivity and febrile acne conglobata. Acta Derm Venereol. 1977;57:51–3.
21. Jemec GBE, Rasmussen I. Bone lesions of acne fulminans: case report and review of the literature. J Am Acad Dermatol. 1989;20:353–7.
22. Nault P, Lassonde M. Acne fulminans with osteolytic lesions. Arch Dermatol. 1985;121:662–4.
23. Hunter LY, Hensinger RN. Destructive arthritis associated with acne fulminans: a case report. Ann Rheum Dis. 1980;39:403–5.
24. Friedlander SF. Effective treatment of acne fulminans-associated granulation tissue with the pulsed dye laser. Pediatr Dermatol. 1998;15:396–8.

Chapter 18
Acne Mechanica

Zoe Diana Draelos

18.1 Introduction

Acne mechanica is a term used to describe the presence of inflammatory papules and pustules caused by friction from repetitive rubbing, stretching, or squeezing of the skin accompanied by heat, pressure, and occlusion.

It can be observed under many different circumstances, which will be discussed in this chapter [1]. Most of the references to acne mechanica in the modern literature come from sports-associated dermatoses [2], but Albert Kligman was present at an NIOSH workshop held in Cincinnati, Ohio, on April 6–8, 1983, that discussed the chronic effects of repeated mechanical trauma to the skin where acne mechanica was discussed in detail [3]. He likened acne mechanica to a category of contact dermatitis only provoked by physical stressors. The goal of the workshop was to define the various categories of superficial skin injuries resulting from repetitive trauma, which led to a clearer understanding of acne mechanica.

18.2 Background

An understanding of acne mechanica demands a discussion of the surface skin architecture. While many might view the skin as a smooth even surface, it is actually a series of mountains and valleys that give rise to skin dermatoglyphics. The mountains are created by the pilosebaceous apparatus sitting higher than the surrounding skin creating the intervening valleys. When the skin is rubbed, the follicular ostia

Z.D. Draelos, M.D. (✉)
Department of Dermatology, Duke University School of Medicine,
2444 North Main Street, High Point, NC 27262, USA
e-mail: zdraelos@northstate.net

J.A. Zeichner (ed.), *Acneiform Eruptions in Dermatology: A Differential Diagnosis*,
DOI 10.1007/978-1-4614-8344-1_18, © Springer Science+Business Media New York 2014

are preferentially mechanically damaged. This chronic irritation is thought to account for acne mechanica; however, several addition factors can worsen the disease. If the skin surface is covered in sweat, the moisture decreases the mechanical resistance of the skin to shear forces and worsens the inflammation. Since the skin is more hydrated when heat is applied, this enhances the susceptibility of the skin to shear forces from rubbing. Finally, if occlusion is present, this hyperhydrates the skin causing further problems in resisting the shear force. Thus, acne mechanica is due to a combination of follicular ostia prominence and skin hydration.

Mills and Kligman developed a model for studying acne mechanica where they sealed acne-bearing skin with adhesive tape for 2 weeks and documented new inflammatory lesions. They believed that the increase in acne resulted from the rupture of microcomedones that were not visible to the human eye [4].

18.3 Clinical Presentation

Acne mechanica can occur in several settings. The most commonly recognized cause of acne mechanica is use of a chinstrap in football [5]. The sweat that accumulates beneath the plastic chin cup macerates the skin that is then subject to continuous rubbing from speaking, mastication, and facial movement. However, acne mechanica can be seen on all body areas where football pads are worn, including the upper back and shoulders [6]. The fact that the pads contacting the skin are causative has been proven by the initiation of acne mechanica with football activities and its spontaneous resolution at the end of the season. Acne mechanica needs to be separated from hormonally induced acne; however, the presentation is similar and both may occur simultaneously. It should be recognized that acne mechanica can occur in the absence of traditional acne.

Another common setting for acne mechanica is under the chinstrap in persons who wear a helmet for equestrian activities [7]. Any helmet or hat that has a chinstrap could potentially cause problems. Acne mechanica is even seen under the chin in violin players from rubbing on the chin rest, a condition known as fiddler's neck [8]. A variety of acne mechanica has been reported from the repeated trauma of a comb and brush on the face [9]. Other causes include rubbing from a backpack or riding in a vehicle for prolonged periods.

18.4 Work-Up

The diagnosis of acne mechanica is primarily made based on clinical appearance and distribution. Moreover, a detailed personal history from the patient should be taken, with particular attention paid to lifestyle factors such as use of products that occlude or mechanically apply trauma to the skin.

18.5 Treatment

The primary treatment for acne mechanica is discontinuation of the trauma to the skin, which may result in spontaneous resolution. However, situations may arise where additional treatment is necessary. Acne mechanica is treated like acne vulgaris with topical and oral therapies. Topical agents useful in treatment include benzoyl peroxide alone or in combination with clindamycin. Benzoyl peroxide possesses antibacterial, anti-inflammatory, and comedolytic effects, all of which may be valuable in the treatment of acne mechanica [10]. When benzoyl peroxide touches the skin, it breaks down into benzoic acid and oxygen. Benzoyl peroxide acts as an anti-inflammatory agent by reducing oxygen radicals. Further, its ability to reduce the *Propionibacterium acnes* (*P. acnes*) population also reduces inflammation due to lessened bacterial induced monocytes producing tumor necrosis factor-alpha, interleukin-1beta, and interleukin-8 [11]. This anti-inflammatory effect is perceived by the patient as reduced redness and pain. Combining benzoyl peroxide with clindamycin also increases antibacterial efficacy. Finally, topical retinoids, such as adapalene, tretinoin, or tazarotene, may be helpful as both anti-inflammatories and comedolytics [12].

Oral antibiotics are appropriate in patients with more painful and inflammatory acne mechanica. The same antibiotics used in traditional acne treatment may be employed here. These include oral tetracycline, doxycycline, minocycline, trimethoprim/sulfamethoxazole, and ciprofloxacin [13]. One treatment regimen is to use the oral antibiotic along with a topical benzoyl peroxide/clindamycin preparation until control is achieved and then discontinue the oral medication while continuing the topical treatment until the activity causing the acne mechanica has been discontinued. Perhaps the most important aspect of acne mechanica treatment is the identification of the source of friction, heat, pressure, and occlusion that is inciting the disease. The patient will then be reassured of the diagnosis and can vary activities to assist in prevention.

A variety of ancillary over-the-counter preparations can also be used for the treatment of acne mechanica. These include triclosan-containing antibacterial soaps and salicylic acid containing cleansers. Removing bacteria and sweat from the skin afflicted with acne mechanica is important. Immediate removal of the sweat-soaked clothing from the body and elimination of the acne causing athletic device as soon as possible may be helpful. Special clothing made of a non-water retaining fabrics, such as polyester, should be selected over cotton to avoid keeping sweat in contact with the skin.

In summary, acne mechanica is a term used to describe the presence of inflammatory papules and pustules caused by friction from repetitive rubbing, stretching, or squeezing of the skin accompanied by heat, pressure, and occlusion. Eliminating the inciting factors is the key to treatment and preventions.

References

1. Basler RSW. Skin injuries in sports medicine. J Am Acad Dermatol. 1989;21(6):1257–62.
2. Levine N. Dermatologic aspects of sports medicine. J Am Acad Dermatol. 1980;3(4):415–24.
3. Kligman AM. The chronic effects of repeated mechanical trauma to the skin. Am J Ind Med. 1985;8:257–64.
4. Mills OH, Kligman A. Acne mechanica. Arch Dermatol. 1975;111(4):481–3.
5. Farber GA, Burks JW, Hegre AM, Brown GR. Football acne—an acneiform eruption. Cutis. 1977;20(3):356–60.
6. Kirkland R, Adams BB. Dermatologic problems in the football player. Int J Dermatol. 2006;4(8):927–32.
7. Freiman A, Barakin B, Elpern DJ. Sports dermatology part 1: common dermatoses. Can Med Assoc J. 2004;7(8):851–3.
8. Peachey RDG, Matthews CAN. Fiddler's neck. Br J Dermatol. 2006;98(6):669–74.
9. Petrozzi W. Comb and brush acne. Cutis. 1980;26(6):568–71.
10. Tanghetti E. The evolution of benzoyl peroxide therapy. Cutis. 2008;82(5):5–11.
11. Kim J, Ochoa M, Krutzik S, Takeuchi O, Uematsu S, Legaspi A, et al. Activation of toll-like receptor 2 in acne triggers inflammatory cytokine responses. J Immunol. 2002;169:1535–41.
12. Pharis DB, Teller C, Wolf JE. Cutaneous manifestations of sports participation. J Am Acad Dermatol. 1997;36(3):448–59.
13. Shalita A. Clinical aspects of acne. Dermatology. 1998;196(1):93–4.

Chapter 19
Cushing's Syndrome

Nick Zilieris, Cheryl J. Gustafson, and Steven R. Feldman

19.1 Introduction

Cushing's syndrome is a constellation of signs and symptoms due to chronic glucocorticoid excess. Glucocorticoids have far-reaching effects that are not only seen within the body but also seen externally affecting the integumentary system. This chapter will review the pathophysiology, epidemiology, clinical cutaneous manifestations, diagnosis, and treatment of Cushing's syndrome.

Harvey Williams Cushing, M.D., an American Neurosurgeon, first described Cushing's syndrome in 1912 as an endocrinological syndrome caused by a malfunction of the pituitary gland, which he termed "polyglandular syndrome" [1]. Today, Cushing's syndrome is defined as a constellation of signs and symptoms due to chronic glucocorticoid excess. The etiology of hypercortisolism can be classified as exogenous or endogenous. Exogenous hypercortisolism typically results from the administration of corticosteroids prescribed by physicians to manage chronic diseases, whereas endogenous hypercortisolism results from an imbalance in the body's regulation of serum cortisol levels. Endogenous forms of Cushing's syndrome can be further subcategorized into adrenocorticotropin (ACTH)-dependent and adrenocorticotropin (ACTH)-independent conditions. ACTH-dependent

N. Zilieris, D.O.
Department of Internal Medicine, Baptist Hospital, Miami Beach, FL, USA

C.J. Gustafson, M.D. (✉)
Department of Dermatology, Wake Forest University Baptist Medical Center, 4618 Country Club Road, Winston-Salem, NC 27104, USA
e-mail: cgustafs@wakehealth.edu

S.R. Feldman, M.D., Ph.D.
Department of Dermatology, Pathology, and Public Health Sciences, Wake Forest University Baptist Medical Center, Winston-Salem, NC, USA

J.A. Zeichner (ed.), *Acneiform Eruptions in Dermatology: A Differential Diagnosis*, DOI 10.1007/978-1-4614-8344-1_19, © Springer Science+Business Media New York 2014

conditions are characterized by high or inappropriately normal ACTH levels, which result in excess production and secretion of cortisol from the adrenal glands. There are three main types of ACTH-dependent conditions: (1) ACTH-secreting pituitary adenomas (i.e., Cushing's disease), (2) ectopic ACTH-secreting tumors (typically bronchogenic or neuroendocrine in origin), and (3) ectopic corticotropin-releasing hormone (CRH). ACTH-independent conditions are characterized by excessive cortisol secretion by the adrenal glands despite a suppressed ACTH level. These conditions include (1) adrenal adenomas, (2) bilateral adrenal hyperplasia, and (3) adrenal carcinoma [2].

19.2 Background

Cushing's syndrome follows a complex pathway within the pituitary–hypothalamic–adrenal axis. The paraventricular nucleus (PVN) of the hypothalamus releases CRH, which stimulates the release of ACTH from the pituitary gland. ACTH travels hematogenously to the adrenal gland to stimulate the release of cortisol and other steroids from the *zona fasciculata* and *reticularis* of the adrenal cortex. Elevated levels of cortisol exert negative feedback on the pituitary gland, thereby decreasing the release of ACTH [3].

Cushing's disease refers specifically to hypercortisolism secondary to excess production of ACTH from a corticotrophic pituitary adenoma. The tumor renders the pituitary gland unresponsive to the negative feedback effect of elevated cortisol levels. As a result, Cushing's disease is characterized by elevated levels of ACTH and cortisol.

In adrenal sources of Cushing's syndrome, excess cortisol is produced by adrenal gland tumors, hyperplastic adrenal glands, or adrenal glands with nodular adrenal hyperplasia. As a result, the serum ACTH level is low and serum cortisol is high. Additionally, ectopic tumors, which are located outside the normal pituitary-adrenal system, can produce ACTH, thereby stimulating excess secretion of cortisol from the adrenal glands. This results in elevated serum levels of ACTH and cortisol.

In all forms of Cushing's syndrome, the effects of excess glucocorticoids may be mixed with the effects of excess mineralocorticoids and androgenic steroids. These effects are seen in many body systems because cortisol is part of the pituitary–hypothalamic–adrenal axis, which affects the higher functioning central nervous system, as well as lower functioning organ systems. Hence, cutaneous manifestations of Cushing's syndrome result from the effects of excess cortisol on the epidermis and dermis. More specifically, hypercortisolism inhibits epidermal cell division and impairs the synthesis of collagen and mucopolysaccharides [4]. As a result, the epidermis becomes thin, shiny, and even scaly.

Cushing's syndrome affects 1–2 individuals per 100,000 each year [3]. Women are affected four times more than men. The disease occurs primarily between the ages 25 and 40, with peak onset during the second and third decades. No ethnic disparities have been identified [5, 6]. Cushing syndrome occurs in 30 % of people with Carney complex, a familial form of micronodular hyperplasia of the adrenal gland that results in an ACTH-independent form of Cushing's syndrome [7].

Iatrogenic Cushing's syndrome, due to the exogenous administration of glucocorticoids, accounts for the majority of Cushing's syndrome cases. However, traditional estimates regarding the prevalence of different forms of Cushing's syndrome do not include iatrogenic cases. This is largely due to the lack of a uniformly accepted definition and/or gold standard diagnostic tests. Despite this fact, exogenous hypercortisolism accounts for more causes of Cushing's syndrome than all causes of endogenous hypercortisolism combined. Although there is no widely accepted definition, most clinicians agree that exogenous Cushing's syndrome is present when symptoms of Cushing's syndrome develop in individuals treated with supraphysiological doses of glucocorticoids [8].

Endogenous Cushing's syndrome results from excessive production of cortisol. Overproduction of cortisol may occur in three ways: (1) Excess production of ACTH from the pituitary (Cushing's disease) accounts for 70 % of these cases. Although pituitary microadenomas are one of the main sources of excess ACTH from the pituitary, 40–60 % of patients with Cushing's disease have no identified tumor [8]. (2) Ectopic corticotropin-producing tumors (typically bronchogenic or pancreatic cancer) are the underlying etiology in 15 % of Cushing's syndrome patients. However, in infants, adrenal carcinoma is the leading cause of Cushing's syndrome [9]. (3) Primary adrenal sources of excess cortisol production (e.g., adrenal hyperplasia, adrenal adenomas) account for the remaining 15 % of endogenous Cushing's syndrome cases.

19.3 Clinical Presentation

Cushing's syndrome, like many endocrine disorders, induces changes in multiple body systems, the extent to which depends on the adrenocortical hormone involved, as well as the duration of exposure [5]. Glucocorticoid excess induces striking changes in body habitus. Central obesity is the most common feature, occurring in 97 % of patients. Fat deposition occurs in the face ("moon" facies), retro-orbital fossa, neck, supraclavicular fossa ("supraclavicular fat pads"), trunk, upper back ("buffalo" hump), and abdomen with loss of subcutaneous fat in the extremities [10]. The exact cause of adipose deposition in Cushing's syndrome remains unknown; however, it is theorized to be secondary to insulin resistance [9]. Central obesity is accompanied by wasting of the extremities. Additionally, increased protein catabolism occurs in peripheral supportive tissue resulting in muscle weakness, fatigability, and osteoporosis.

A variety of cutaneous manifestations are seen in Cushing's syndrome. Violaceous, atrophic striae on the abdomen and thighs is a classic finding. Striae and easy bruisability result from rupture of weakened collagen fibers in the dermis [9]. Thinning of the epidermis is another common skin manifestation. It is often

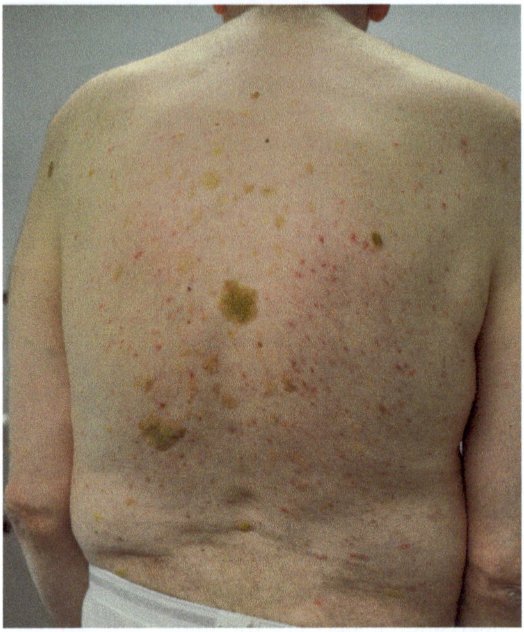

Fig. 19.1 The back of a man diagnosed with Cushing's disease. The patient presented with acne on his back. On close examination, he showed signs of a small prominence of fat on the upper back, the so-called buffalo hump. After his primary care doctor discovered he suffered from osteoporosis, a work-up revealed an ACTH-secreting pituitary adenoma leading to hypercortisolism. The tumor was subsequently surgically removed (Photo credit: Joshua A. Zeichner, M.D.)

described as a fine "cigarette paper" wrinkling and primarily involves the dorsal surfaces of the hands and elbows [11]. In severe cases, the epidermis can peel off after being covered with adhesive tape, a finding referred to as the Liddle sign [12]. Likewise, the dermis becomes thin and loose in areas of reduced subcutaneous fat [13]. Overall, the skin becomes friable and easily damageable with markedly impaired wound healing. Subsequently, other complications may result, such as infections (e.g., dermatophyte, bacterial, fungal, and opportunistic) and ulcerations [14]. Another common cutaneous manifestation of Cushing's syndrome is plethora of the face, neck, and chest, which is not accompanied by an increase in red blood cell concentration.

Acneiform eruptions occur with Cushing's syndrome because sebaceous gland activity and sebum production are intricately involved acne formation and are hormonally regulated (Fig. 19.1). The hormones specifically related to Cushing's syndrome that affect the sebaceous glands include androgens, CRH, ACTH, and glucocorticoids [15]. Androgen receptors have been localized to the basal layer of the sebaceous gland and the outer root sheath of the hair follicle. When activated, these receptors stimulate the sebaceous gland to secrete sebum, which can potentially clog the follicle and result in pimples [15]. When glucocorticoid excess is accompanied by androgen excess, acne and oily skin can develop. In Cushing's syndrome, acneiform eruptions are typically monomorphic, perifollicular papules produced by hyperkeratosis of follicular openings typically on the face, chest, and back. Mild pustule formation can be seen; however, deep cystic lesions and comedo formation, which are features characteristic of adolescent acne, are uncommon in Cushing's syndrome [15]. Additionally, the pimples of steroid acne are usually more uniform in size unlike acne vulgaris [16].

CRH's main effect on the skin is at the level of the sebaceous gland where it inhibits sebaceous proliferation, promotes sebaceous differentiation, and induces sebaceous gland lipogenesis by enhancing androgen bioavailability. Clinical and experiment evidence implicates the involvement of CRH in the development of acne [17]. Other skins changes include cutis xerosis, purpura, ecchymoses, livedo reticularis, and poikiloderma-like changes [9]. Hyperpigmentation may be seen secondary to the production of ACTH and related peptides, such as melanocyte-stimulating hormone (MSH). MSH is derived from the same prohormone, pro-opiomelanocortin, as is ACTH [14].

In addition to the classical cutaneous manifestations, Cushing's syndrome is characterized by a diversity of systemic manifestations. In regard to the endocrine system, hypercortisolism induces increased hepatic gluconeogenesis and insulin resistance, which can subsequently lead to impaired glucose tolerance [18]. Ultimately, less than 20 % of patients develop diabetes mellitus type II. In association with impaired glucose tolerance, acanthosis nigricans can be seen in patients with Cushing's syndrome [19]. Hypertension is a common cardiovascular manifestation of Cushing's syndrome and occurs in 82 % of patients due to sodium and water retention. Interestingly, in people diagnosed with primary hypertension, 0.5–1 % have Cushing's syndrome [9]. Other common systemic manifestations of Cushing's syndrome include proximal myopathy, oligomenorrhea/amenorrhea, personality changes, osteoporosis, and edema [9].

19.4 Work-Up

The overnight dexamethasone suppression test is the initial screening test of choice as it has a sensitivity of 97 % and a specificity of 80 %, if the cortisol level is >3 μg/dl [3]. A 24-h urine free cortisol level can be used as an alternative screening test. A level >140 nmol is suggestive of Cushing's syndrome with 90–95 % specificity and sensitivity [18]. Definitive diagnosis is confirmed with a standard low-dose dexamethasone suppression test done over 48 h. The test is positive when urinary cortisol stays >25 nmol/L or plasma cortisol remains >140 nmol/L.

Determining the etiology of Cushing's syndrome is complicated secondary to the fact that tests lack specificity. Additionally, tumors producing this syndrome are prone to spontaneous and often dramatic changes in hormone secretion (periodic hormonogenesis) [3]. Hence, a combination of laboratory and imaging tests is often needed to determine the specific cause.

Plasma ACTH levels can be useful in determining the specific etiology of Cushing's syndrome, particularly in regard to differentiating ACTH-dependent from ACTH-independent causes. Evaluating the response of cortisol output upon administration of high-dose dexamethasone can help distinguish ACTH-secreting pituitary microadenomas or hypothalamic–pituitary dysfunction from other etiologies of Cushing's syndrome. The metyrapone and CRH infusion tests function under the rationale that the hypothalamic–pituitary axis will be suppressed by steroid hypersecretion by an adrenal tumor or ectopic production of ACTH, thereby resulting in inhibition of ACTH release by the pituitary. As a result, patients with pituitary–hypothalamic dysfunction and/or a microadenoma have an increase in steroid or ACTH secretion in response to metyrapone or CRH administration.

The diagnosis of adrenal carcinoma is suggested by a palpable abdominal mass and by markedly elevated baseline values of both urine 17-ketosteroids and plasma DHEA sulfate. Plasma and urine cortisol levels are variably elevated. Adrenal carcinoma is usually resistant to both ACTH stimulation and dexamethasone suppression. Imaging modalities include brain MRI to evaluate the pituitary, high-resolution chest CT to evaluate ectopic ACTH, and abdominal CT to evaluate the adrenals [9].

19.5 Treatment

Treatment is directed at correcting the source of the hypercortisolism, thus restoring hormone balance. The gold standard for Cushing's disease is transsphenoidal surgery with an initial cure rate of 70–80 % [9]. For adrenal tumors, the treatment is typically surgical resection of the tumor. Once the tumor causing the hypercortisolism is removed, the HPA axis typically remains suppressed. Therefore, hydrocortisone replacement therapy is needed postsurgery until there is physiologic adaptation to normal cortisol levels, which may require many months or even years of therapy [9].

In some cases adjuvant therapy, such as radiation therapy, chemotherapy, and/or drug therapy, is required to suppress cortisol synthesis [7]. Oral agents with established efficacy in regard to inhibition of steroid synthesis in Cushing's syndrome include metyrapone, ketoconazole, and mitotane.

References

1. Deacon SP. Pituitary-dependent Cushing's disease. BMJ. 1977;1:1409.
2. Boscaro M et al. Cushing's syndrome. Lancet. 2001;357:783.
3. Arlt Wiebke. Disorders of the adrenal cortex (chapter 342). In: Fauci AS, Braunwald E, Kasper DL, Hauser SL, Longo DL, Jameson JL, Loscalzo J, editors. Harrison's principles of internal medicine, 18th ed. http://www.accessmedicine.com/content.aspx?aID=9140931.
4. Fisher LB, Maibach HI. The effect of corticosteroids on human epidermal mitotic activity. Arch Dermatol. 1971;103:39–44.
5. Wilkins L. Professional guide to diseases. 9th ed. 2009;11:631–37.
6. Humes H, et al. Kelley's textbook of internal medicine, 4th edn. 2000;407:2721–27.
7. James W, Berger T, Elston D. Andrews' Diseases of the skin: clinical dermatology, vol. 24. 10th ed. London: Saunders; 2005. p. 500–1.
8. Carroll TB, Findling JW.Curr Opin Endocrinol Diabetes Obes. 2009;16(4):308–15. Review Erratum in: Curr Opin Endocrinol Diabetes Obes. 2010;17(5):492.

9. Fauci AS, Braunwald E, Kasper DL, Hauser SL, Longo DL, Jameson JL, Loscalzo J.In: Disorders of the adrenal cortex (chapter 336). Fauci AS, Braunwald E, Kasper DL, Hauser SL, Longo DL, Jameson JL, Loscalzo J, editors. Harrison's Principles of internal medicine, 17th ed.
10. Freinkel RK. Cutaneous manifestations of endocrine diseases. In: Fitzpatrick TB, Eisen AZ, Wolff K, et al., editors. Dermatology in general medicine. 4th ed. New York: McGraw-Hill; 1993. p. 2113–31.
11. Yanovski JA, Cutler GB. Glucocorticoid action and the clinical features of Cushing's syndrome. Endocrinol Metab Clin North Am. 1994;23(3):487–509.
12. Orth DN, Kovacs WJ. The adrenal cortex. In: Wilson JD, Foster DW, Kronenberg HM, et al., editors. William's textbook of endocrinology. 9th ed. Philadelphia: Saunders; 1998. p. 565–9.
13. Rokowski K, Sheehy J, Cutroneo KR. Glucocorticoid-mediated selective reduction of functioning collagen messenger ribonucleic acid. Arch Biochem Biophys. 1981;210:74–81.
14. Findling JW, Raff H. Diagnosis and differential diagnosis of Cushing's syndrome. Endocrinol Metab Clin North Am. 2001;30(3):729–47.
15. Lolis MS, Bowe WP, Shalita AR. Acne and systemic disease. Med Clin N Am. 2009;93:1161–81.
16. Ross EJ, Linch DC. Cushing's syndrome-killing disease: discriminatory value of signs and symptoms aiding early diagnosis. Lancet. 1982;2:646–9.
17. Shome B, Saffran M. Peptides of the hypothalamus. J Neurochem. 1966;13(5):433–48.
18. Meier CA, Biller BM. Clinical and biochemical evaluation of Cushing's syndrome. Endocrinol Metab Clin North Am. 1997;26:741–62.
19. Winkelmann RK, Scheen RS, Underhal LO. Acanthosis nigricans and endocrine disease. JAMA. 1960;174(9):1145–52.

Chapter 20
PAPA Syndrome

Fan Liu and Kanade Shinkai

Abbreviations

ASC	Apoptosis-associated speck-like protein with a caspase recruitment domain
C3	Complement component 3
CAPS	Cryopyrin-associated periodic syndromes
CD2BP1	CD2-binding protein 1
DMARDs	Disease-modifying antirheumatic drugs
FMA	Familial Mediterranean fever
IgM	Immunoglobulin M
IL	Interleukin
IL-1β	Interleukin-1-beta
kD	Kilodalton
NLRP3	Nucleotide oligomerization domain-like receptor family pyrin domain containing 3
NSAIDs	Nonsteroidal anti-inflammatory drugs
PAPA	Pyogenic sterile arthritis, pyoderma gangrenosum, and acne
PSTPIP1	Proline-serine-threonine phosphatase interacting protein 1
PTP-PEST	Proline-glutamic acid-serine-threonine-rich family of protein tyrosine phosphatases
TNFα	Tumor necrosis factor alpha

F. Liu, B.A., M.D. • K. Shinkai, M.D., Ph.D. (✉)
Department of Dermatology, University of California, San Francisco, 1701 Divisadero Street, 3rd Floor, San Francisco, CA 94115, USA
e-mail: shinkaik@derm.ucsf.edu

J.A. Zeichner (ed.), *Acneiform Eruptions in Dermatology: A Differential Diagnosis*,
DOI 10.1007/978-1-4614-8344-1_20,

20.1 Introduction

The pyogenic sterile arthritis, pyoderma gangrenosum, and acne (PAPA) syndrome was first recognized in 1997 when ten family members in three generations manifested with variable expression of juvenile-onset arthritis and subsequent presentation of pyoderma gangrenosum and cystic acne in adolescence and adulthood [1]. This inherited disorder stems from dysregulation of the innate immune system, presenting with symptoms of seemingly unprovoked episodes of synovial tissue and skin inflammation [1]. Recurrent inflammation seen in PAPA syndrome typifies that classically seen in autoinflammatory disorders. Autoinflammatory disorders, though lacking clear diagnostic criteria, are marked by chronic and intermittent episodes of fever, cytokine dysregulation, and organ inflammation; skin and joint involvement is a prominent feature [2, 3]. Unlike autoimmune diseases, autoinflammatory disorders lack high-titer autoantibodies and autoreactive T lymphocytes [2]. Genes associated with inherited syndromes of autoinflammation encode for protein mediators of apoptosis, inflammation, and cytokine processing (Table 20.1) [3].

Table 20.1 Inherited autoinflammatory disorders

Inherited autoinflammatory disorders	Associated genetic mutation	OMIM#
Familial Mediterranean fever (FMF)	Pyrin (MEFV)	249100
Cryopyrin-associated periodic syndromes [Muckle-Wells syndrome (MWS), familial cold autoimmune syndrome (FCAS), neonatal-onset multisystem inflammatory disease (NOMID)]	Nucleotide oligomerization domain-like receptor family, pyrin domain containing 3 (NLRP3, also known as Nalp3 or cryopyrin)	191900, 120100, 607115
Tumor necrosis factor receptor-associated periodic syndrome (TRAPS)	Tumor necrosis factor receptor superfamily member 1A (TNFRSF1A)	142680
Hyper-immunoglobulin D syndrome (HIDS)	Mevalonate kinase (MVK)	260920
Blau syndrome	Caspase recruitment domain family, member 15/nucleotide-binding oligomerization domain protein 2 (CARD15/NOD2)	186580
Deficiency of interleukin 1 receptor antagonist (DIRA)	Interleukin 1 receptor antagonist (IL1RN)	612852
Generalized pustular psoriasis (GPP)	Interleukin 36 receptor antagonist (IL-36RN)	614204
Crohn's disease	Caspase recruitment domain family, member 15/nucleotide-binding oligomerization domain protein 2 (CARD15/NOD2)	266600
Japanese autoinflammatory syndrome with lipodystrophy (JASL)	Proteasome subunit, β type 8 (PSMB8)	256040

20.2 Background

Five years after the first cases of PAPA was described, a gene mutation associated with this syndrome was localized to the CD2-binding protein 1 (CD2BP1) gene on chromosome 15q. CD2BP1 and its murine ortholog, proline-serine-threonine phosphatase interacting protein 1(PSTPIP1), are cellular signaling adaptors known to play integral roles in cellular distribution of proteins, including actin reorganization [2]. Indeed, cultured macrophages from patients with PAPA syndrome demonstrate abnormal podosome structures and focal adhesion complexes, leading to defects in chemotaxis and migration [4].

CD2BP1 also activates innate immune responses by regulating inflammatory cytokine production, especially interleukin-1-beta (IL-1β). Key members of the signaling cascade upstream of IL-1β activation include pyrin (the susceptibility gene for Familial Mediterranean fever, FMF) and the Nalp3 inflammasome, a multi-protein signaling complex comprised of cryopyrin (also known as nucleotide oligomerization domain-like receptor family pyrin domain containing 3, NLRP3), apoptosis-associated speck-like protein with a caspase recruitment domain (ASC) and caspase 1[4, 5].

Mutations in CD2BP1 seen in association with PAPA syndrome result in enhanced IL-1β production through its effects on critical upstream regulatory pathways. Specifically, known mutations of CD2BP1 abrogate binding to proline-glutamic acid-serine-threonine-rich family of protein tyrosine phosphatases (PTP-PEST), an interaction essential for CD2BP1 dephosphorylation [3, 6]. Hyperphosphorylation of CD2BP1 in turn augments its interaction with pyrin, downregulating the inhibitory effect of pyrin on activation of the Nalp3 inflammasome, the multi-protein signaling complex that mediates the catalytic cleavage of pro-IL-1β to its active form [4, 7]. While the direct mechanism by which pyrin interacts with the inflammasome remains unclear, mutations in CD2BP1 associated with PAPA syndrome may enhance recruitment of CD2BP1 to ASC aggregates, potentially augmenting inflammasome signaling [8]. An alternative hypothesis postulates that mutations in CD2BP1 activate pathways leading to cell death and cytokine release, including IL-1β [4, 9]. Taken in sum, mutations in CD2BP1 impact many important aspects of immunity: immune cell adhesion, migration, activation, signaling, cytokine production, and apoptosis.

The importance of the IL-1 regulatory pathway in inflammation is highlighted by the emerging knowledge that several inherited autoinflammatory syndromes are associated with IL-1 dysregulation, including FMF, cryopyrin-associated periodic syndromes (CAPS), and deficiency of IL-1 receptor antagonist (DIRA). It is unknown whether enhanced IL-1 production seen in autoinflammatory diseases results from aberrant activation (i.e., activation of the pathway in the absence of physiologic triggers such as infection) or an inability to turn off normal inflammatory responses due to mutations in key signaling or regulatory components [10]. The aforementioned IL-1 signaling cascade is highly expressed in both skin and synovial tissue, possibly explaining the common involvement of these tissues in autoinflammatory disorders.

20.3 Clinical Presentation

To date there are eight families with PAPA syndrome reported in the literature, with a total of 37 affected family members (Table 20.2) [1, 11–17]. The syndrome is inherited in an autosomal dominant pattern, with clinical manifestations typically presenting in childhood. The most common clinical feature of PAPA syndrome is chronic, recurrent, sterile arthritis with prominent neutrophilic synovial infiltrate with onset in childhood. Skin involvement is variable and presents in adolescence or adulthood after joint signs have resolved or subsided; cutaneous manifestations include pyoderma gangrenosum, severe acne, and ulcerations (Figs. 20.1 and 20.2) [1, 16].

20.3.1 Joint Manifestations of PAPA Syndrome

Patients with PAPA syndrome present with asymmetric, destructive, and inflammatory poly-arthropathy with onset usually by 5 years of age. The natural history of this arthritis is chronic and intermittent. Some patients recall an initiating monoarticular traumatic event [1, 13–17]. Recurrent episodes of synovial inflammation fluctuate with periods of inactivity and eventually enter remission by late adolescence. While the most commonly affected joints are the ankle, knee, and elbow, cases of jaw and axial involvement, specifically the cervical spine, have been reported [14]. Diagnostic imaging often reveals diffuse joint space narrowing, osteophyte formation, subchondral sclerosis, cyst formation, periosteal proliferation, and ankylosis (Fig. 20.3) [1, 14].

20.3.2 Cutaneous Manifestations of PAPA Syndrome

Skin manifestations of PAPA syndrome present in adolescence, as the inflammatory joint disease subsides. A majority of patients with PAPA syndrome develop acne, usually severe. The acne seen in these individuals has been described in the literature as cystic in morphology, early in onset (including infancy), and persistent into adulthood (oldest reported age was 63 years) [1, 11]. The anatomic distribution resembles that commonly seen in patients with acne vulgaris, with predominant facial and truncal involvement. Acne associated with PAPA syndrome is often scarring. Other acneiform eruptions, including hidradenitis suppurativa, pustulosis, and pustular rosacea, have also been reported in patients with PAPA syndrome [1, 14, 17].

Pyoderma gangrenosum was observed in a total of 11 of 37 reported patients with PAPA syndrome. Sites most commonly affected include the upper and lower extremities, face, and neck. Several cases of pyoderma gangrenosum have been

Table 20.2 Clinical features of 37 patients with PAPA syndrome reported in the literature

Family	Family member	Arthritis		Pyoderma gangrenosum		Acne		Other
		Age of onset (years)	Joints involved	Age of onset (years)	Site	Age of onset (years)	Clinical description	Clinical description
Family 1 [1]	1	4	Elbow, hand, hip, knee	19	Legs	13	Severe, cystic	Sterile abscess at injection site, hidradenitis suppurativa
	2	16	Elbow	52	Legs	12	[a]	None
	3	2	Elbow, hand, knee	None	None	12	[a]	Sterile abscess at injection site
	4	3	Elbow, knee, ankle	None	None	12	[a]	Sterile abscess at injection site
	5	1.5	Wrist, hip, ankle	11	Face, cesarean section scar	11	[a]	Sterile abscess at injection site
	6	None	None	None	None	11	[a]	None
	7	1.5	Elbow, knee	12	Face	11	[a]	None
	8	5	Elbow, knee	None	None	None	None	None
	9	1	Shoulder, elbow, ankle	None	None	None	None	None
	10	8	Knee, ankle	None	None	None	None	None

(continued)

Table 20.2 (continued)

Family	Family member	Arthritis		Pyoderma gangrenosum		Acne		Other
		Age of onset (years)	Joints involved	Age of onset (years)	Site	Age of onset (years)	Clinical description	Clinical description
Family 2 [11]	1	Infancy	Elbow, knee, ankle	8	Arms, legs	Infancy	Cystic	None
	2	Infancy	Elbow, knee, ankle	None	None	[a]	[a]	None
	3	Infancy	Elbow, knee, ankle	None	None	[a]	[a]	None
	4	Between 3 months and 5 years of age	[a]	None	None	Yes	Severe	None
	5		[a]	None	None	[a]	[a]	None
	6		[a]	None	None	[a]	[a]	None
	7		[a]	None	None	[a]	[a]	None
	8		[a]	None	None	[a]	[a]	None
	9		[a]	None	None	[a]	[a]	None
Family 3 [12]	1	2	Shoulder, wrist, hand, hip, knee, ankle	2	Arm	[a]	[a]	None
	2	[a]	[a]	[a]	[a]	Adolescence	Severe, necrotic; face, trunk	None
	3	Childhood	Multiple	[a]	[a]	[a]	[a]	None

Family 4 [13]	1	16	Knee, ankle	[a]	[a]	Yes	Mild; peri-nasal	None
	2	Yes	[a]	[a]	[a]	Yes	Mild; peri-nasal	None
	3	Yes	[a]	[a]	[a]	Yes	Mild; peri-nasal	None
	4	Yes	[a]	[a]	[a]	Yes	Mild; peri-nasal	None
	5	Yes	[a]	[a]	[a]	Yes	Mild; peri-nasal	None
Family 5 [14]	1	5	Cervical spine, jaw, hip, knee, ankle	Probable	Legs	Yes	Mild	Psoriasis
	2	5	Jaw, shoulder, hip, knee, foot	None	None	Yes	Severe	Pustular rosacea
	3	2	Cervical spine, jaw, elbow, hand, hip, knee	Yes	[a]	Yes	Severe	None
	4	Before age 5	Jaw, shoulder, elbow, wrist, hand, hip, knee, ankle	Probable	[a]	Yes	Mild, cystic	None
	5	Before age 5	Jaw, elbow, wrist, hand, knee, ankle, foot	None	None	Yes	Mild	None
Family 6 [15]	1	Adolescence	Elbow, knee, ankle	Before age 42	Neck, leg	Adolescence	Severe; face, upper back	None
Family 7 [16]	1	22	Knee	12	Legs	16	Nodulocystic; face	[a]
Family 8 [17]	1	3	Ankle	None	None	None	None	Pustulosis
	2	33	Ankle	None	None	18	[a]	Abscess, hidradenitis suppurativa
	3	26	[a]	None	None	16	[a]	Abscess

[a]Data not reported

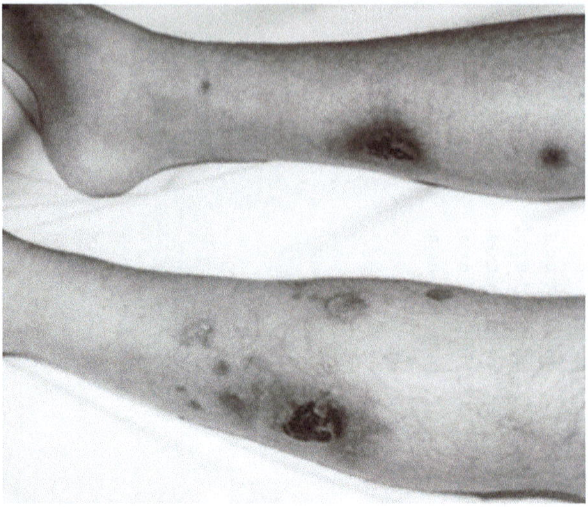

Fig. 20.1 Biopsy-confirmed lesions of pyoderma gangrenosum on bilateral lower extremities of a patient with PAPA syndrome [1]

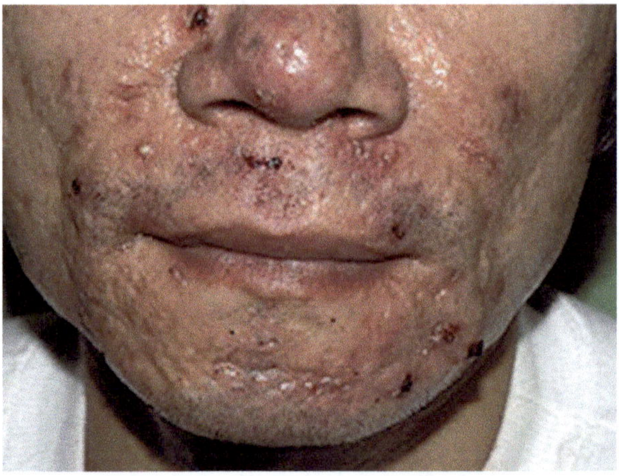

Fig. 20.2 Scarring, papulopustular, and nodulocystic acne on the face of a patient with PAPA syndrome [16]

reported to develop after a pathergy-like reaction to mild trauma. In some cases, lesions begin as erythematous or violaceous sterile papules or pustules with subsequent evolution to persistent, deep inflammatory ulcerations [1, 11, 14, 15].

20.4 Work-Up

The unique constellation of clinical features and natural history of PAPA syndrome often make it a clinical diagnosis. However, fever, arthralgias, elevated markers of systemic inflammation, acneiform or neutrophilic dermatoses, and ulcers may be

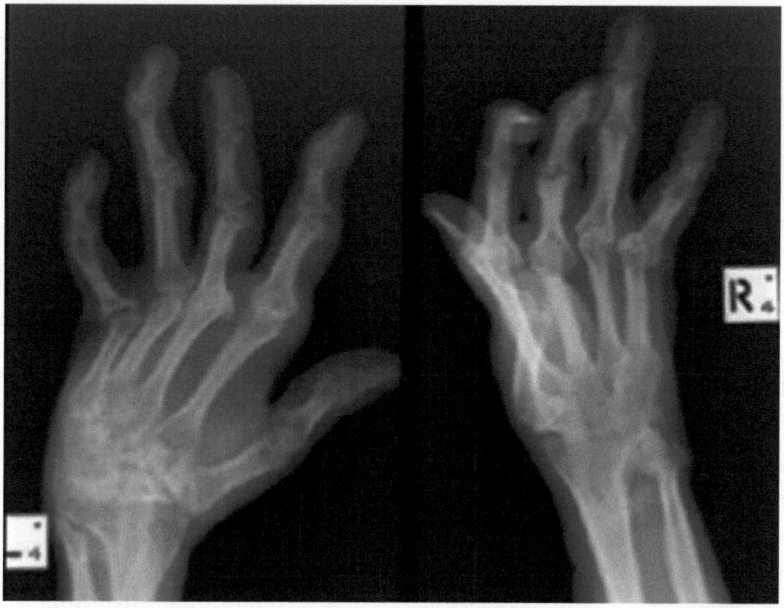

Fig. 20.3 X-ray of the hands of a patient with PAPA syndrome demonstrating advanced arthritis with joint space narrowing, osteophyte formation, and subchondral sclerosis [14]

seen in a broad spectrum of conditions; the differential diagnosis of PAPA syndrome with distinguishing clinical features is presented in Table 20.3. Commercially available genetic testing for common CD2BP1 coding mutations associated with PAPA syndrome is helpful in confirming the diagnosis and is currently the only specific diagnostic test [4]. Of note, there is one reported patient with all of the classical clinical features of PAPA syndrome without an identifiable mutation in the CD2BP1 gene [16].

Common laboratory findings include elevated serum markers of general systemic inflammation, such as erythrocyte sedimentation rate (ESR) and C-reactive protein (CRD). More specifically, elevated IL-1β and tumor necrosis factor alpha (TNFα) have also been observed [1, 11]. A 160 kD yet-unidentified streaking leukocyte factor is also seen; it is so named for its ability to enhance migration of mononuclear cells [4]. In vitro stimulation of patients' peripheral blood mononuclear cells with lipopolysaccharide showed increased IL-1α, IL-1β, TNFα, and IL-10 production [17].

Synovial biopsies typically reveal a nonspecific pattern of neutrophilic infiltrate. Skin biopsies of ulcerations or pyoderma gangrenosum lesions also reveal dense neutrophilic infiltrates with dermal inflammation, hemorrhage, and signs of wound healing [1, 11, 16]. Immunofluorescence of both skin and synovium lack immunoglobulin M (IgM), complement component 3 (C3), or fibrinogen deposition. Cultures of synovial fluid are sterile. Serum rheumatoid factor and antinuclear antibodies are also absent [11, 14].

Table 20.3 Differential diagnoses of PAPA syndrome

Disease	Age of onset	Skin involvement	Bone and joint involvement	Associated genetic mutation	OMIM #
PAPA (pyogenic sterile arthritis, pyoderma gangrenosum, and acne)	Childhood	Acne, pyoderma gangrenosum	Pyogenic sterile arthritis	CD2BP1 (autosomal dominant)	604416
DIRA (deficiency of the interleukin-1-receptor antagonist)	Infancy	Pustulosis	Periostitis, osteomyelitis	IL1RN (autosomal recessive)	612852
SAPHO (synovitis, acne, pustulosis, hyperostosis, and osteitis)	Childhood or adulthood	Acne, pustulosis	Synovitis, hyperostosis, osteomyelitis	unknown	
Majeed syndrome	Childhood	Acne, Sweet's syndrome	Recurrent multifocal osteomyelitis	LPIN2 (autosomal recessive)	609628
Acne inversa (hidradenitis suppurativa)	Adolescence	Acne, cysts, sinus tracts, pyoderma gangrenosum	Arthralgias	NCSTN, PSENEN, and PSEN1 (familial form)	142690
PASH (pyoderma gangrenosum, acne, and suppurative hidradenitis)	Adolescence	Acne, pyoderma gangrenosum, suppurative hidradenitis	None	unknown	
PAPASH (Pyogenic arthritis, pyoderma gangrenosum, acne, and hidradenitis suppurativa	Adulthood	Acne, pyoderma gangrenosum, suppurative hidradenitis	Pyogenic arthritis	PSTPIP1	None

CD2BP1 CD2-binding protein 1, *IL1RN* interleukin-1 receptor antagonist, *LPIN2* lipin 2, *NCSTN* nicastrin, *PSENEN* presenilins, *PSEN1* presenilin 1

20.5 Treatment

Given PAPA syndrome is so rare, there is limited evidence supporting the efficacy of treatments for this condition. Treatments for pyogenic arthritis have been reported in the literature with variable success. These therapies include aspirin, ibuprofen, methotrexate, leflunomide, sulfasalazine, hydroxychloroquine, antibiotics, osteotomy, and bone grafting. High-dose intra-articular and systemic corticosteroids may be effective in controlling arthritic flares [1, 11, 13]. Disease-modifying antirheumatic drugs (DMARDs) have also been used early in the treatment course in an attempt to prevent full expression of the PAPA syndrome with inconclusive results. Patients with aggressive joint disease may require joint replacements [14].

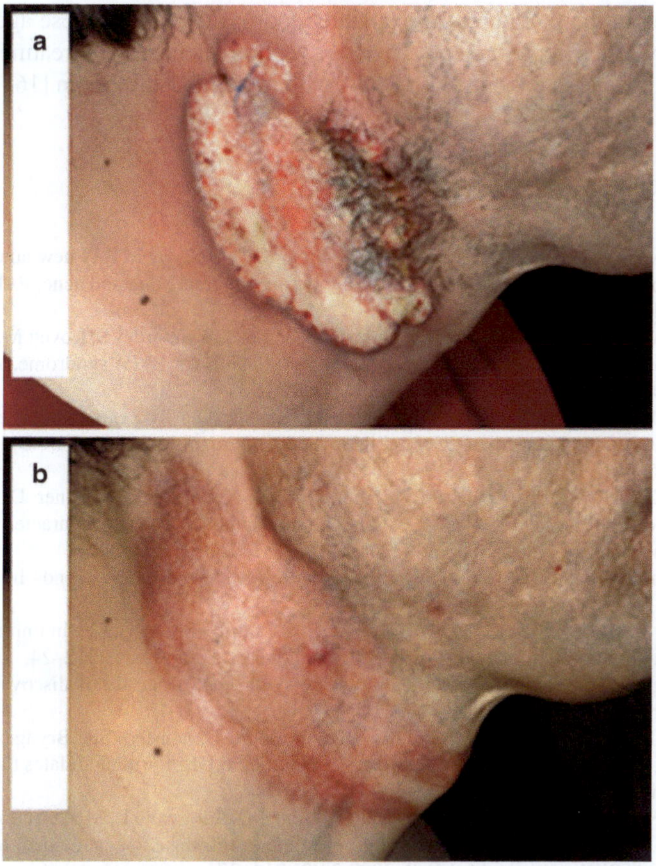

Fig. 20.4 Patient with PAPA syndrome and pyoderma gangrenosum of the neck before (**a**) and 1 month after (**b**) anakinra therapy [15]

For the treatment of pyoderma gangrenosum, a combination of topical steroids and systemic DMARDs such as azathioprine, methotrexate, and hydroxychloroquine have been shown to be effective in some patients with PAPA [1, 11, 14, 17]. Because IL-1β and TNFα levels are elevated in patients with PAPA, and because of important role of TNFα in the pathogenesis of pyoderma gangrenosum, these cytokines have emerged as new therapeutic targets. Anakinra, a recombinant IL-1 receptor antagonist requiring daily subcutaneous injection, has been reported to be effective in treating three patients with PAPA syndrome, improving active arthritic flares, severe cystic acneiform eruptions, and chronic pyoderma gangrenosum lesions (Fig. 20.4) [13, 15, 17, 18]. The duration of anakinra treatment for these patients ranged from 1 week to 8 months in reported cases. Anti-TNFα blockade, including infliximab and etanercept, have also been reported to be effective in treating some of the symptoms of PAPA syndrome, with dramatic resolution of pyoderma gangrenosum in one patient [4, 12, 19]. While the impact of these biologic therapies on acne is not well documented in the literature, the available reports suggest that these agents are less consistently efficacious for acne. There are reports of successful treatment of severe nodulocystic acne in patients with PAPA with systemic isotretinoin [16, 17].

References

1. Lindor NM, Arsenault TM, Solomon H, Seidman CE, McEvoy MT. A new autosomal dominant disorder of pyogenic sterile arthritis, pyoderma gangrenosum, and acne: PAPA syndrome. Mayo Clin Proc. 1997;72(7):611–5.
2. Wise CA, Gillum JD, Seidman CE, Lindor NM, Veile R, Bashiardes S, Lovett M. Mutations in CD2BP1 disrupt binding to PTP PEST and are responsible for PAPA syndrome, an autoinflammatory disorder. Hum Mol Genet. 2002;11(8):961–9.
3. Hull KM, Shoham N, Chae JJ, Aksentijevich I, Kastner DL. The expanding spectrum of systemic autoinflammatory disorders and their rheumatic manifestations. Curr Opin Rheumatol. 2003;15(1):61–9.
4. Smith EJ, Allantaz F, Bennett L, Zhang D, Gao X, Wood G, Kastner DL, Punaro M, Aksentijevich I, Pascual V, Wise CA. Clinical, molecular, and genetic characteristics of PAPA syndrome: a review. Curr Genomics. 2010;11(7):519–27.
5. McDermott MF. A common pathway in periodic fever syndromes. Trends Immunol. 2004; 25(9):457–60.
6. Veillette A, Rhee I, Souza CM, Davidson D. PEST family phosphatases in immunity, autoimmunity, and autoinflammatory disorders. Immunol Rev. 2009;228(1):312–24.
7. Goldfinger S. The inherited autoinflammatory syndrome: a decade of discovery. Trans Am Clin Climatol Assoc. 2009;120:413–8.
8. Waite AL, Schaner P, Richards N, Balci-Peynircioglu B, Masters SL, Brydges SD, Fox M, Hong A, Yilmaz E, Kastner DL, Reinherz EL, Gumucio DL. Pyrin modulates the intracellular distribution of PSTPIP1. PLoS One. 2009;4(7):e6147.
9. Yu JW, Fernandes-Alnemri T, Datta P, Wu J, Juliana C, Solorzano L, McCormick M, Zhang Z, Alnemri ES. Pyrin activates the ASC pyroptosome in response to engagement by autoinflammatory PSTPIP1 mutants. Mol Cell. 2007;28(2):214–27.
10. Shinkai K, McCalmont TH, Leslie KS. Cryopyrin-associated periodic syndromes and autoinflammation. Clin Exp Dermatol. 2008;33(1):1–9.
11. Wise CA, Bennett LB, Pascual V, Gillum JD, Bowcock AM. Localization of a gene for familial recurrent arthritis. Arthritis Rheum. 2000;43(19):2041–5.
12. Cortis E, De Benedetti F, Insalaco A, Cioschi S, Muratori F, D'Urbano LE, Ugazio AG. Abnormal production of tumor necrosis factor (TNF) alpha and clinical efficacy of the TNF inhibitor etanercept in a patient with PAPA syndrome. J Pediatr. 2004;145(6):851–5.
13. Dierselhuis MP, Frenkel J, Wulffraat NM, Boelens JJ. Anakinra for flares of pyogenic arthritis in PAPA syndrome. Rheumatology. 2005;44(3):406–8.
14. Tallon B, Corkill M. Peculiarities of PAPA syndrome. Rheumatology. 2006;45(9):1140–3.
15. Brenner M, Ruzicka T, Plewig G, Thomas P, Herzer P. Targeted treatment of pyoderma gangrenosum in PAPA (pyogenic arthritis, pyoderma gangrenosum and acne) syndrome with the recombinant human interleukin-1 receptor antagonist anakinra. Br J Dermatol. 2009;161(5):1199–201.
16. Hong JB, Su YN, Chiu HC. Pyogenic arthritis, pyoderma gangrenosum, and acne syndrome (PAPA syndrome): report of a sporadic case without an identifiable mutation in the CD2BP1 gene. J Am Acad Dermatol. 2009;61(3):533–5.
17. Schellevis MA, Stoffels M, Hoppenreijs EP, Bodar E, Simon A, van der Meer JW. Variable expression and treatment of PAPA syndrome. Ann Rheum Dis. 2011;70(6):1168–70.
18. Lolis MS, Bowe WP, Shalita AR. Acne and systemic diseases. Med Clin North Am. 2009; 93(6):1161–81.
19. Stichweh DS, Punaro M, Pascual V. Dramatic improvement of pyoderma gangrenosum with infliximab in a patient with PAPA syndrome. Pediatr Dermatol. 2005;22(3):262–5.

Chapter 21
Polycystic Ovary Syndrome

Joslyn Kirby

21.1 Introduction

Polycystic ovary syndrome (PCOS) was first described in 1935 by Stein and Leventhal [1]. They described several women with amenorrhea, hirsutism, obesity, and polycystic ovaries. Today, PCOS is one of the most common endocrine diseases in women. It is also one of the most common causes of infertility and menstrual irregularity. Acne is common in women with PCOS and may be the initial reason women with occult PCOS seek medical attention. Inquiring about menstrual irregularity and/or hirsutism in women with acne may facilitate referral to a gynecologist or endocrinologist for early intervention on fertility issues and medical comorbidities.

21.2 Background

PCOS is one of the most common endocrine disorders in women. In a study of unselected black and white women, the prevalence was 6–12 % [2]. The prevalence is higher in women with obesity, diabetes mellitus (type 1, type 2, or gestational), and those with first-degree family members with PCOS [3]. The variability in the reported prevalence is in part due to the inherent variability among patient populations (black, Caucasian, Latina, etc.) and the method of diagnosis (which diagnostic criteria are used) [4].

J. Kirby, M.D. (✉)
Department of Dermatology, Penn State Hershey, 500 University Drive, Hershey, PA 17033, USA
e-mail: jkirby@hmc.psu.edu

J.A. Zeichner (ed.), *Acneiform Eruptions in Dermatology: A Differential Diagnosis*,
DOI 10.1007/978-1-4614-8344-1_21,

The principle characteristics of PCOS are anovulation, polycystic ovaries, and hyperandrogenism. PCOS is likely a multifactorial condition with genetic as well as environmental contributions. Studies have shown women with PCOS have abnormal function of the hypothalamic–pituitary–ovary endocrine axis as well as other tissues and organs. The hypothalamus in women with PCOS secretes gonadotropin-secreting hormone (GnRH) at an elevated frequency. It is not known what factor(s) incites the abnormal pulse frequency, be it an intrinsic abnormality in the hypothalamus or faulty feedback mechanisms at the ovary [5]. This increased frequency favors the production of lutenizing hormone (LH) over follicle-stimulating hormone (FSH). This results in an elevated LH to FSH ratio and excess LH results in the overproduction of androgens by the ovarian theca cells.

Acne has been shown to be more common in women with high levels of androgens. Androgen overproduction in PCOS likely contributes to acne by triggering excessive sebum production. Conversely, acne is less common in women with elevated levels of sex-hormone binding globulin (SHBG) [6]. This protein binds the hormones and reduces the amount of free androgens available in the serum. Oral contraceptive pills have been shown to increase levels of SHBG, partially explaining their efficacy in treating acne [7]. In addition to overproduction of androgens, acne may be more common in these patients due to the influence of 5-α-reductase. This enzyme is found in facial hair follicles and converts testosterone to dihydrotestosterone (DHT), a more potent androgen. DHT production via 5-α-reductase is stimulated by excess androgens, insulin, and insulin-like growth factor, which are all elevated in women with PCOS [8, 9].

21.3 Clinical Presentation

PCOS is a spectrum disorder due to hyperandrogenism with a variety of possible symptoms and signs, some of which may be absent and others expressed with variable severity. Menstrual irregularity, hirsutism (Fig. 21.1), and polycystic ovaries are common features; however the diagnosis does not hinge on any single feature [10, 11]. Though not strictly a feature of the cutaneous exam, women with PCOS are frequently at least overweight or more frequently obese; obesity is found in 30–75 % of women with PCOS [12]. The most common cutaneous features of PCOS are hirsutism, acne, and androgenetic alopecia [5].

Acne affects an estimated 10–34 % of women with PCOS (Fig. 21.2) [13]. Compared to age-matched controls, acne has been shown to be at least three times more prevalent in women with PCOS [14]. Facial acne is most common, but 50 % of women with PCOS also have involvement of their chest and back [8]. In one study, 37 % (19/51) of women presenting with acne met criteria for PCOS [15]. The diagnosis of PCOS was based on menstrual disturbances, cutaneous signs of hyperandrogenism (acne, hirsutism, seborrhea), presence of ovarian cysts, and elevated LH to FSH ratio. This study supports the practice of asking women presenting with acne about their menstrual cycles. This may facilitate referral of appropriate patients to a gynecologist or endocrinologist for work-up and diagnosis.

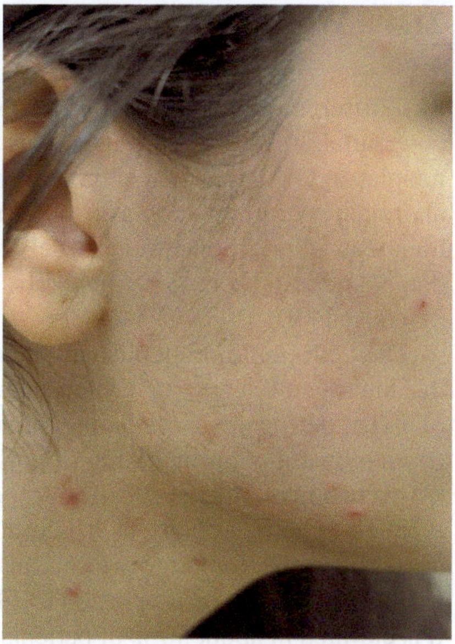

Fig. 21.1 Hirsutism in the sideburn and neck of a woman with polycystic ovary syndrome. She also suffered from mild acne along the lower 1/3 of the face (Photo credit: Joshua A. Zeichner, M.D.)

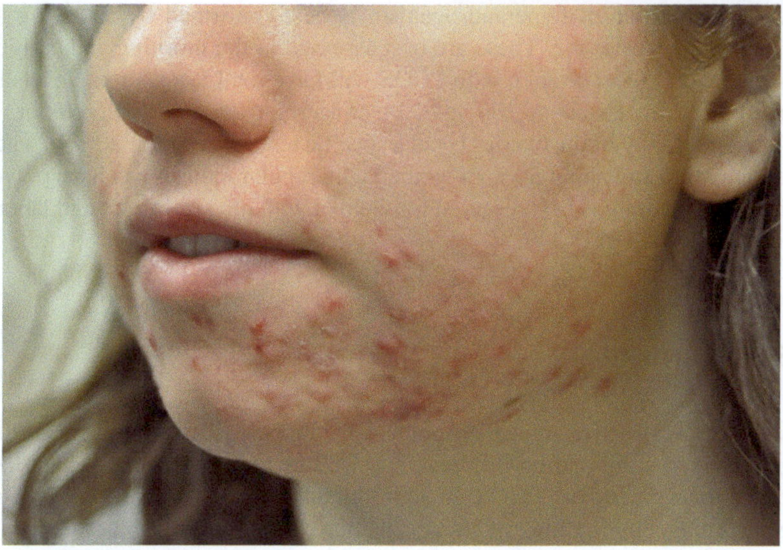

Fig. 21.2 Typical appearance of acne along the chin of the a woman with polycystic ovary syndrome (Photo credit: Joshua A. Zeichner, M.D.)

Given the high prevalence of obesity, it is not surprising women with PCOS have an elevated prevalence of other systemic metabolic diseases. Impaired glucose tolerance is found in 30–40 % [16]. Women are also more likely to develop endometrial hyperplasia and carcinoma [17], lipid abnormalities (including hypertriglyceridemia, elevated LDL, and low HDL) [18], obstructive sleep apnea [19], and cardiovascular disease [20].

21.4 Work-Up

The differential diagnosis of PCOS includes hyperprolactinemia, acromegaly, congenital adrenal hyperplasia, Cushing's syndrome, and an androgen-secreting neoplasm. Of these, congenital adrenal hyperplasia, Cushing's syndrome, and an androgen-secreting neoplasm are the most likely to present with acne and/or hirsutism in addition to menstrual irregularity or infertility [5]. The most recent diagnostic criteria require the exclusion of these conditions before PCOS can be diagnosed [10].

There are multiple published diagnostic criteria for PCOS [4, 11, 21]. In 2006, the Androgen Excess Society suggested that PCOS be diagnosed based on (1) signs of hyperandrogenism including hirsutism and hyperandrogenemia, (2) signs of ovarian dysfunction including oligo-anovulation or polycystic ovaries, and finally (3) exclusion of other states of androgen excess [21]. If the practitioner is suspicious a patient has the condition, it is prudent to refer the patient to a gynecologist or endocrinologist. Laboratory tests can be ordered in anticipation of this consultation. LH is elevated out of proportion to FHS, resulting in an elevated LH to FSH ratio. It is elevated in about 50 % of patients with PCOS [5]. LH and FSH should be tested during the early follicular phase of the menstrual cycle, before the midcycle LH surge. The presence of hyperandrogenism is best confirmed by assessing serum total and free testosterone. These are best assessed in the morning and early in the menstrual cycle. Most women with PCOS will have total testosterone levels below 150 ng/dl [22]. Levels above 200 ng/dl are concerning for a virilizing tumor.

Ultrasonography of the ovaries is not a specific test, since about 20 % of a general adult population and about 50 % of women with regular menses can have polycystic ovaries [23]. Imaging is best reserved for women with physical exam and laboratory findings suggestive of PCOS.

21.5 Treatment

Typical therapies such as topical retinoids, benzoyl peroxide, and topical antibiotics (singly or fixed-combination products), as well as oral antibiotics, are utilized to treat acne for women with PCOS. In addition, due to the hyperandrogenism underlying the cutaneous findings of PCOS (namely, acne, androgenetic alopecia, and hirsutism), therapy is aimed at reducing androgen production and the efficacy of their hormones at their targets (e.g., hair follicle, sebaceous glands) [13].

One of the most common treatments is hormonal birth control. Combination hormonal birth control, containing both an estrogen and progestin, has been shown to decrease ovarian production of androgens and increase levels of sex-hormone-binding globulin [24]. Oral contraceptives with 30–35 mcg of ethinyl estradiol and a progestin with minimal androgenicity such as norethindrone norgestimate, desogestrel, or drospirenone are favored [25].

Spironolactone can be an effective therapy alone or in combination with hormonal contraceptives [26, 27]. Spironolactone is an aldosterone antagonist with antiandrogenic properties. It has been commonly used to treat hirsutism. The mechanism of action includes competition for the androgen receptor, suppression of cytochrome P450, and inhibition of steroidogenesis, as well as reduction in 5-α-reductase activity. In an open-label study, 27 women with severe facial acne were treated with a hormonal birth control containing drospirenone and spironolactone 100 mg daily. 85 % of subjects were entirely clear of acne lesions or had excellent improvement. In another study, 35 women with acne of various severities received spironolactone 100 mg daily for 16 days per month for 3 months. Twenty-four patients (85.71 %) had significant improvement. The patients with clinical response also had a decrease in their mean DHEAS level; however, there was no change in the mean total testosterone levels [28].

Other therapies with androgen-mitigating effects include flutamide, an androgen-receptor antagonist, and 5-α-reductase inhibitor, a 5-α-reductase inhibitor. Both have demonstrated efficacy for therapy of acne but fewer studies have been done with these agents in comparison to spironolactone [29, 30].

Metformin is an insulin-sensitizing agent commonly used to treat PCOS. Along with other insulin-sensitizing agents (e.g., thiazolidinediones), metformin has been shown to decreased androgen production. One study demonstrated improvement of mild acne after 12 months of metformin therapy [31]. More research is needed before these drugs can be recommended to treat acne in the PCOS population.

References

1. Stein I. Amenorrhea associated with bilateral polycystic ovaries. Am J Obstet Gynecol. 1935;29:181.
2. Knochenhauer ES, Key TJ, Kahsar-Miller M, Waggoner W, Boots LR, Azziz R. Prevalence of the polycystic ovary syndrome in unselected black and white women of the southeastern United States: a prospective study. J Clin Endocrinol Metab. 1998;83(9):3078–82.
3. Yildiz BO, Knochenhauer ES, Azziz R. Impact of obesity on the risk for polycystic ovary syndrome. J Clin Endocrinol Metab. 2008;93(1):162–8.
4. Broekmans FJ, Knauff EA, Valkenburg O, Laven JS, Eijkemans MJ, Fauser BC. PCOS according to the Rotterdam consensus criteria: change in prevalence among WHO-II anovulation and association with metabolic factors. BJOG. 2006;113(10):1210–7.
5. Ehrmann DA. Polycystic ovary syndrome. N Engl J Med. 2005;352(12):1223–36.
6. Karrer-Voegeli S, Rey F, Reymond MJ, Meuwly JY, Gaillard RC, Gomez F. Androgen dependence of hirsutism, acne, and alopecia in women: retrospective analysis of 228 patients investigated for hyperandrogenism. Medicine (Baltimore). 2009;88(1):32–45.
7. Walton S, Cunliffe WJ, Keczkes K, et al. Clinical, ultrasound and hormonal markers of androgenicity in acne vulgaris. Br J Dermatol. 1995;133(2):249–53.
8. Archer JS, Chang RJ. Hirsutism and acne in polycystic ovary syndrome. Best Pract Res Clin Obstet Gynaecol. 2004;18(5):737–54.
9. Falsetti L, Gambera A, Andrico S, Sartori E. Acne and hirsutism in polycystic ovary syndrome: clinical, endocrine-metabolic and ultrasonographic differences. Gynecol Endocrinol. 2002; 16(4):275–84.

10. Azziz R, Carmina E, Dewailly D, et al. The Androgen Excess and PCOS Society criteria for the polycystic ovary syndrome: the complete task force report. Fertil Steril. 2009;91(2):456–88.
11. Revised 2003 consensus on diagnostic criteria and long-term health risks related to polycystic ovary syndrome (PCOS). Hum Reprod. 2004;19(1):41–7.
12. Azziz R, Ehrmann D, Legro RS, et al. Troglitazone improves ovulation and hirsutism in the polycystic ovary syndrome: a multicenter, double blind, placebo-controlled trial. J Clin Endocrinol Metab. 2001;86(4):1626–32.
13. Chuan SS, Chang RJ. Polycystic ovary syndrome and acne. Skin Therapy Lett. 2010; 15(10):1–4.
14. Kelekci KH, Kelekci S, Incki K, Ozdemir O, Yilmaz B. Ovarian morphology and prevalence of polycystic ovary syndrome in reproductive aged women with or without mild acne. Int J Dermatol. 2010;49(7):775–9.
15. Timpatanapong P, Rojanasakul A. Hormonal profiles and prevalence of polycystic ovary syndrome in women with acne. J Dermatol. 1997;24(4):223–9.
16. Legro RS, Kunselman AR, Dodson WC, Dunaif A. Prevalence and predictors of risk for type 2 diabetes mellitus and impaired glucose tolerance in polycystic ovary syndrome: a prospective, controlled study in 254 affected women. J Clin Endocrinol Metab. 1999;84(1):165–9.
17. Hardiman P, Pillay OC, Atiomo W. Polycystic ovary syndrome and endometrial carcinoma. Lancet. 2003;361(9371):1810–2.
18. Talbott E, Guzick D, Clerici A, et al. Coronary heart disease risk factors in women with polycystic ovary syndrome. Arterioscler Thromb Vasc Biol. 1995;15(7):821–6.
19. Gopal M, Duntley S, Uhles M, Attarian H. The role of obesity in the increased prevalence of obstructive sleep apnea syndrome in patients with polycystic ovarian syndrome. Sleep Med. 2002;3(5):401–4.
20. Orio Jr F, Palomba S, Spinelli L, et al. The cardiovascular risk of young women with polycystic ovary syndrome: an observational, analytical, prospective case-control study. J Clin Endocrinol Metab. 2004;89(8):3696–701.
21. Azziz R, Carmina E, Dewailly D, et al. Positions statement: criteria for defining polycystic ovary syndrome as a predominantly hyperandrogenic syndrome: an Androgen Excess Society guideline. J Clin Endocrinol Metab. 2006;91(11):4237–45.
22. Derksen J, Nagesser SK, Meinders AE, Haak HR, van de Velde CJ. Identification of virilizing adrenal tumors in hirsute women. N Engl J Med. 1994;331(15):968–73.
23. Codner E, Villarroel C, Eyzaguirre FC, et al. Polycystic ovarian morphology in postmenarchal adolescents. Fertil Steril. 2011;95(2):702–6. e701-702.
24. Azzizz R. The evaluation and management of hirsutism. Obstet Gynecol. 2003;101(5): 995–1007.
25. Arowojolu AO, Gallo MF, Lopez LM, Grimes DA, Garner SE. Combined oral contraceptive pills for treatment of acne. Cochrane Database Syst Rev. 2009;3, CD004425.
26. Goodfellow A, Alaghband-Zadeh J, Carter G, et al. Oral spironolactone improves acne vulgaris and reduces sebum excretion. Br J Dermatol. 1984;111(2):209–14.
27. Krunic A, Ciurea A, Scheman A. Efficacy and tolerance of acne treatment using both spironolactone and a combined contraceptive containing drospirenone. J Am Acad Dermatol. 2008; 58(1):60–2.
28. Yemisci A, Gorgulu A, Piskin S. Effects and side-effects of spironolactone therapy in women with acne. J Eur Acad Dermatol Venereol. 2005;19(2):163–6.
29. Cusan L, Dupont A, Gomez JL, Tremblay RR, Labrie F. Comparison of flutamide and spironolactone in the treatment of hirsutism: a randomized controlled trial. Fertil Steril. 1994; 61(2):281–7.
30. Carmina E, Lobo RA. A comparison of the relative efficacy of antiandrogens for the treatment of acne in hyperandrogenic women. Clin Endocrinol (Oxf). 2002;57(2):231–4.
31. Harborne L, Fleming R, Lyall H, Sattar N, Norman J. Metformin or antiandrogen in the treatment of hirsutism in polycystic ovary syndrome. J Clin Endocrinol Metab. 2003; 88(9):4116–23.

Chapter 22
Pomade Acne

Oge Onwudiwe and Valerie D. Callender

22.1 Introduction

Pomade acne (aka acne venenata) is considered a clinically distinct entity from the more common acne vulgaris. It is caused by the use of pomades applied to the hair and scalp in individuals of African descent with tight curly hair. Pomades are oil- or ointment-based hair care products used to lubricate the scalp and improve manageability of the hair. Pomade acne consists mainly of uniform, closely set comedones predominantly of the forehead and temple region. Involvement of the cheeks and ears has been documented as well [1]. It is said to be associated with little to no inflammation [2] which is in stark contrast with the comedones of acne vulgaris in which Halder et al. histologically found a marked inflammatory response in individuals with skin of color [3]. These lesions are primarily follicular and considered to be of very slow onset. Characteristically, pomade acne is limited to the comedonal stage but inflammatory papules, pustules, miliary cyst, and an erythematous and edematous phase have all been documented [1, 2].

22.2 Background

In 1954, Berlin described an acneiform eruption of predominantly the cheeks and secondly the forehead which was seen in children who applied paraffin oil to their scalp. The eruption consisted of uniform pinhead-sized papules, confined to the follicles. Some showed black points in the center while others a perifollicular inflammatory process. Few cysts and pitted scars were also seen. The disease was readily

O. Onwudiwe, M.D. (✉) • V.D. Callender, M.D.
Callender Dermatology and Cosmetic Center, 12200 Annapolis Road,
Ste 315, Glenn Dale, MD 20769, USA
e-mail: oconwudiwe@yahoo.com

J.A. Zeichner (ed.), *Acneiform Eruptions in Dermatology: A Differential Diagnosis*,
DOI 10.1007/978-1-4614-8344-1_22, © Springer Science+Business Media New York 2014

distinguished from the adolescent type of acne by the age of onset, the uniformity of the eruption, the overwhelming predominance of comedones, and finally the lack of seborrhea and lack of involvement of back and chest. Improvement was seen upon discontinuation of the use of paraffin oil to the scalp as well as the use of a comedo extractor and benzine to dissolve the oil [1].

In 1970, Plewig et al. described a similar eruption. This was seen in African American men who applied various grooming substances to the face and scalp. The observations in this study were confined to Negro male prisoners. The mean age was 30 but ranged from 21 to 53 years of age. Six products were found to be in common use among them: Noxzema, Wildroot, Dixie Peach, Royal Crown, and mineral oil. Common to these are high melting hydrocarbons. In the small study conducted, five of these pomades were applied to the backs of three African Americans and three Caucasian subjects for a period of 8 weeks. The formulation was applied every other day to a 4 cm square area. Occlusion was primarily maintained via the use of a polyethylene film. The control site consisted of a similar occlusive dressing without application of any agents or vehicles. After 8 weeks, 6 mm full thickness punch biopsies were obtained. Clinically, only two of the six subjects displayed follicular papules. The observed lesions were not dense in number and a few were mildly inflammatory. In decreasing order, Dixie Peach, Wildroot, and Noxzema had the highest frequency of pomade acne occurrence. Not surprisingly, histologic accumulation of horny material in the follicular lumen was most evident in the three aforementioned formulations [2].

Plewig et al. showed that a number of chemicals can induce an acneiform eruption upon contact with human skin [2]. Some of these agents contain various mixtures of petrolatum; lanolin; and vegetable, mineral, or animal oils [2, 4–6]. It has been shown that cultural practices play a role in the development of pomade acne. Due to the tight and curly nature of the hair of some individuals of skin of color, hair pomades or "hair grease" and other products are placed on the scalp and hair regularly for more manageability. These agents are usually rubbed into the scalp, hair shaft, and at times directly applied to the face. In addition, the many artistic hairstyles being worn by the same population, requires gels and other products to help keep such styles in place. In one study, skin manifestations related to cultural practices were seen in more than 20 % of patients and most prevalent were alopecia and hypertrophic scars followed by pomade acne [7].

The underlying etiopathogenesis is believed to be occlusion of sebaceous and follicular openings [7]. Pomades which have been implicated are usually thought to be cheaper products in which the acneigenic components are impurities [2]. The question remains whether other factors such as differences in gland size, sebaceous activity, or follicular hyperkeratinization among races are predisposing factors. The true etiology is likely multifactorial. The pomades that typically cause pomade acne are weak acneigens as it generally takes a year or more of daily use to produce the eruption clinically [2]. In addition, human skin is not considered conducive or the optimal host for testing comedogenecity. Plewig et al. were able to produce clinically significant comedones with all six agents in the ear canal of rabbits [2].

The true prevalence of pomade acne is not known. It is, however, less common than acne vulgaris and typically limited to patients of skin of color. The eruption occurs in all age groups and is not restricted to the adolescent or young adult [2]. A survey conducted by Taylor et al. showed that 46.2 % of black individuals admitted to hair pomade use. Of them, 70.3 % presented with lesions clinically consistent with pomade acne [8]. Likewise, Arfan-aul bari et al. reported pomade acne in 103 South African patients or 3.4 % of their study population [7].

22.3 Clinical Presentation

Pomade acne occurs characteristically in African American adults who apply various grooming substances to the scalp and hair. The lesions are typically uniform follicular-based comedones that are in close proximity to one another (Fig. 22.1). Expression of the contents of lesions with an acne extractor yields a firm material with a cheesy consistency [2]. Some comedonal lesions show inflammatory changes. The main ingredients are thought to be materials/hydrocarbons with a high melting point. These pomades are considered to be weak acneigens as a clinically apparent eruption isn't evident after limited use. It generally takes a year or more of daily use to produce the eruption [2] and this may be in part due to the fact that the finished products using comedogenic ingredients are not necessarily comedogenic [7]. In addition, human skin is not a very suitable host for testing comedogenicity [2]. The disease is considered to be relatively mild and typically leaves no scars [2]. On the contrary, due to the inflammatory nature of some of the comedones, pigmentary alterations have been identified.

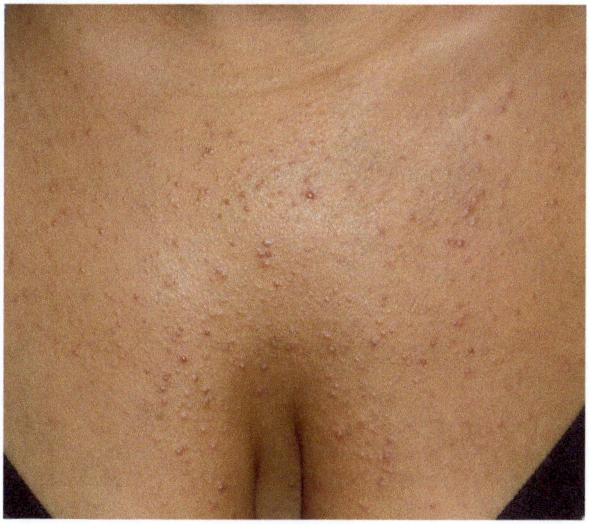

Fig. 22.1 While most common on the face, especially around the hair line and forehead, pomade acne may occur in other areas where pomades were used. This middle aged woman developed this monomorphic acneiform eruption on the chest after starting to use a new pomade body moisturizer (Photo credit: Joshua A. Zeichner, M.D.)

The histologic picture of pomade acne is indistinguishable from acne vulgaris. Plewig et al. showed that the comedones contained numerous gram-positive diphtheroids, marked thinning of the surrounding epithelium, and partial involution of the sebaceous glands. Few comedones showed inflammatory changes [2]. It is important to note that comedones in skin of color, when compared to clinical photographs, the histological inflammatory reaction can be out of proportion from what is seen clinically. Halder et al. and Davis et al. showed that there was always some degree of inflammation around simple comedones which were not clinically inflamed [3, 4].

22.4 Treatment

Discontinuation of the offending agent can lead to resolution in 4–6 months [2]. So therefore, a discussion of the use of current hair and skin care products should be done to determine if these practices are involved in the etiology of pomade acne and should be avoided [4]. Lighter hair moisturizing agents that are less occlusive, such as silicone-based products (dimethacone) should replace the thicker pomades [4, 9–12]. In addition, hair mositurizers should be applied to the hair shaft only, avoid scalp application and the hair should be kept off of the face.

For patients with skin of color, optimal treatment for comedones should include an agent with anti-inflammatory effects to help combat possible pigmentary alterations. As mentioned earlier, in a study conducted by Halder et al., marked inflammation with infiltrates of polymorphonuclear leukocytes was noted in comedonal lesions of African Americans. Of note, these findings were not seen in the Caucasian group that was studied [3]. Topical retinoids are seemingly the drug of choice as it combats follicular hyperkeratosis and concurrently treats post-inflammatory hyperpigmentation (PIH). Other topical regimens solo or in combination with retinoids include azelaic acid, topical dapsone, salicylic acid, benzoyl peroxide, and topical antibiotics. Hydroquinone-containing medications should also be considered in the treatment of acne-induced PIH [10, 12].

Comedone extraction and superficial chemical peels, in particular salicylic acid peels, are useful adjunctive methods of treating open and closed comedones in patients with pomade acne [13].

References

1. Berlin C. Acne comedo in children due to paraffin oil applied on the head. AMA Arch Derm Syphilol. 1954;69(6):683–7.
2. Plewig G, Fulton JE, Kligman AM. Pomade acne. Arch Dermatol. 1970;101(5):580–4.
3. Halder RM, Holmes YC, Bridgeman-Shah S, Kligman AM. A clinicohistopathologic study of acne vulgaris in black females (abstract). J Invest Dermatol. 1996;106:888.
4. Draelos ZD. Black individuals require special products for hair care. Cosmet Dermatol. 1993; 6:19–20.

5. Goode ST. Hair pomades. Cosmet Toil. 1979;94:71–4.
6. Wilborn WS. Disorders in hair growth in African Americans. In: Olsen EA, editor. Disorders of hair growth. New York: McGraw-Hill Inc.; 1994. p. 389–407.
7. Arfan-ul-Bari, Khan MB. Dermatological disorders related to cultural practices in black Africans of Sierra Leone. J Coll Physicians Surg Pak. 2007;17(5):249–52
8. Taylor SC, Cook-Bolden F, Rahman Z, et al. Acne vulgaris in skin of color. J Am Acad Dermatol. 2002;46 Suppl 2:S98–106.
9. Draelos ZD, DiNardo JC. A re-evaluation of the comedogenicity concept. J Am Acad Dermatol. 2006;54(3):507–12.
10. Davis EC, Callender VD. A review of acne in ethnic skin: pathogenesis, clinical manifestations, and management strategies. J Clin Aesthetic Dermatol. 2010;3(4):24–38.
11. Callender VD, Davis EC. Cosmetic applicatins. In: Taylor SC, Badreshia-Bansal S, Callender VD, Cochran-Gathers R, Rodriquez DA, editors. Treatments for skin of color. New York: Elsevier Saunders; 2011. p. 289–308.
12. Callender VD. Acne in ethnic skin: special considerations for therapy. Dermatol Ther. 2004;17:184–95.
13. Grimes PE, Rendon MI, Pellerano J. Superficial chemical peels. In: Grimes PE, editor. Aesthetics and cosmetic surgery for darker skin types. Philadelphia, PA: Lippincott Williams & Wilkins; 2008. p. 154–69.

Chapter 23
Post-adolescent Female Acne

Gillian Heinecke and Diane Berson

23.1 Introduction

While acne has been traditionally considered an adolescent disorder, recent studies show a significant prevalence among adults. The mean age of presentation for acne treatment is 24 years with 21 % of acne office visits by patients 25–34 years old and 15 % of these visits by patients 35 years and older [1]. In adults, acne occurs more frequently among women than men [2]. The characteristic clinical picture is mild to moderate deep-seated inflammatory papules and nodules on the face, especially the chin, jawline, and neck. Most commonly, this is "persistent" acne, which began in adolescence and has continued to adulthood, although a "late-onset" form also occurs. Recognizing acne in this population and providing treatment is essential since acne scarring can be correlated with duration of disease [3].

23.2 Background

Community-based clinical examination of adults found that 54 % of women over 25 years have physiological acne and 12 % have clinical acne [2]. The prevalence of clinical acne in adults does not substantially decrease until after age 45 [2, 4]. While most adults report that the severity of their acne actually improved after teenage years, 13.3 % of women report worsening of their acne in adulthood, and for 9.8 % of women, the acne severity stayed the same [5]. Among the adults with post-adolescent acne, 50 % had a first-degree relative who also had post-adolescent acne [6].

G. Heinecke B.S. (✉)
Department of Dermatology, Mount Sinai, New York, NY, USA
e-mail: Gillian.Heincecke@gmail.com

D. Berson, M.D.
Department of Dermatology, Weill Cornell Medical College, New York, NY, USA

J.A. Zeichner (ed.), *Acneiform Eruptions in Dermatology: A Differential Diagnosis*,
DOI 10.1007/978-1-4614-8344-1_23,

23.3 Pathophysiology

The reason acne persists into adulthood is multifactorial. The most common form of adult acne is persistence of acne that began in adolescence, and this form appears to share the same pathogenic features of increased sebum production, follicular hyperkeratinization, inflammation, and increased *Propionibacterium acnes* colonization as seen in adolescent acne [7]. Women with post-adolescent acne have significantly higher sebum excretion rate compared to women without acne [8]. Since androgens play a role in stimulating the sebaceous gland, the roles of both systemic and local tissue-derived androgens have been explored. While most women with post-adolescent acne have androgen levels in the normal range, several studies report lower levels of sex hormone-binding globulin (SHBG) and higher levels of free testosterone and dehydroepiandrosterone sulfate (DHEA-S) in adult female acne patients compared to controls [9–11]. However, the severity of the acne is not positively correlated with these levels [9–12]. In patients with signs of hyperandrogenism, the presence of an underlying endocrine disorder such as polycystic ovarian syndrome or late-onset adrenal hyperplasia should be explored.

The skin and sebaceous gland can produce and metabolize androgens. The presence of several key steroidogenic enzymes, 3β-hydroxysteroid dehydrogenase (3β-HSD), 17β-HSD, and 5α-reductase, enables the conversion of inactive adrenal precursors to potent androgens in the sebaceous gland. Excess local tissue androgens produced through increased sebaceous steroidogenic enzyme activity and therefore increased androgen synthesis has been proposed as a cause of the elevated sebum production seen in adult acne patients [13–15].

Other etiological factors include genetic predisposition, smoking, and stress. The role of heredity in acne vulgaris is well established by several twin and cross-sectional studies [16, 17]. The post-adolescent variant also appears to have a genetic component since 50 % of patients were found to have a first-degree relative also with post-adolescent acne [6]. While the correlation between smoking and acne in the general population remains controversial [18, 19], there appears to be a strong correlation between smoking and the comedonal post-adolescent (CPAA) variant of acne in adult females [20]. Nicotine has been shown to have a hyperkeratizing effect by stimulating the acetylcholine receptors on epidermal keratinocytes while also being anti-inflammatory and vasoconstrictive. This correlates with the clinical picture of CPAA, a predominance of micro- and macrocomedones with few inflammatory lesions [21]. Chronic stress activating the hypothalamic-pituitary-adrenal (HPA) axis has also been purported to exacerbate acne. Activation of HPA axis leads to both enhanced secretion of adrenal androgens and neuropeptides such as corticotrophin-releasing hormone (CRH). Recent studies demonstrate that CRH promotes lipid synthesis in the sebaceous gland and that the CRH system is abundantly expressed in acne-involved skin [22].

While antibacterial resistance of *P. acnes* and use of cosmetics were initially proposed as potential etiological factors, the current evidence suggests that they do not play a significant role in the pathophysiology of post-adolescent female acne.

When the cutaneous microbiology and serum P. *acne* antibody levels of patients with either persistent or late-onset post-adolescent acne were compared to adolescent acne patients, no differences were found between the acne variants [23]. Initially the use of cosmetics was the attributed etiological factor in the majority of adult females presenting with a mild acneiform eruption, leading Kligman to coin the condition "acne cosmestica" [24]. While a variety of cosmetic ingredients are known to be comedogenic including lanolin, petrolatum, types of vegetable oils, butyl stearate, lauryl alcohol, and oleic acid, many cosmetic companies now replace these ingredients with non-comedogenic alternatives [24, 25]. Recent studies suggest that external factors such as cosmetics, drugs, and occupation are less important etiological factors [6].

23.4 Clinical Features

Classically post-adolescent acne has been divided into two clinical types: persistent and late onset. Persistent acne represents a continuation of adolescent acne into adulthood. It is the more prevalent of the two types occurring in 82 % of cases [2]. Late-onset acne occurs for the first time after age 25. The characteristic clinical picture for both types is mild to moderate deep-seated, tender inflammatory papules predominantly involving the lower third of the face, jaw line and neck. The shoulders and back may also be affected. Comedonal lesions may occur on the forehead or lateral margins of the face but they are not prominent. Acne flares that occur premenstrually or at times of increased psychological stress are common.

Several clinical variants have been described. Comedonal post-adolescent acne (CPAA) has been documented in darker skin types (type III and IV) and is characterized by the predominance of retention lesions and micro- and macrocomedones, with fewer than 5 % inflammatory lesions. The comedones are homogenously distributed over the entire face [20]. While acne scarring is usually attributed to inflammatory lesions [26], ice pick scars occur in CPAA patients, and in severe cases numerous ice pick scars can coalesce into carters [20]. "Chin acne" is a clinical variant in mature females, which is characterized by premenstrual flares of inflammatory papules on the chin and perioral region (see Fig. 23.1). "Sporadic acne" consists of unpredictable sudden outbreaks of inflammatory papules and pustules in usually one but sometimes several locations in middle aged and older adults. These outbreaks usually coincide with a systemic illness or surgical operation, although inciting events are not always found [27].

23.5 Work-Up

While routine endocrinologic evaluation is not indicated for the majority of acne patients, this evaluation can be helpful in adult women with recalcitrant or late-onset acne or those with symptoms of hyperandrogenism including irregular

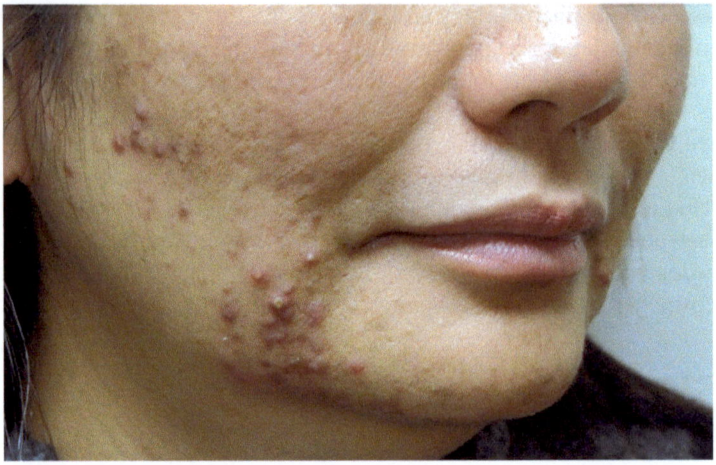

Fig. 23.1 Pustules and inflammatory papules on the cheeks and chin of an adult woman. She has been suffering from acne since her teenage years

menses, hirsutism, alopecia, infertility, deepening of voice, increased libido, acanthosis nigricans, and truncal obesity [28]. Features of hyperandrogenism are not uncommon in adult female acne patients, occurring in 37 % [6] of patients, and should be sought out by a focused medical history and physical examination. Polycystic ovarian syndrome (PCOS) is the most common cause of hyperandrogenism in women and is important to be identified since it may impart an increased risk for type 2 diabetes mellitus and cardiovascular disease [29]. The screening laboratory tests for an underlying endocrine disorder consist of serum DHEA-S, total testosterone, free testosterone, and luteinizing hormone/follicle-stimulating hormone (LH/FSH) ratio (Table 23.1) [31]. Since the hormone surge that occurs with ovulation can cause an inaccurate assessment, these tests should be drawn either just before or during the menstrual period. Oral contraceptives may mask underlying hyperandrogenism, therefore the oral contraceptives should be discontinued 4–6 weeks prior to laboratory assessment [31].

23.6 Treatment

The general principles of treating female post-adolescent acne are not significantly different from treating other acne populations, though there are some subtle differences that should be considered. Older skin tends to be more sensitive to the potential irritant effects of topical retinoids but more resistant to the irritant effects of benzoyl peroxide [27]. Acne is a chronic condition for many of these patients with 81 % of women reporting failures with systemic antibiotics and 15–30 % having

Table 23.1 Typical results of screening laboratory tests in women with endocrine abnormalities [30–32, 35]

Endocrine abnormality	Typical screening test abnormalities
Polycystic ovarian syndrome	LH/FSH ratio greater than 2–3 Serum total testosterone 70–120 ng/dL Androstenedione 3–5 ng/mL 50 % of women also have elevation in DHEA-S
Late-onset congenital adrenal hyperplasia	DHEAS 4,000–8,000 ng/mL 17-Hydroxyprogesterone greater than 200 ng/dL
Cushing's syndrome	Overnight dexamethasone suppression test >5 μg/100 mL
Ovarian tumor	Serum total testosterone greater than 150–200 ng/dL Normal serum DHEAS
Adrenal tumor	DHEAS >8,000 ng/mL Serum total testosterone greater than 150–200 ng/dL

Table 23.2 Hormonal modifying treatments of acne [30, 31, 35]

Drug	Standard dose	Side effects
Androgen receptor blockers		
Spironolactone	50–200 mg daily	Menstrual irregularities, breast tenderness, hyperkalemia, birth defects, hypotension, headache, dizziness, downiness, confusion, nausea, vomiting, anorexia, diarrhea
Cyproterone acetate	50–100 mg daily or 2 mg with 35 μg of ethinyl estradiol	Breast tenderness, headache, nausea, breakthrough bleeding, fatal hepatotoxicity Birth defects
Flutamide	62.5–500 mg daily	Breast tenderness, gastrointestinal upset, hot flashes, decreased libido, fatal hepatitis, birth defects
Ovarian androgen production blocker		
Oral contraceptives	Varies depending on specific pill (see Table 23.3)	Menstrual irregularities, breast tenderness, gastrointestinal upset, weight gain, thromboembolic events, myocardial infarction
Adrenal androgen production blocker		
Glucocorticoids—preferably prednisone	2.5–5 mg daily (at bedtime)	Adrenal suppression (higher risk with dexamethasone)

had recurrence after isotretinoin treatment [30]. Hormonal therapies can be a useful therapeutic approach and can be effective even in patients with normal serum androgen levels [31]. These include androgen receptor blockers, which block the effect of the androgens on the sebaceous gland, and inhibitors of androgen production either by oral contraceptives which block ovarian production or glucocorticoids which block adrenal production (Table 23.2). Glucocorticoids are most commonly used to treat patients with late-onset adrenal hyperplasia.

Table 23.3 Oral contraceptives used in treatment of female acne

Trade name	Ethinyl estradiol (μg)	Progesterone (mg)
FDA approved		
Estrostep (Warner Chilcott Company Inc., Fajardo, Puerto Rico)	20/30/35	Norethindrone 1
Ortho Tri-Cyclen (Ortho-McNeil Pharmaceutical Inc., Raritan, NJ)	35	Norgestimate 0.18/0.215/0.25
Yaz (Bayer Healthcare Pharmaceuticals Inc., Wayne, NJ)	30	Drospirenone 3
Non-FDA approved		
Alesse (Wyeth Pharmaceuticals Inc. A Wyeth-Ayerst Company Philadelphia, PA)	20	Levonorgestrel 0.1
Desogen (N.V. Organon, Oss, Holland or Organon (Ireland) Ltd., *Swords, Co. Dublin, Ireland)	30	Desogestrel 0.15
Diane-35 (Bayer Schering Pharma, Berlin, Germany)	35	Cyproterone 2
Femodene/Femovan (Bayer HealthCare Pharmaceuticals Inc. Wayne, NJ)	30	Gestodene .75
Mircette (Duramed Pharmaceuticals Inc., subsidiary of Barr Pharmaceutical, Inc., Pomona, NY)	20/10	Desogestrel 0.15
Nordette/Microgynon/Levlen (Duramed Pharmaceuticals Inc., subsidiary of Barr Pharmaceutical, Inc., Pomona, NY)	30	Levonorgestrel 0.15
Ortho Cyclen (Ortho-McNeil Pharmaceutical Inc. Raritan, NJ)	35	Norgestimate 0.25
Triphasil (Wyeth Laboratories, A Wyeth-Ayerst Company Philadelphia, PA)	30/40/30	Levonorgestrel 0.5/0.75/0.125
Yasmin (Bayer Healthcare Pharmaceuticals Inc., Wayne, NJ)	30	Drospirenone 3

The class of androgen receptor blockers includes spironolactone, cyproterone acetate, and flutamide. In the United States, none of these agents are FDA approved for the treatment of acne, and cyproterone acetate is not available [31]. Spironolactone is the most commonly used and has been shown to effectively control female acne at dosages of 25–200 mg daily [33, 34]. Side effects are dose dependent with the most common in women being menstrual irregularities and breast tenderness/enlargement. Hyperkalemia can occur and it is generally recommended to check potassium levels in older patients with comorbidities or 1 month into therapy when high doses are utilized [30]. Spironolactone is contraindicated in pregnancy due to the risk of hypospadias and feminization of the male fetus with prenatal exposure. Due to the risk of birth defects and to minimize side effects spironolactone is usually used in combination with an oral contraceptive pill [35].

Combination estrogen and progestin oral contraceptives reduce the production of ovarian androgens and sebum through the inhibition of LH and FSH. They are particularly useful in women with acne who also desire the contraceptive benefits. While several oral contraceptives have been studied specifically for the treatment of acne (Table 23.3), only four (Ortho Tri-Cyclen®, Estrostep®, Yaz®, and Beyaz®) are FDA approved for this purpose [35]. While the use of oral contraceptives is generally considered safe, potential adverse events must be considered before prescribing. The most serious potential side effects are thromboembolic events and myocardial infarction, however in healthy nonsmokers under 35 years of age the risk is low. Contraindications to oral contraceptives include pregnancy, history of thromboembolic or heart disease, smoking, liver disease, hypertension, diabetes, migraine, breast feeding and certain malignancies including current breast and liver cancer [36]. Oral contraceptives are usually used in combination with other modalities for the treatment of female acne.

23.7 Conclusion

Acne vulgaris is a disease that affects not only teenagers but also adults. It can be a source of significant psychological impairment and interfere with interpersonal and professional activities. A full work-up is important in evaluating these patients to rule out potential endocrine abnormalities. While many of the same treatments can be used in adult women as other patients with acne, an additional option includes the use of hormonal and anti-androgen therapies.

References

1. McConnell RC, Fleischer Jr AB, Willford PM, Feldman SR. Most topical tretinoin treatment is for acne vulgaris through the age of 44 years: an analysis of the national ambulatory medical care survey, 1990–1994. J Am Acad Dermatol. 1998;38:221–6.
2. Goulden V, Stables GI, Cunliffe WJ. Prevalence of facial acne in adults. J Am Acad Dermatol. 1999;41:577–80.
3. Layton AM, Henderson K, Cunliffe WJ. A clinical assessment of acne scarring. Clin Exp Dermatol. 1994;4:303–8.
4. Cunliffe WJ, Gould DJ. Prevalence of facial acne vulgaris in late adolescence and in adults. Br Med J. 1979;1:1109–10.
5. Collier CN, Harper JC, Cafardi JA, et al. The prevalence of acne in adults 20 years and older. J Am Acad Dermatol. 2008;58:56–9.
6. Goulden V, Clark SM, Cunliffe WJ. Post-adolescent acne: a review of clinical features. Br J Dermatol. 1997;136:66–70.
7. Gollnick H, Cunliffe W, Berson D, et al. Management of acne: a report from a global alliance to improve outcomes in acne. J Am Acad Dermatol. 2003;49:S1–37.
8. McGeown CH, Goulden V, Holland DB, et al. Sebum excretion rate in post-adolescent acne compared to controls and adolescence acne. J Invest Dermatol. 1997;108:386.
9. Aizawa H, Niimura M. Adrenal androgen abnormalities in women with late onset and persistent acne. Arch Dermatol Res. 1993;284:451–5.

10. Darley CR, Kirby JD, Besser GM et al. Circulating testosterone, sex hormone binding globulin and prolactin in women with late onset or persistent acne vulgaris
11. Seirafi H, Farnaghi F, Vasheghani-Farahani A, et al. Assessment of androgens in women with adult-onset acne. Int J Dermatol. 2007;46:1188–91.
12. Cibula D, Hill M, Vohradnikova O, Kuzel D, Fanta M, Zivny J. The role of androgens in determining acne severity in adult women. Br J Dermatol. 2000;143:399–404.
13. Lookingbill DP, Horton R, Demers LM, Egan N, Marks Jr JG, Santen RJ. Tissue production of androgens in women with acne. J Am Acad Dermatol. 1985;12:481–7.
14. Carmina E, Lobo RA. Evidence for increased androsterone metabolism in some normandrogenic women with acne. J Clin Endocrinol Metab. 1993;76:1111–4.
15. Carmina E, Godwin AJ, Stanczyk FZ, Lippman JS, Lobo RA. The association of serum androsterone glucuronide with inflammatory lesions in women with adult acne. J Endocrinol Invest. 2002;25:765–8.
16. Cunliffe WJ. Natural history of acne. In: Plewig G, Marks R, editors. Acne and related disorders. London: Martin Dunitz; 1989. p. 4–6.
17. Ballanger F, Baudry P, N'Guyen JM, Khammari A, Dréno B. Heredity: a prognostic factor for acne. Dermatology. 2006;212:145–9.
18. Schäfer T, Nienhaus A, Vieluf D, Berger J, Ring J. Epidemiology of acne in the general population: the risk of smoking. Br J Dermatol. 2001;145:100–4.
19. Mills CM, Peters TJ, Finlay AY. Does smoking influence acne? Clin Exp Dermatol. 1993;18:100–1.
20. Capitanio B, Sinagra JL, Bordignon V, Cordiali Fei P, Picardo M, Zouboulis CC. Underestimated clinical features of post-adolescent acne. J Am Acad Dermatol. 2010;63:782–8.
21. Misery L. Nicotine effects on the skin: are they positive or negative? Exp Dermatol. 2004; 13:665–70.
22. Ganceviciene R, Graziene V, Fimmel S, Zouboulis CC. Involvement of the corticotropin-releasing hormone system in the pathogenesis of acne vulgaris. Br J Dermatol. 2009;160:345–52.
23. Till AE, Goulden V, Cunliffe WJ, Holland KT. The cutaneous microflora of adolescence, persistent and late-onset acne patients does not differ. Br J Dermatol. 2000;142:885–92.
24. Kligman AM, Mills Jr OH. Acne Cosmetica. Arch Dermatol. 1975;106:843–50.
25. Nelson FP, Rumsfield J. Cosmetics. Content and function. Int J Dermatol. 1988;27:665–72.
26. Rivera AE. Acne scarring: a review and current treatment modalities. J Am Acad Dermatol. 2008;59:659–76.
27. Marks R. Acne and its management beyond the age of 35 years. Am J Clin Dermatol. 2004; 5:459–62.
28. Strauss JS, Krowchuk DP, Leyden JJ, et al. Guidelines of care for acne vulgaris management. J Am Acad Dermatol. 2007;56:651–63.
29. Goudas VT, Dumesic DA. Polycystic ovary syndrome. Endocrinol Metab Clin North Am. 1997;26:893–912.
30. Ebede TL, Arch EL, Berson D. Hormonal treatment of acne in women. J Clin Aesthetic Dermatol. 2009;2:16–22.
31. Thiboutot D. Acne: hormonal concepts and therapy. Clin Dermatol. 2004;22:419–28.
32. Lobo RA. Hyperandrogenism: physiology, etiology, differential diagnosis, management. In: Katz VL, Lentz GM, Lobo RA, Gershenson DM, editors. Comprehensive gynecology. 5th ed. Philadelphia, PA: Elsevier; 2007. p. 983–92.
33. Goodfellow A, Alaghband-Zadeh J, Carter G, et al. Oral spironolactone improves acne vulgaris and reduces sebum excretion. Br J Dermatol. 1984;111:209–14.
34. Saint-Jean M, Ballanger F, Nguyen JM, Khammari A, Dreno B. Importance of spironolactone in the treatment of acne in adult women. J Eur Acad Dermatol Venereol. 2011;25:1480–1.
35. George R, Clarke S, Thiboutot D. Hormonal therapy for acne. Semin Cutan Med Surg. 2008; 27:188–96.
36. Frangos JE, Alavian CN, Kimball AB. Acne and oral contraceptives: update on women's health screening guidelines. J Am Acad Dermatol. 2008;58:781–6.

Chapter 24
SAPHO Syndrome

Caroline L. LaRosa and Andrea L. Zaenglein

24.1 Introduction

SAPHO syndrome is a chronic rheumatologic disorder that involves the skin, bone, and joints. The name SAPHO is an acronym for the primary manifestations associated with this disorder: synovitis, acne, pustulosis, hyperostosis, and osteitis. It is listed by the National Institutes of Health as a rare disease, but it is an important one for physicians to include in their differential diagnosis for acne as it is often misdiagnosed and under-recognized.

24.2 Background

As a result of the lack of awareness and difficulty in diagnosing SAPHO syndrome, it may be unrecognized or misdiagnosed, and therefore, the exact prevalence is unknown [1, 2]. SAPHO typically affects children and young to middle-aged adults [3]. There is no sexual predilection. Familial cases have been reported but are rare.

The etiology of SAPHO syndrome is still largely unknown, but it is likely the result of a complex interaction between various genetic and immunologic factors. Inflammation, particularly abnormal neutrophil function and response, affects the skin and bones.

Genetic predisposition plays a prominent role in patients with SAPHO syndrome. Certain genes have been suspected as having a role in SAPHO due to their association with other inflammatory disorders. These candidate genes include the proline-serine-threonine phosphatase-interacting protein 2 gene (PSTPIP2), which

C.L. LaRosa, B.S. • A.L. Zaenglein, M.D. (✉)
Department of Dermatology and Pediatrics, Penn State/Milton S. Hershey Medical Center, 500 University Drive, Hershey, PA 17033, USA

J.A. Zeichner (ed.), *Acneiform Eruptions in Dermatology: A Differential Diagnosis*, DOI 10.1007/978-1-4614-8344-1_24, © Springer Science+Business Media New York 2014

encodes a protein expressed on macrophages and is involved in macrophage motility. In addition, the LPIN2 gene may be involved, as it encodes a protein involved in lipid metabolism and inflammation [4]. Mutations of the LPIN2 gene also play a role in Majeed syndrome, which shares the SAPHO feature of chronic recurrent multifocal osteomyelitis. Finally, the NOD2 gene is also a candidate, as it is involved in the development of bacterial recognition and inflammation. NOD2 is also strongly associated with Crohn's disease. While no variants in any of these genes have been found consistently in SAPHO patients, two rare variants of LPIN2 have been associated in SAPHO patients with psoriasis. The LPIN2 locus is weakly associated with the psoriasis susceptibility locus, PSORS10, and therefore may account for the psoriasis component of SAPHO in some patients. While there is similarity between psoriasis and SAPHO, affected individuals do not show a predominance of class II HLA genes (HLA-B27, HLA-Cw6, or HLA-DR) typical for psoriasis [3]. Evidence for the genetic basis of a SAPHO-like phenotype was found in the observance of neutrophil defects in patients with SAPHO [5]. A significant reduction in oxidant production in neutrophils was observed in one patient with SAPHO syndrome, and the same reduced internal oxidative burst was observed in neutrophils isolated from the patient's mother, who had a similar SAPHO-like phenotype. This example of familial SAPHO-like syndrome showed a response to anti-inflammatory medications, suggestive of an autoinflammatory disorder.

Due to the association between acne and SAPHO syndrome, *Propionibacterium acnes* (*P. acnes*), a follicular gram-positive anaerobic bacterium that plays a substantial role in the pathogenesis of acne, is being investigated as a causative agent. *P. acnes* can be strong inducer of innate immunity through the Toll-like receptor 2 pathway. To what extent its role is in SAPHO is unclear. Bone biopsies performed on six patients with SAPHO only found *P. acnes* in one specimen, indicating that it is not often found in bone lesions of patients with SAPHO [6]. It is thought that *P. acnes* may be a trigger for global neutrophil activation and a widespread inflammatory response [7]. Two immunomodulators, interleukin (IL)-8 and tumor necrosis factor (TNF)-α, were found at higher levels in patients with SAPHO syndrome. Yet *P. acnes*-induced production of IL-8 and TNF-α in polymorphonuclear neutrophils was impaired in patients with SAPHO as compared to those with rheumatoid arthritis and psoriatic arthritis [7]. Taken together, this evidence suggests that SAPHO syndrome may be triggered by the effects of *P. acnes* in initiating a strong cellular inflammatory response.

24.3 Clinical Presentation

The clinical course of the SAPHO syndrome has great variability between patients. Proposed diagnostic criteria require one of the three following criteria [8]:

1. Chronic recurrent multifocal osteomyelitis
   (a) Usually sterile
   (b) Spine may be involved
   (c) With or without skin condition

Table 24.1 Cutaneous presentations of SAPHO syndrome

Commonly associated	Less commonly associated
Palmoplantar pustulosis	Sneddon-Wilkinson disease
Acne fulminans	Linear IgA bullous dermatosis
Acne conglobata	Behçet's disease
Psoriasis	Sweet's syndrome
Pustular psoriasis	Pyoderma gangrenosum
Hidradenitis suppurativa	

2. Acute, subacute or chronic arthritis associated with any of the following:
   (a) Palmoplantar pustulosis
   (b) Pustular psoriasis
   (c) Severe acne
3. Any sterile (or *P. acnes*-positive) osteitis associated with any of the following:
   (a) Palmoplantar pustulosis
   (b) Pustular psoriasis
   (c) Psoriasis vulgaris
   (d) Severe acne

The main dermatologic findings of SAPHO syndrome include severe acne and neutrophilic, pustular dermatoses. Palmoplantar pustulosis (PPP), the most common skin manifestation, presents as chronic, yellowish intradermal sterile pustules on the palms and soles. Acne is generally more severe, such as acne fulminans or acne conglobata, but can be mild in some cases. Hidradenitis suppurativa and dissecting cellulitis of the scalp have also been reported. Psoriasis, especially pustular psoriasis, is also associated with SAPHO syndrome. Sweet's syndrome and pyoderma gangrenosum has also been described in a patient with SAPHO syndrome highlighting the overlap of neutrophilic disorders [9]. Table 24.1 lists the cutaneous disorders associated with SAPHO syndrome.

Skin lesions do not always present at the time of the osteoarticular manifestations. They may precede, occur simultaneously, or follow the bone and joint symptoms. Skin lesions usually appear within a 2-year time period, though some report onset 20 years following initial diagnosis [10], a study of 120 patients revealed 66 % with PPP, 31 % with psoriasis, and 25 % with severe acne [3]. Approximately 16 % of patients did not exhibit any cutaneous manifestations.

Musculoskeletal findings associated with SAPHO syndrome are characterized by osteitic and hyperostotic bone lesions [8, 11]. Most patients experience pain, soft tissue swelling, and limitations in mobility of the involved area. The osteoarticular findings often display an age-dependent pattern. In adults, synovitis affects the joints of the anterior chest wall, sacroiliac joins, and, to a lesser extent, the peripheral joints. Other typical osteoarthritic manifestations include hyperostosis and osteitis, both symptoms of a chronic inflammatory reaction. Hyperostosis sometimes, though rarely, involves the pelvis and the long bones. In children and young adults, osteomyelitis has a preference for the anterior chest wall, particularly the clavicle, and often displays multiple, symmetric lesions along the metaphyses of long bones.

Chronic recurrent multifocal osteomyelitis (CRMO), a chronic nonbacterial osteomyelitis, manifests as recurrent flares of inflammatory bone pain, typically involving the metaphyses of long bones, and may present with or without fever. Some consider CRMO to be the pediatric equivalent of SAPHO syndrome or at least in the same spectrum of disease [11, 12].

Though usually confined to the skin, bone, and joints, systemic symptoms such as fever sometimes occur [13]. Inflammatory bowel disease, both Crohn's disease and ulcerative colitis, have been associated [3, 14].

24.4 Work-Up

Laboratory blood tests are often useful but rarely diagnostic in SAPHO syndrome. The erythrocyte sedimentation rate (ESR) is usually elevated, indirectly indicative of the inflammation associated with synovitis, acne, pustulosis, and osteitis. The ESR is a screening test and cannot be used to diagnose SAPHO syndrome but may be used for monitoring the degree of inflammation in patients. Similarly, elevated C-reactive protein (CRP) values may also indicate degree of inflammation in the condition.

Definitive diagnosis is difficult and often requires confirmation by scintigraphy or histopathology of bony lesions. Bone metastasis cannot completely be ruled out by scintigraphy alone, and fluorodeoxyglucose positron emission tomography (FDG-PET) is used for definitive exclusion of metastatic bone tumors [15, 16].

Bone scans, CT scans, and even full-body MRI are also helpful diagnostically in establishing sites of bone involvement. Radiological features of SAPHO syndrome are mainly hyperostosis and osteitis. Multiple skeletal sites may be involved and the lesions can occur simultaneously or successively. Hyperostosis is characterized by a chronic periosteal reaction and cortical thickening that results in narrowing of the medullary canal and leads to hypertrophy.

Bone biopsy may be performed to confirm a diagnosis of CRMO or to distinguish unifocal CRMO from a tumor or infection. Histopathological analysis of the biopsy specimen may show Paget-like hyperostosis and inflammatory cell infiltration. Inflammation characterizes the acute phase, which shows polymorphonuclear leukocytes, plasma cells, edema, and prominent periostitis. The later phase has less evident inflammation but displays enlarged and sclerotic trabeculae and increased marrow fibrosis.

Skin biopsy will reveal the histopathologic findings characteristic of the associated skin finding such as acne or pustular psoriasis. Polymorphonuclear leukocytes characteristically predominate the various skin lesions associated with SAPHO syndrome.

24.5 Treatment

Treatment for SAPHO syndrome is based on the severity of presentation and generally aimed at reducing the associated inflammation in the affected organ system, bone, or skin. Treatment options and effects are listed in Table 24.2.

If severe acne is seen, prompt and aggressive systemic treatment with oral tetracyclines or isotretinoin should be started to prevent scarring. The addition of oral corticosteroids may be necessary to control inflammation when starting isotretinoin. Etanercept has been used in severe refractory cases.

For the psoriatic manifestations (palmoplantar pustulosis, pustular psoriasis, or pustular psoriasis), topical corticosteroids may be used to control mild and limited presentations. The addition of phototherapy with narrowband UVB is typically considered second-line therapy for most patients with psoriatic skin lesions. For extensive, severe, or refractory disease, oral retinoids, methotrexate, or anti-TNF-α agents or PUVA could be employed depending on the age of the patient and comorbid factors as well as the severity of joint disease. Combinations of these therapies may be required in those patients unresponsive to monotherapy.

Table 24.2 Treatment of SAPHO syndrome

Treatment of skin manifestations	
Disorder	Treatment
Acne conglobata Acne fulminans	Oral tetracyclines (tetracycline, doxycycline, minocycline) Isotretinoin Oral corticosteroids
Palmoplantar pustulosis Pustular psoriasis Psoriasis	Mid to high potency topical corticosteroids Methotrexate Etanercept or other anti-TNF-α agents Phototherapy
Hidradenitis suppurativa	Oral tetracyclines (tetracycline, doxycycline, minocycline) Isotretinoin Etanercept or other anti-TNF-α agents
Treatment of joint manifestations	
Medication	Effect
NSAIDs	Pain relief and anti-inflammatory
Corticosteroids (intralesional or oral)	Anti-inflammatory
Methotrexate	Anti-inflammatory
Oral antibiotics (doxycycline, azithromycin, clindamycin)	Antibiotic (in P. acnes-positive joint cultures)
Etanercept or other anti-TNF-α agents	Anti-inflammatory
Pamidronate or other bisphosphonates	To prevent bone loss
Colchicine	Anti-inflammatory
Sulfasalazine	Anti-inflammatory

For the joint disease, a variety of standard therapies are used. Nonsteroidal anti-inflammatory drugs (NSAIDs), such as aspirin, ibuprofen, and naproxen are first-line drugs used to provide relief from bone pain. Corticosteroids, including oral or intralesional injection, as well as topical cold applications, are also used to treat the inflammatory symptoms. Successful prolonged antibiotic therapy has also been reported for cases where bone biopsy is positive for P. acnes, but flaring occurs with discontinuation [17]. Sulfasalazine and methotrexate are used for more severe cases or for patients with persistent joint pain. Etanercept, an anti-TNF-α biological agent, has shown success in several case reports as well [18, 19]. Of note, life-threatening disseminated tuberculosis was observed as a complication of TNF-α blockade in a 17-year-old female with SAPHO, highlighting the need for careful screening of patients prior to initiating systemic biologic therapies [20]. Combination therapy is often required to control the disease. Pamidronate or other bisphosphonates have demonstrated success in some uncontrolled series and case reports in preventing bone loss [21].

24.6 Conclusion

Dermatologists should be familiar with the association between cutaneous neutrophilic disorders and sterile arthritis. An understanding of SAPHO syndrome is useful in providing a link between several idiopathic disorders that share clinical, radiological, and pathologic characteristics. Proper identification of patients with SAPHO will help by unifying the diagnosis and establishing a cohesive treatment plan for affected individuals.

References

1. Karadag-Saygi E, et al. SAPHO syndrome: misdiagnosed and operated. Acta Reumatol Port. 2008;33(4):460–3.
2. Van Doornum S, et al. SAPHO: rare or just not recognized? Semin Arthritis Rheum. 2000;30(1):70–7.
3. Hayem G, et al. SAPHO syndrome: a long-term follow-up study of 120 cases. Semin Arthritis Rheum. 1999;29(3):159–71.
4. Hurtado-Nedelec M et al. Genetic susceptibility factors in a cohort of 38 patients with SAPHO syndrome: a study of PSTPIP2, NOD2, and LPIN2 genes. J Rheumatol. 2010;37(2):401–9.
5. Ferguson PJ, et al. Neutrophil dysfunction in a family with a SAPHO syndrome-like phenotype. Arthritis Rheum. 2008;58(10):3264–9.
6. Colina M, et al. Propionibacterium acnes and SAPHO syndrome: a case report and literature review. Clin Exp Rheumatol. 2007;25(3):457–60.
7. Hurtado-Nedelec M, et al. Characterization of the immune response in the synovitis, acne, pustulosis, hyperostosis, osteitis (SAPHO) syndrome. Rheumatology. 2008;47(8):1160–7.
8. Kahn M-F, Khan MA. The SAPHO syndrome. BailliÃ¨re's Clin Rheumatol. 1994;8(2):333–62.
9. Bachmeyer C, et al. Overlapping neutrophilic dermatosis in a patient with SAPHO syndrome. Arch Dermatol. 2007;143(2):275–6.

10. Davies AM, et al. SAPHO syndrome: 20-year follow-up. Skeletal Radiol. 1999;28(3):159–62.
11. Earwaker JW, et al. SAPHO: syndrome or concept? Imaging findings. Skeletal Radiol. 2003; 32(6):311–27.
12. Tlougan BE, et al. Chronic recurrent multifocal osteomyelitis (CRMO) and synovitis, acne, pustulosis, hyperostosis, and osteitis (SAPHO) syndrome with associated neutrophilic dermatoses: a report of seven cases and review of the literature. Pediatr Dermatol. 2009;26(5):497–505.
13. Beretta-Piccoli BC, et al. Synovitis, acne, pustulosis, hyperostosis, osteitis (SAPHO) syndrome in childhood: a report of ten cases and review of the literature. Eur J Pediatr. 2000; 159(8): 594–601.
14. Colina M, et al. Clinical and radiologic evolution of synovitis, acne, pustulosis, hyperostosis, and osteitis syndrome: a single center study of a cohort of 71 subjects. Arthritis Rheum. 2009;61(6):813–21.
15. Quirico Rodriguez M et al. The importance of bone scintigraphy in the diagnosis of SAPHO syndrome. Rev Esp Med Nucl. 2010;29(3):127–30.
16. Salles M et al. The SAPHO syndrome: a clinical and imaging study. Clin Rheumatol. 2011;30(2):245–9.
17. Assmann G, et al. Efficacy of antibiotic therapy for SAPHO syndrome is lost after its discontinuation: an interventional study. Arthritis Res Ther. 2009;11(5):R140.
18. Vilar-Alejo J et al. SAPHO syndrome with unusual cutaneous manifestations treated successfully with etanercept. Acta Derm Venereol. 2010;90(5):531–2.
19. Ben Abdelghani K et al. Tumor necrosis factor-alpha blockers in SAPHO syndrome. J Rheumatol. 2010;37(8):1699–704.
20. Hess S et al. Life-threatening disseminated tuberculosis as a complication of TNF-α blockade in an adolescent. Eur J Pediatr. 2011;170(10):1337–42.
21. Ichikawa J, et al. Successful treatment of SAPHO syndrome with an oral bisphosphonate. Rheumatol Int. 2009;29(6):713–5.

Part IV
Genetic Syndromes Mimicking Acne Vulgaris

Chapter 25
Apert Syndrome

Yasser Albahrani and Joshua A. Zeichner

25.1 Introduction

Apert syndrome is a condition characterized by skeletal abnormalities as well as acne. It was first described in two cases by Wheaton in 1894 [1, 2] and by renowned French pediatrician Eugène Charles Apert, who in 1906 reported several individuals with congenital malformations of the skull and syndactyly of the hands and feet [3].

25.2 Background

Also known as acrocephalosyndactyly type I (ACS1), Apert syndrome is a rare congenital disorder that affects males and females equally. While generally considered to have an autosomal dominant inheritance pattern, the majority of cases are due to sporadic mutations. Apert syndrome incidence ranges from 1 in 160,000 to 1 in 2,000,000 live births [4, 5].

A missense germ-line mutation in the fibroblast growth factor receptor 2 (FGFR2) gene mapped to chromosome 10q25-10q26 has been identified in Apert syndrome. This gain-of-function mutation leads to increased FGF binding, upregulation of PI3K/Akt, and a resulting reduction of FoxO1, a transcription factor suggested to play an important role in sebaceous gland activity [6–11]. Thus, patients with Apert syndrome may have an atypical sensitivity to normal levels of circulating androgens rather than an excess number of androgen receptors [12].

Y. Albahrani M.D. • J.A. Zeichner, M.D. (✉)
Department of Dermatology, Mt. Sinai School of Medicine, New York, NY, USA

J.A. Zeichner (ed.), *Acneiform Eruptions in Dermatology: A Differential Diagnosis*,
DOI 10.1007/978-1-4614-8344-1_25,

25.3 Clinical Presentation

Apert syndrome is part of the acrocephalosyndactyly spectrum, which is classified into five subtypes:

Type I Apert syndrome
Type II Vogt Cephalosyndactyly
Type III Saethre-Chotzen syndrome
Type IV Waardenburg syndrome
Type V Pfeiffer syndrome

Cutaneous manifestations of Apert syndrome include moderate to severe resistant acne, oily skin, hyperhidrosis, interrupted eyebrows, excessive forehead wrinkling, lateral plantar hyperkeratosis, skin dimpling over joints, and oculocutaneous hypopigmentation [13–15].

Acne in Apert syndrome typically begins in early puberty in the form of comedones, papules, pustules, nodules, and cysts. Patients suffer from extensive post-inflammatory pigment alteration and scarring of varying severity. The distribution is usually widespread affecting face, chest, back, arms, buttocks, and thighs [1, 16, 17].

The severity of the clinical features of Apert syndrome is varied. Patients suffer from bony abnormalities of the head including craniosynostosis (premature fusion of one or more of the skull fibrous sutures), midfacial hypoplasia, broad nasal bridge, micrognathia, and a cleft palate. In addition, they have a prominent forehead, proptosis, and low-set ears. Other bony changes include vertebral fusion, severe symmetric syndactyly (fusion of digits), and symphalangism (fusion of phalanges to the digits). Craniosynostosis often leads to elevated cranial pressure and variable degrees of mental impairment [1].

25.4 Work-Up

Diagnosis of Apert syndrome is made based on the clinical constellation of findings. A thorough history should be obtained with a complete list of medications that can cause acneiform eruptions. A laboratory work-up should be performed to evaluate endocrine function. Skin cultures may be performed to evaluate pustular lesions.

25.5 Treatment

Management of Apert syndrome is shared among different medical specialties. Surgical interventions may be necessary to address bony abnormalities of the skull and face. Evaluation for chronic infections of airways and ears with possible continuous positive airway pressure (CPAP) machines and placement of ear tubes must be performed. Finally behavioral and psychological interventions may be necessary for social and intellectual impairments.

For cutaneous disease, topical therapy may suffice in mild to moderate cases of acne. In resistant or more severe patients, oral therapies may be added. Oral isotretinoin has been reported to be successful in treating severe, nodulocystic acne in patients with Apert syndrome [18–22]. One published report describes a female patient with Apert syndrome put on an oral contraceptive pill to treat a large ovarian cyst, who experienced a significant improvement of her acne [23].

References

1. Cunningham ML, Seto ML, Ratisoontorn C, Heike CL, Hing AV. Syndromic craniosynostosis: from history to hydrogen bonds. Orthod Craniofac Res. 2007;10(2):67–81.
2. Wheaton SW. Two specimens of congenital cranial deformity in infants associated with fusion of the fingers and toes. Trans Pathol Soc Lond. 1894;45:238.
3. Steffen C. The man behind the eponym. Eugene Apert (1868–1940). Am J Dermatopathol. 1984;6:223–4.
4. Boulet SL, Rasmussen SA, Honein MA. A population-based study of craniosynostosis in metropolitan Atlanta, 1989–2003. Am J Med Genet A. 2008;146A:984–91.
5. Blank CE. Apert's syndrome (a type of acrocephalosyndactyly)—observations on British series of 39 cases. Ann Hum Genet. 1950;24:151–63.
6. Melnik BC. Role of FGFR2-signaling in the pathogenesis of acne. Dermatoendocrinol. 2009;1(3):141–56.
7. Melnik BC. FoxO1- the key for the pathogenesis and therapy of acne? J Dtsch Dermatol Ges. 2010;8:105–14.
8. Melnik BC. Is nuclear deficiency of FoxO1 due to increased growth factor/PI3K/Akt-signalling in acne vulgaris reversed by isotretinoin treatment? Br J Dermatol. 2010;162:1398–400.
9. Wilkie AO, Slaney SF, Oldridge M, et al. Apert syndrome results from localized mutations of FGFR2 and is allelic with Crouzon syndrome. Nat Genet. 1995;9:165–72.
10. Melnik BC, Schmitz G, Zouboulis CC. Anti-acne agents attenuate FGFR2 signal transduction in acne. J Investig Dermatol. 2009;129:1868–77.
11. Chen W, Obermayer-Pietsch B, Hong JB, et al. Acne-associated syndromes; models for better understanding of acne pathogenesis. J Eur Acad Dermatol Venereol. 2011;25:637–46.
12. Henderson CA, Knaggs H, Clark A, Highet AS, Cunliffe WJ. Apert's syndrome and androgen receptor staining of the basal cells of sebaceous glands. Br J Dermatol. 1995;132:139–43.
13. Freiman A, Tessler O, Barankin B. Apert syndrome. Int J Dermatol. 2006;45:1341–3.
14. Cohen MM, Kreiborg S. Cutaneous manifestations of Apert syndrome. Am J Med Genet. 1995;58:94–6.
15. Cohen Jr MM, Kreiborg S. Visceral anomalies in the Apert syndrome. Am J Med Genet. 1993;45:758–60.
16. Solomon LM, Fretzin D, Pruzansky S. Pilosebaceous abnormalities in Apert's syndrome. Arch Dermatol. 1970;102:381–5.
17. Atherton DJ, Rebello T, Wells RS. Apert's syndrome with severe acne vulgaris. Proc Roy Soc Med. 1976;69:517–8.
18. Downs AMR, Condon CA, Tan R. Isotretinoin therapy for antibiotic-refractory acne in Apert's syndrome. Clin Exp Dermatol. 1999;24:461–3.
19. Robinson D, Wilms NA. Successful treatment of the acne of Apert syndrome with isotretinoin. J Am Acad Dermatol. 1989;21:315–6.

20. Campanati A, Marconi B, Penna L, Paolinelli M, Offidani A. Pronounced and early acne in Apert's syndrome: a case successfully treated with oral isotretinoin. Eur J Dermatol. 2002; 12:496–8.
21. Gilaberte M, Puig L, Alomar A. Isotretinoin treatment of acne in a patient with Apert syndrome. Pediatr Dermatol. 2003;20:443–6.
22. Parker TL, Roth JG, Esterly NB. Isotretinoin for acne in Apert syndrome. Pediatr Dermatol. 1992;9:298–300.
23. Hsieh T, Ho N. Resolution of acne following therapy with an oral contraceptive in a patient with Apert syndrome. J Am Dermatol. 2005;53(1):173–4.

Chapter 26
Birt-Hogg-Dubé Syndrome

Kristina Goldenberg and Gary Goldenberg

26.1 Introduction

Birt-Hogg-Dubé syndrome (BHD), also known as fibrofolliculomas with trichodiscomas and acrochordons syndrome, is an autosomal dominant genodermatosis [1]. Internal tumors, such colonic polyps and renal carcinomas, have also been described in these patients. This condition was originally described in 1977, when Birt, Hogg, and Dubé described a family in which 15 of 70 members over three generations exhibited multiple, skin-colored, dome-shaped papules distributed over the face, neck, and upper trunk [2, 3]. It has been shown that BHD is caused by a germline mutation in the *FLCN* (folliculin) gene (Online Mendelian Inheritance in Man #135150) [4].

26.2 Background

The gene locus for BHD was identified in 2001, localized to chromosome 17p11.2 by linkage analysis [5, 6]. Nickerson and colleagues later described a truncating germline mutation in a novel gene, the FLCN (BHD) gene, coding for a protein of unknown function called folliculin (FLCN) [7]. Chromosome 17p11.2 contains 14 exons and encodes folliculin. This evolutionary conserved protein of 579 amino acids that has no major homology to any other human protein and its function is unknown. Tumor suppressor function for FLCN was noted in BHD-associated renal tumors, consistent with somatic second-hit mutations [8], and loss of FLCN

K. Goldenberg, M.D. (✉)
Department of Dermatology, Mt. Sinai School of Medicine, New York, NY, USA

G. Goldenberg, M.D. (✉)
Department of Dermatology, The Mount Sinai Hospital, New York, NY, USA

J.A. Zeichner (ed.), *Acneiform Eruptions in Dermatology: A Differential Diagnosis*, DOI 10.1007/978-1-4614-8344-1_26, © Springer Science+Business Media New York 2014

mRNA expression was found in renal tumors from patients with BHD [9]. Interestingly, Van Steensel and colleagues did not detect loss of FLCN mRNA in fibrofolliculomas, suggesting that mechanisms of tumorigenesis might differ in renal and skin tumors [10].

Pathogenesis of Birt-Hogg-Dubé syndrome has also been associated with the energy-sensing mammalian target of rapamycin (mTOR) pathway [11, 12]. A 130-kDa FLCN-interacting protein, FNIP1, interacts with 5′AMP-activated protein kinase (AMPK), a protein involved in the mTOR pathway [13]. Hasumi and colleagues and Tagaki and colleagues showed an interaction between an FNIP homologue, FNIP2, with FLCN and AMPK [14, 15].

Some clinical overlap between BHD and tuberous sclerosis exists, such as skin hamartomas, pulmonary cysts, pneumothorax, and renal tumors [4]. The tuberous sclerosis complex genes *TSC1* and *TSC2* encode proteins that regulate the mTOR pathway. It has been shown that downregulation of FLCN leads to mTOR inhibition and downregulation of TSC proteins leads to mTOR activation [16]. Therefore, it seems likely that folliculin has several functions and its role in the mTOR pathway is still under investigation [4].

Birt-Hogg-Dubé is a rare condition and its epidemiology is largely unknown. Some authors suggest that it may be underdiagnosed [17].

26.3 Clinical Presentation

26.3.1 Dermatologic Manifestation

The original description by Birt, Hogg, and Dubé included fibrofolliculomas, trichodiscomas, and acrochordons as a triad of skin lesions that characterize BHD syndrome [3]. The lesions usually appear in the late teens or early twenties. These are usually flesh-colored to reddish dome-shaped papules on the face, with nose and cheeks being the most common locations (see Fig. 26.1) [4]. Lesions can also be seen on the neck, upper trunk, and ears. The lesions are typically 2–4 mm in size and have been described as waxy, white, opaque, and smooth [18]. Acrochordon-like papillomatous lesions have also been described in this syndrome and are usually seen on the eyelids, around the eyes, neck, and skin folds.

Histopathology of lesions found in BHD syndrome ranges from fibrofolliculomas and trichodiscomas to fibroepithelial polyps with or without cystic features. While the diagnosis of fibrofolliculoma or trichodiscoma is not specific to BHD, presence of multiple biopsy-proven lesions in a single patient should alert the clinician to this possibility. Therefore, multiple biopsies are usually needed.

Histopathology of fibrofolliculoma shows a central distorted hair follicle from which numerous thin, anastomosing, basaloid bands of follicular epithelium extend into the surrounding stroma. The surrounding stroma is fibrous and somewhat basophilic. The central hair follicle may be dilated or cystic and a connection to the epidermis is not seen in every case.

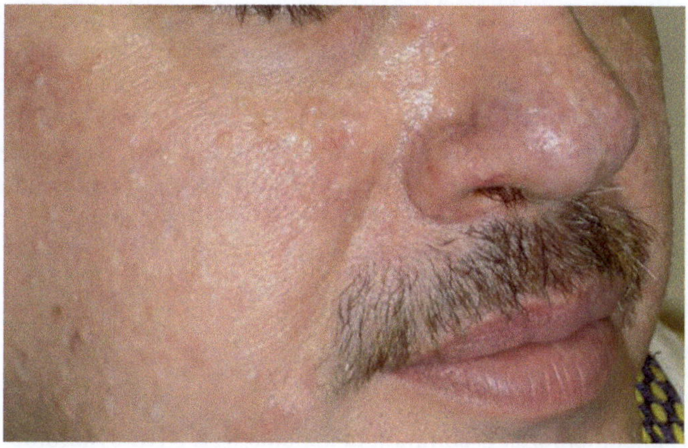

Fig. 26.1 Monomorphic, flesh-colored to white, dome-shaped papules on the face of a patient with Birt-Hogg-Dubé syndrome. Histologically these lesions reveal fibrofolliculomas and trichodiscomas, which can be difficult to distinguish clinically

Trichodiscomas are thought to represent hamartomas of the mesodermal component of hair disk. Histopathology of trichodiscomas shows area of fine, eosinophilic, fibrilar connective tissue stroma with dilated blood vessels. The overlying epidermis is usually attenuated and a collarette surrounding the central fibrilar stroma may be seen. A follicular structure is usually found at the edge of the lesion, although multiple step sections may be required to find it. Some authors, including authors of this chapter, consider fibrofolliculomas and trichodiscomas to be lesions on the same spectrum. In fact, oftentimes features of both lesions can be seen in different areas of the same biopsy specimen.

The clinical differential diagnosis of BHD syndrome is broad. It includes other adnexal tumors, such as syringomas, trichoepitheliomas, and trichoblastomas; vascular tumors, such as angiofibromas and capillary hemangiomas; acne vulgaris; rosacea; vellus hair cysts; and milia. Other familial cancer syndromes are also on the differential diagnosis, including Cowden syndrome, Brooke-Spiegler syndrome, and Basal cell nevus (Gorlin's) syndrome [18, 19].

26.3.2 Renal Manifestations

The risk of a renal neoplasm in patients with BHD syndrome ranges from 20 to 30 %, with equal male and female distribution [20, 21]. This differs from general population, where renal cell carcinoma is more prevalent in men. The average age of presentation is around 50 year old, which is younger than patients with spontaneous renal cell carcinoma usually present [22]. Multiple renal cysts have also been reported in patients with BHD and these are usually seen after the age of 40 [23].

FLCN is thought to be a tumor suppressor gene in the kidneys [18]. Somatic mutations or loss of heterozygosity of the FLCN gene causes different renal tumors in patients with BHD [8]. Therefore, BHD differs from other hereditary renal cancer syndromes in the diversity of histological subtypes of renal cell tumors these patients develop.

The most common and characteristic tumor types in BHD syndrome are hybrid chromophobe/oncocytic (50 %) and chromophobe (33 %) renal cancer, clear cell carcinomas (9 %), oncocytoma (5 %), and papillary carcinomas [24]. These tumors can be solitary and unilateral or multifocal and bilateral.

26.3.3 Pulmonary Manifestations

Spontaneous pneumothorax is common in patients with BHD syndrome, with prevalence of 25 %, occurring most commonly during the fifth decade of life [25]. Lung cysts are another common (90 %) findings in patients with BHD syndrome. Pulmonary manifestations may be seen in absence of dermatologic or renal disease.

The differential diagnosis of cystic lung disease in BHD includes lymphangioleiomyomatosis; pulmonary Langerhans' cell histiocytosis, lymphocytic interstitial pneumonitis, and pneumocystis pneumonia; smoking-related interstitial lung disease; and rarely metastatic neoplasms, such as adenocarcinomas and low-grade sarcomas [18].

26.4 Work-Up

Diagnosis of BHD is based on the presence of the following criteria [4]:

Major Criteria

At least five fibrofolliculomas or trichodiscomas, at least one histologically confirmed, of adult onset
Pathogenic FLCN germline mutation

Minor Criteria

Multiple lung cysts with or without spontaneous primary pneumothorax
Renal cancer: early onset (<50 years) or multifocal or bilateral renal cancer, or renal cancer of mixed chromophobe and oncocytic histology
A first-degree relative with BHD

Several laboratory and radiologic tests aid in the diagnosis of BHD syndrome. DNA-based testing for FLCN gene is recommended for patients with a clinical diagnosis of BHD syndrome [4]. Counseling and testing the relative of patients with positive test should also be considered. Ultrasound, computated tomography (CT), and magnetic resonance imaging (MRI) can all be used to evaluate and diagnose renal tumors in patients with BHD. Chest X-ray, CT, and MRI can be used to evaluate lung disease.

26.5 Treatment

26.5.1 Dermatologic Manifestations

The treatment options for patients with fibrofolliculomas and trichodiscomas are limited. Treatment is largely surgical, with excision, shave and cautery, electrodessication, and curettage reported [4]. Laser ablation with erbium-YAG or fractional CO_2 laser has also been reported [26, 27]. Although the treatment is not curative, the psychological burden of multiple facial lesions should be conserved and treatment offered to the patients.

26.5.2 Renal Manifestations

Patients with known BHD syndrome should undergo an annual renal MRI, with renal ultrasound also an option [18]. Surveillance for renal tumors is also indicated for carriers of FLCN germline mutations and for relatives of patients with known BHD syndrome. Once renal cancer is diagnosed, staging and treatment should follow standard procedure [28]. It has also been suggested that rapamycin and its derivatives can be used, since FLCN mutation can result in deregulation on mTOR [18].

26.5.3 Pulmonary Manifestations

The treatment of pneumothorax in patients with BDH is the same as spontaneous pneumothorax. Smoking should be strongly discouraged in these patients. Patients should also be counseled regarding changes in ambient pressure, flying, and deep-sea diving [18].

26.6 Conclusion

Skin changes may be the first manifestation of the Birt-Hogg-Dubé syndrome. This condition affects several organ systems in the body, and recognition of the unique presenting skin changes can lead to early diagnosis and work-up. Given the potentially severe renal and pulmonary manifestations, full work-ups should be performed for patients in which this condition is suspected. Referral to the appropriate specialists, including genetic counselors, is important to properly manage this syndrome.

References

1. Toro JR, Glenn G, Duray P, Darling T, Weirich G, Zbar B, Linehan M, Turner ML. Birt-Hogg-Dubé syndrome: a novel marker of kidney neoplasia. Arch Dermatol. 1999;135(10):1195–202.
2. Warwick G, Izatt L, Sawicka E. Renal cancer associated with recurrent spontaneous pneumothorax in Birt-Hogg-Dubé syndrome: a case report and review of the literature. J Med Case Rep. 2010;4:106.
3. Birt AR, Hogg GR, Dube WJ. Hereditary multiple fibrofolliculomas with trichodiscomas and acrochordons. Arch Dermatol. 1977;113:1674–7.
4. Menko FH, van Steensel MA, Giraud S, Friis-Hansen L, Richard S, Ungari S, Nordenskjöld M, Hansen TV, Solly J, Maher ER, European BHD Consortium. Birt-Hogg-Dubé syndrome: diagnosis and management. Lancet Oncol. 2009;10(12):1199–206.
5. Khoo SK, Bradley M, Wong FK, Hedblad M-AM, Nordenskjöld BT. The Birt-Hogg-Dubé syndrome: mapping of a novel hereditary neoplasia gene to chromosome 17p12–q11.2. Oncogene. 2001;20:5239–42.
6. Schmidt LS, Warren MB, Nickerson ML, et al. Birt-Hogg-Dubé syndrome, a genodermatosis associated with spontaneous pneumothorax and kidney neoplasia, maps to chromosome 17p11.2. Am J Hum Genet. 2001;69:876–82.
7. Nickerson ML, Warren MB, Toro JR, et al. Mutations in a novel gene lead to kidney tumors, lung wall defects, and benign tumors of the hair follicle in patients with the Birt-Hogg-Dubé syndrome. Cancer Cell. 2002;2:157–64.
8. Vocke CD, Yang Y, Pavlovich CP, et al. High frequency of somatic frameshift BHD gene mutations in Birt-Hogg-Dubé-associated renal tumors. J Natl Cancer Inst. 2005;97:931–5.
9. Warren MB, Torres-Cabala CA, Turner ML, et al. Expression of Birt-Hogg-Dubé gene mRNA in normal and neoplastic human tissues. Mod Pathol. 2004;17:998–1011.
10. van Steensel MA, Verstraeten VL, Frank J, et al. Novel mutations in the BHD gene and absence of loss of heterozygosity in fibrofolliculomas of Birt-Hogg-Dubé patients. J Invest Dermatol. 2007;127:588–93.
11. Inoki K, Corradetti MN, Guan K-L. Dysregulation of the TSC-mTOR pathway in human disease. Nat Genet. 2005;37:19–24.
12. van Steensel MA, van Geel M, Badeloe S, Poblete-Gutiérrez P, Frank J. Molecular pathways involved in hair follicle tumor formation: all about mammalian target of rapamycin. Exp Dermatol. 2009;18:185–91.
13. Baba M, Hong S-B, Sharma N, et al. Folliculin encoded by the *BHD* gene interacts with a binding protein, FNIP1, and AMPK, and is involved in AMPK and mTOR signaling. Proc Natl Acad Sci U S A. 2006;103:15552–7.
14. Hasumi H, Baba M, Hong SB, et al. Identification and characterization of a novel folliculin-interacting protein FNIP2. Gene. 2008;415:60–7.
15. Takagi Y, Kobayashi T, Shiono M, et al. Interaction of folliculin (Birt-Hogg-Dubé gene product) with a novel Fnip1-like (FnipL/Fnip2) protein. Oncogene. 2008;27:5339–47.
16. Hartman TR, Nicolas E, Klein-Szanto A, et al. The role of the Birt-Hogg-Dubé protein in mTOR activation and renal tumorigenesis. Oncogene. 2009;28:1594–604.
17. Lindor NM, et al. Birt-Hogg-Dube syndrome: an autosomal dominant disorder with predisposition to cancers of the kidney, fibrofolliculomas, and focal cutaneous mucinosis. Int J Dermatol. 2001;40(10):653–6.
18. Reese E, Sluzevich J, Kluijt I, Teertstra HJ, De Jong D, Horenblas S, Ryu J. Birt-Hogg-Dubé syndrome. In: Riegert-Johnson DL, Boardman LA, Hefferon T, Roberts M, editors. Cancer syndromes [Internet]. Bethesda, MD: National Center for Biotechnology Information (US); 2009.
19. Vincent A, et al. Birt-Hogg-Dube syndrome: a review of the literature and the differential diagnosis of firm facial papules. J Am Acad Dermatol. 2003;49(4):698–705.
20. Pavlovich CP, et al. Renal tumors in the Birt-Hogg-Dube syndrome. Am J Surg Pathol. 2002;26(12):1542–52.

21. Toro JR, et al. BHD mutations, clinical and molecular genetic investigations of Birt-Hogg-Dube syndrome: a new series of 50 families and a review of published reports. J Med Genet. 2008;45(6):321–31.
22. Schmidt LS, et al. Germline BHD-mutation spectrum and phenotype analysis of a large cohort of families with Birt-Hogg-Dube syndrome. Am J Hum Genet. 2005;76(6):1023–33.
23. Gupta P, et al. Radiological findings in Birt-Hogg-Dube syndrome: a rare differential for pulmonary cysts and renal tumors. Clin Imaging. 2007;31(1):40–3.
24. Linehan WM, et al. Identification of the genes for kidney cancer: opportunity for disease-specific targeted therapeutics. Clin Cancer Res. 2007;13(2 Pt 2):671s–9.
25. Ayo DS, et al. Cystic lung disease in Birt-Hogg-Dube syndrome. Chest. 2007;132(2):679–84.
26. Gambichler T, Wolter M, Altmeyer P, Hoffman K. Treatment of Birt-Hogg-Dubé syndrome with erbium: YAG laser. J Am Acad Dermatol. 2000;43:856–8.
27. Kahle B, Hellwig S, Schulz T. Multiple mantelome bei Birt-Hogg-Dubé-Syndrom. Erfolchreiche therapie mit dem CO_2-laser. Hautarzt. 2001;52:43–6.
28. Ng CS, Wood CG, Silverman PM, Tannir NM, Tamboli P, Sandler CM. Renal cell carcinoma: diagnosis, staging, and surveillance. Am J Roentgenol. 2008;191:1220–32.

Chapter 27
Brooke-Spiegler Syndrome

Bradley Glodny and Joshua A. Zeichner

27.1 Introduction

Brooke-Spiegler syndrome (BSS) is an autosomal dominant (AD) inherited syndrome predisposing those affected, to the development of multiple hamartomas/neoplasms derived from skin appendage structures. These tumors include cylindromas, trichoepitheliomas, and spiradenomas. In the setting of BSS, these lesions most often appear as multiple papules or nodules on the head and neck region during adolescence or early adulthood. BSS may be mistaken for the eruption of acne vulgaris [1, 2]. While BSS was initially described as a unique entity, it is now thought to exist as part of a spectrum of AD appendage tumor syndromes allelic for germline mutations within the Cylindromatosis (CYLD) gene. This group includes two other syndromes: familial cylindromatosis (FC) and multiple familial trichoepithelioma (MFT) [2]. As indicated by their name, MFT is characterized by trichoepitheliomas, while FC is characterized by cylindromas [3]. Therefore, MFT and FC represent two ends of a spectrum with BSS falling within the middle [4].

27.2 Background

BSS is a rare AD syndrome, occurring secondary to a germline mutation in the tumor suppressor gene CYLD, located on chromosome 16q12-q13 [4]. To date, 73 families have been identified with CYLD mutations without an identifiable racial or ethnic predilection [4]. These CYLD mutations have been associated with BSS, MFT, as well as FC.

B. Glodny, M.D. (✉)
Department of Dermatology, Mt. Sinai, New York, NY, USA
e-mail: Bglodny@gmail.com

J.A. Zeichner, M.D.
Department of Dermatology, Mt. Sinai School of Medicine, New York, NY, USA

J.A. Zeichner (ed.), *Acneiform Eruptions in Dermatology: A Differential Diagnosis*,
DOI 10.1007/978-1-4614-8344-1_27, © Springer Science+Business Media New York 2014

More than 50 mutations have been described within exons 9–20 of the CYLD gene. The CYLD tumor suppressor protein product functions by negatively regulating the nuclear factor (NF)-kB and c-Jun N-terminal kinase pathways [1, 4]. Approximately 86 % of these mutations lead to a truncated CYLD protein, while the remaining 14 % are missense mutations leading to a dysfunctional CYLD protein [4]. CYLD is thought to be involved in regulating many cellular functions, including cell proliferation [4]. CYLD expression has found to be exceptionally high in the outer root sheath of human scalp hair follicles [5]. Recently, animal models have been developed to study the effects of the CYLD gene mutation, including those in "immunity, lipid metabolism, spermatogenesis, antimicrobial defense, and inflammation" [4]. Dysfunction of the CYLD gene in BSS is limited to the skin adnexa, with resulting appendageal tumors. Cylindromas and spiradenomas are thought to develop from the secretory portion of the sweat gland, while trichoepitheliomas from hair follicles [2].

27.3 Clinical Presentation

Neoplasms in BSS include cylindromas, trichoepitheliomas, and less often spiradenomas. These tumors may develop individually in sporadic cases. However, when many of these neoplasms occur in the same patient, a syndrome like BSS, FC, or MFT should be considered. However, given the common folliculosebaceous-apocrine lineage, even patients without BSS have been found to develop individual cylindromas, trichoepitheliomas, and spiradenomas [6].

In the setting of BSS, these tumors commonly present on the head and neck during childhood or early adulthood and continue to develop later in life [4]. Patients may confuse these lesions with acne, but there is a lack of comedones or acne papules or pustules. Rarely, cylindromas many coalesce to form a large plaque covering the scalp, referred to as a "turban tumor" [7]. Trichoepitheliomas present as papules on the nasolabial folds, nose, and upper lips, but can cover large surface areas of the face [1, 2]. Spiradenomas are clinically indistinct papules affecting non-glabrous skin. Patient may experience spontaneous pain, which can be a clue to its diagnosis. Additionally, spiradenomas may have a blue hue [1]. While these are the most common cutaneous neoplasms of BSS, these patients also can develop syringomas and basal cell cancers (BCC) [8]. These neoplasms are frequently numerous, becoming aesthetically bothersome to the patient.

While most tumors in BSS are benign, malignant transformation is a risk. More than 25 cases of cylindrocarcinomas developing from cylindromas have been reported [9–11]. Likewise, trichoepithelioma must be followed as they may degenerate into BCC [12]. Over 35 cases of carcinomatous or sarcomatous transformation from spiradenomas have also been described [13]. Both cylindrocarcinomas and malignant spiradenomas have been found to be more aggressive compared to BCC's, posing a great risk for both local destruction and metastasis [9, 14]. In addition to cutaneous neoplasms, patients with BSS are at risk for neoplasms of the salivary and parotid glands [9, 15]

27.4 Work-Up

All patients with multiple, fixed facial papules of unclear etiology should be worked up, as definite diagnosis by clinical inspection is difficult. While dermoscopic evaluation may provide a consistent appearance with telangiectasia and blue structures [16], histopathology is often necessary [2]. Trichoepitheliomas represent an over proliferation of follicular germinative, basaloid cells organized in a cribriform pattern surrounded by a coarse, fibrous stroma [1, 17, 18]. As opposed to BCCs, there is no clefting between basaloid cells and the stroma [19]. Cylindromas are well-circumscribed nodules in the dermis or subcutis comprised of compact lobules of basaloid cells that form a "jigsaw puzzle" arrangement [1]. Spiradenomas appear as dermal or subcutaneous multinodular growths with pale-staining cells in trabecular pattern, with basophilic cells at the periphery. A clue to the diagnosis is the presence of lymphocytes scattered throughout the lesion [1].

Patients with multiple trichoepitheliomas, spiradenomas, and/or cylindromas should be referred to genetics to be screened for CYLD gene mutations. The differential diagnosis for trichoepitheliomas and trichoepitheliomas includes Bazex and Rombo syndromes, but the patients also develop epidermoid cysts, milia, hypotrichosis, BCCs, atrophoderma vermiculatum, and peripheral cyanosis [1]. Patients should also be referred to otolaryngology for evaluation for salivary or parotid tumors.

27.5 Treatment

Most of the cutaneous neoplasm in BSS are benign in nature and pose more of a cosmetic challenge than medical necessity. However, close monitoring for malignant transformation is prudent. Biopsies should be performed lesions that are growing or ulcerating [1, 9]. When lesions grow so large that they cause functional derangements, they may require treatment. Individual lesions may be surgically excised, but surgery may not be a realistic option for BSS patients with large numbers of lesions [1, 20], Alternative therapies include electrosurgery, cryosurgery, photodynamic therapy, imiquimod, or laser ablation that can be used alone or in combination [20].

27.6 Conclusion

Brooke-Spiegler syndrome is a condition characterized by the development of many adnexal neoplasms. While cosmesis is usually the primary concern for these patients, functional impairments from large growing lesions must be addressed. Moreover, these patients must be continually monitored because of the risk for malignant transformation.

References

1. Bolognia JL, Jorizzo JL, Schaffer JV. Dermatology. 3rd ed. Saunders; June 4, 2012. Ch 111; 1834–1835.
2. Lee DA, Grossman ME, Schneiderman P, Celebi JT. Genetics of skin appendage neoplasms and related syndromes. JMEd Genet. 2005;42:811–9.
3. Welch JP, Wells RS, Kerr CB. Ancell-Spiegler cylindromas (turban tumors) and Brooke-Fordyce trichoepitheliomas: evidence for a single genetic entity. J Med Genet. 1968;5:29–35.
4. Blake PW, Toro JR. Update of cylindromatosis gene (CYLD) Mutations in Brooke-Spiegler syndrome: novel insights into the role of deubiquitination in cell signaling. Hum Mutat. 2009;30(7):1025–36.
5. Massoumi R, Podda M, Fassler R, Paus R. Cylindroma as tumor of hair follicle origin. J Invest Dermatol. 2006;126:1182–4.
6. Michal M, Lamovec J, Mukensnabl P, Pizinger K. Spiradenocylindromas of the skin: tumors with morphological features of spiradenoma and cylindroma in the same lesion: report of 12 cases. Pathol Int. 1999;49:419–25.
7. Nerad JA, Folberg R. Multiple cylindromas. "The turban tumor". Arch Opthalmol. 1987;105:1137.
8. Uede K, Yamamoto Y, Furukawa F. Brooke-Spiegler syndrome associated with cylindroma, trichoepithelioma, spiradenoma, and syringoma. J Dermatol. 2004;31:32–8.
9. Gerretsen A, van der Putte S, Deenstra W. Cutaneous cylindroma with malignant transformation. Cancer. 1993;72:1618–23.
10. Durani BK, Kurzen H, Jaeckel A, Kuner N, Naeher H, Hartschuh W. Malignant transformation of multiple dermal cylindromas. Br J Dermatol. 2001;145(4):653–6.
11. Pizinger K, Michal M. Malignant cylindroma in Brooke-Spiegler Syndrome. Dermatology. 2000;201(3):255–7.
12. Ayhan M, Adanali G, Senen D, Gorgu M, Erdogan B. Rarely seen cutaneous lesions in an elderly patient: malignant transformation of multiple trichoepithelioma. Ann Plast Surg. 2001; 47:98–9.
13. Ishikawa M, Nakanishi Y, Yamazaki N, Yamamoto A. Malignant eccrine spiradenoma: a case report and review of the literature. Dermatol Surg. 2001;27:67–70.
14. Lo JS, Snow SN, Reizner GT, Mohs FE, Larson PO, Hruza GJ. Metastatic basal cell carcinoma: report of twelve cases with a review of the literature. J Am Acad Dermatol. 1991;24: 715–9.
15. Jungehulsing M, Wagner M, Damm M. Turban tumor with involvement of the parotid gland. J Laryngol Otol. 1999;113:779–83.
16. Jarret R, Walker L, Bowling J. Dermoscopy of Brooke-Spiegler syndrome. Arch Dermatol. 2009;145(7):854.
17. Ackerman AB, Reddy VB, Soyer HP. Neoplasms with follicular differentiation. 2nd ed. New York: Ardor Scribendi; 2001. p. 1109.
18. Elston D, Ferringer T, Ko C, Peckham S, High W, DiCaudo D, Bhuta S. Requisites in dermatology: dermatopathology. New York, Saunders Elsevier; 2008. p. 70–1.
19. Bettencourt MS, Preito VG, Shea CR. Trichoepithelioma: a 19-year clinicopathologic re-evaluation. J Cutan Pathol. 1999;26:398–404.
20. LoPiccolo M, Sage R, Kouba D. Comparing ablative fractionated resurfacing, photodynamic therapy, and topical imiquimod in the treatment of trichoblastomas of Brooke-Spiegler syndrome: a case study. Dermatol Surg. 2011;37:1047–50.

Chapter 28
Cowden Syndrome

Rita V. Linkner and Joshua A. Zeichner

28.1 Introduction

Cowden syndrome (CS) is an autosomal dominant genodermatosis and represents one of the clinical disorders on the spectrum linked to the germline mutation in the phosphatase and tensin homolog gene (PTEN). Located on chromosome 10, the PTEN gene is a dual specificity phosphatase which plays various roles in cell migration, apoptosis, and all processes that are important in the regulation of normal cellular growth [1]. Mutations in PTEN have been associated with various other disorders including Bannayan-Riley-Ruvalcaba syndrome, Proteus syndrome, adult L'hermitte-Duclos disease, and autism-like disorders associated with macrocephaly [2].

Cowden syndrome was first described by in the 1960s in a case report involving a patient named Rachel Cowden who presented with multiple hamartomas, unusual cutaneous findings, abnormal CNS findings, and fibrocystic breast disease [3]. Years later, Weary et al further reported the existence of this disorder with the first case series involving five subjects with similar clinical findings [4]. The PTEN mutation was finally found to be the cause in 1996. Currently, the clinical definition of CS has not only been widened to include multiple hamartomas involving any and sometimes all of the three embryonic germ cell layers but also now incorporates the significant risk of developing breast and/or non-medullary thyroid malignancy [5].

28.2 Background

With identification of the PTEN mutation, the estimated incidence of CS is between 1 in 200,000 and 1 in 250,000 [6]. Studies report a Caucasian female predominance. The age of diagnosis is variable, ranging from 13 to 65 years of age [7].

R.V. Linkner, M.D. (✉) • J.A. Zeichner, M.D.
Department of Dermatology, Mount Sinai School of Medicine, New York, NY, USA
e-mail: Rita.Linkner@mountsinai.org

J.A. Zeichner (ed.), *Acneiform Eruptions in Dermatology: A Differential Diagnosis*,
DOI 10.1007/978-1-4614-8344-1_28, © Springer Science+Business Media New York 2014

Cowden syndrome is inherited autosomal dominantly with incomplete penetrance and variable expressivity. The PTEN gene was localized to chromosome 10q22-23 by an extensive linkage family study involving 12 separate families [5]. PTEN is a 9-exon tumor suppressor gene that acts as a lipid phosphatase to negatively regulate the mTOR pathway [8]. Studies have shown the involvement of PTEN in a large number of sporadic tumors such as glioblastomas, prostate cancer, melanoma, thyroid, and endometrial tumors. Germline coding sequence mutation in PTEN is reported in 80 % of those with CS [9].

28.3 Clinical Presentation

Cowden syndrome affects various organs and increases the risk for overgrowth of different tissues. Mucocutaneous lesions are found in nearly all cases of CS [10]. While the age of onset of these characteristic lesions is quite variable, the lesions most commonly associated with CS include trichilemmomas, oral papillomas, and acral keratoses. Trichilemmomas are benign hamartomatous lesions of the follicle outer root sheath that end to be slow growing and skin colored and most commonly found on the face or neck (Fig. 28.1) [11]. Oral papillomas are benign lesions that can occur on the oral mucosa, primarily on the tongue (Fig. 28.2) [12]. Acral keratoses are clinically seen as verrucous papules on the dorsal surfaces of the hands and feet (Fig. 28.3).

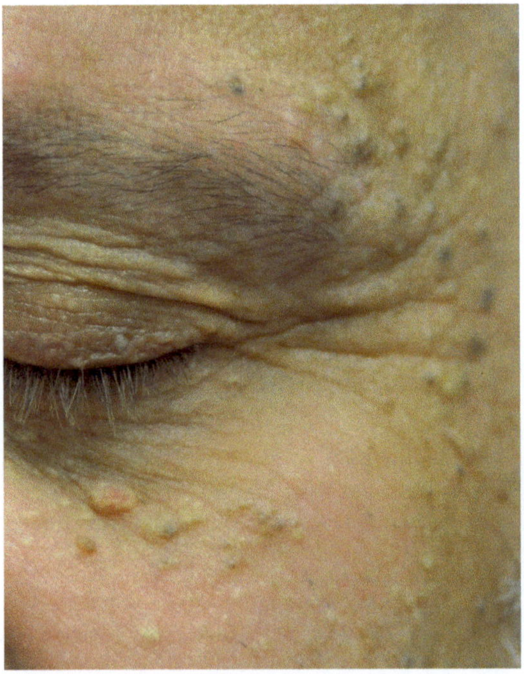

Fig. 28.1 Flesh-colored papules on the face, which histologically were revealed to be trichilemmomas. In addition, he also suffered from comedones (Photo credit: Joshua A. Zeichner, M.D.)

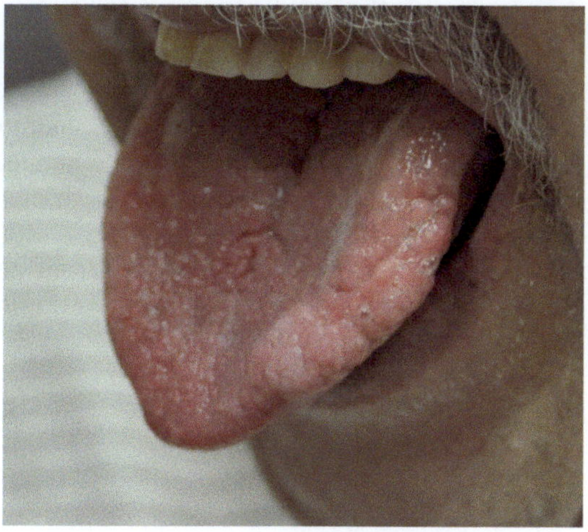

Fig. 28.2 Flesh-colored papules along the border of the tongue, consistent with the oral papillomas observed in Cowden syndrome (Photo credit: Joshua A. Zeichner, M.D.)

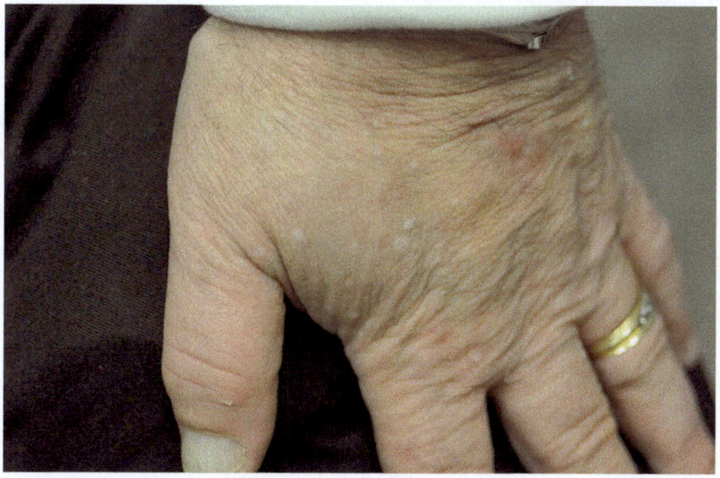

Fig. 28.3 Acral keratoses on the dorsal hands, which clinically appear as warty, stuck on papules (Photo credit: Joshua A. Zeichner, M.D.)

Strict mucosal involvement, which typically occurs after cutaneous involvement, is seen in over 80 % of cases and is described when either the gingival or buccal mucosa is developing a "cobblestone" appearance [13].

The most common malignancy associated with CS is breast cancer, with a lifetime risk of 25–50 % and an average age of diagnosis of 36–46 years old [14]. Similar to what is observed in the general population, ductal adenocarcinoma is most commonly diagnosed in patients with CS [15]. Other benign breast disorders are increased in CS, including fibroadenomas, apocrine metaplasia, and mammary hamartomas. These benign entities have not been associated with malignant transformation these patients [16].

Other cancers observed in CS include follicular thyroid carcinoma, malignant testicular seminoma, mixed germ cell tumors, and endometrial cancers [17]. Melanoma, renal cell carcinoma, and colon cancer have also been reported as well [18]. L'hermitte-Duclos disease is pathognomonic for CS. This indolent, benign hamartomatous overgrowth of the cerebellum leads to headaches, ataxia, and visual disturbances. The diagnosis may be made through MRI and surgical excision can be curative [19].

Patients with CS commonly suffer from periodontitis, dental caries, skeletal abnormalities, and a high arched palate. Additionally, mental retardation occurs in up to 20 % of patients [20–23].

28.4 Work-Up

Patients with fixed facial papules or oral lesions of unclear diagnosis should be evaluated with a biopsy for histologic evaluation, as they may be a presenting sign of CS. The United States National Comprehensive Cancer Network (NCCN) has published screening criteria, outlined in Table 28.1. Clinical diagnostic criteria for CS are met if the patient has adult L'hermitte-Duclos disease or a requisite number of mucocutaneous lesions, macrocephaly plus one other major criterion, one major and three minor criteria, or four minor criteria. Any patient who fits the screening criteria, should be referred to genetics for PTEN gene testing [24]. Patients should also be evaluated for the presence of internal malignancies, including breast and thyroid disease.

Table 28.1 Cowden syndrome NCCN guidelines, 2009 [24]

Pathognomonic criteria	Adult L'hermitte-Duclos disease
	Mucocutaneous lesions
	Facial trichilemmomas
	Acral keratoses
	Papillomatous papules
Major criteria	Breast carcinoma
	Non-medullary thyroid carcinoma
	Macrocephaly
	Endometrial carcinoma
Minor criteria	Other thyroid lesions
	Mental retardation (IQ<75)
	GI hamartomas
	Fibrocystic disease of the breast
	Lipomas
	Fibromas
	Genitourinary tumors (especially renal cell carcinoma)
	Genitourinary structural abnormalities
	Uterine fibroids

28.5 Treatment

A multidisciplinary approach must be employed in treating CS. These patients require the resources of dermatology, endocrinology, gynecology, and genetics. Women should conduct monthly self breast examinations, starting at 18 years old. A physician clinical breast examination should be initiated at age 25 or 10 years prior to the earliest known breast cancer in the family, whichever occurs first. Mammography along with breast MRI should commence at 30 years old or 5 years prior to the earliest known breast cancer in the family, whichever occurs first. Prophylactic mastectomy should be discussed on a case by case basis with familial history being taken into account [24].

For both males and females, a full physical examination should be started at the age of 18 or 5 years before to the diagnosis of a component cancer in the family, whichever occurs first. At the age of 18, thyroid ultrasounds should be initiated annually. A dermatologist conducting a total body skin check should also be recommended. Genetic counseling is another important topic to be broached with the patient and those relatives whom are deemed to be at high risk [24].

Treatment of cutaneous lesions is largely cosmetic in nature, as these lesions are benign. However, larger lesions affecting the mouth or acral areas may lead to functional impairment requiring intervention. Physical modalities such as surgical excision or laser ablation may be of use.

28.6 Conclusion

It is important for the dermatologist to be familiar with Cowden syndrome, considering the malignant potential of this disorder. The various unique skin manifestations potentially offer early clues to screen, properly diagnose, and treat patients early in the course of the disease to improve patients' quality of life.

References

1. Tamguney T, Stokoe D. New insights into PTEN. J Cell Sci. 2007;120(23):4071–9.
2. Pilarski R. Cowden syndrome: a critical review of the literature. J Genet Counsel. 2009; 18:13–27.
3. Lloyd KM, Denis M. Cowden disease: a possible new symptom complex with multiple symptom involvement. Ann Inten Med. 1963;58:136–42.
4. Weary PE, Gorlin RJ, Gentry WC, Comer JE, Greer KE. Multiple hematoma syndrome (Cowden disease). Arch Dermatol. 1972;106(5):682–90.
5. Nelen MR, Kremer H, Konigns IBM, Schoute F, van Essen AJ, Koch R, et al. Novel PTEN mutations in patients with Cowden disease: absence of clear genotype phenotype correlations. Eur J Human Genet. 1999;7:267–73.

6. Starlink T, Cander Veen J, Artwert F, Erikson AW. The Cowden syndrome: a clinical and genetic study in 21 patients. Clin Genet. 1986;29:222–33.
7. Salem OS, Steck WD. Cowden's disease. A case report and review of the English literature. J Am Acad Dermatol. 1983;8(5):686–96.
8. Pilarski R, Eng C. Will the real Cowden syndrome please stand up (again)? Expanding mutational and clinical spectra of the PTEN hamartoma tumour syndrome. J Med Genet. 2004; 41(5):323–6.
9. Guldberg P, Thor Straten P, Birck A, Ahrenkiel V, Kirkin AF, Zeuthen J. Disruption of the MMAC1/PTEN gene by deletion of mutation is a frequent event in malignant melanoma. Cancer Res. 1997;57(17):3660–3.
10. Fistarol SK, Marc D, Anliker MS, Peter H. Cowden disease or multiple hamartoma syndrome—cutaneous clue to internal malignancy. Eur J Dermatol. 2002;12(5):411–21.
11. Brownstein MH, Mehregan AH, Bilowski JB. Trichilemmomas on Cowden's disease. J Am Med Assoc. 1977;238(1):26.
12. Devlin MF, Barrie R, Ward-Booth RP. Cowden's disease: a rare but important manifestation of oral papillomatosis. Br J Oral Maxillofacial Surg. 1992;30:335–6.
13. Blumenthal GM, Dennis PA. PTEN hamartoma tumor syndromes. Eur J Human Genet. 2008;16:1289–300.
14. Nusbaum R, Vogel JK, Ready K. Susceptibility to breast cancer: hereditary syndromes and low penetrance genes. Breast Dus. 2007;27:21–50.
15. Schrager CA, Schneider D, Gruener AC. Clinical and pathological features of breast disease in Cowden's syndrome: an under-recognized syndrome with an increased risk of breast cancer. Human Pathol. 1998;29:47–53.
16. Brownstein MH, Wolf M, Bikowski JB. Cowden's disease: a cutaneous marker of breast cancer. Cancer. 1978;41:2393–8.
17. Farooq A, Walker LJ, Bowling J, Audisio RA. Cowden syndrome. Cancer Treat Rev. 2010;8: 577–83.
18. Pilariski R. Cowden syndrome: a critical review. J Genet Counsel. 2009;18:13–27.
19. Lok C, Viseux V, Avril MF, Richard MA, Gondry-Jouet C, Deramond H, et al. Brain magnetic resonance imaging in patients with Cowden syndrome. Medicine. 2005;84(2):129–36. doi:10.1097/01.md.0000158792.24888.d2.
20. Bagan JV, Penarrocha M, Vera-Sempere F. Cowden syndrome: clinical and pathological considerations in two new cases. J Oral Maxillofacial Surg. 1989;47(3):291–4. doi:10.1016/0278-2391(89)90234-6.
21. Starink TM. Cowden's disease: analysis of fourteen new cases. J Am Acad Dermatol. 1984;11(6):1127–41. doi:10.1016/S0190-9622(84)70270-2.
22. Salem OS, Steck WD (1983) Cowden's disease (multiple hamartoma and neoplasia syndrome). A case report and review of the English literature. J Am Acad Dermatol. 8(5):686–96.aa
23. Parisi M, Dinulos MB, Leppid KA, Sybert VP, Eng C, Hudgins L. The spectrum and evolution of phenotypic findings in PTEN mutation positive cases of Bannayan-Riley-Ruvalcaba syndrome. J Med Genet. 2001;38:52–7.
24. The NCCN 1.2009 Cowden syndrome clinical practice guidelines in oncology. National Comprehensive Cancer Network, 2009. Available from: http://www.nccn.org. Adapted with permission from NCCN [accessed 10.06.09]. (To view the most recent and complete version of the guideline, go online to www.nccn.org).

Chapter 29
Gardner Syndrome

Alexandra Golant and Joshua A. Zeichner

29.1 Introduction

Gardner syndrome (GS) is a phenotypic variant of familial adenomatous polyposis (FAP). The syndrome is characterized by premalignant intestinal polyposis and distinct extraintestinal features, such as multiple epidermoid cysts, osteomas, and desmoid or fibrous tumors of the skin and soft tissue [1].

29.2 Background

FAP and GS are caused by mutations in the adenomatous polyposis coli (*APC*) tumor suppressor gene on chromosome 5q21–22 [2]. There is a correlation between the site of the mutation on the APC gene and the clinical phenotype [3]. Specifically, APC mutations between codon 1395 and 1493 are frequently associated with features of GS [4]. APC gene mutations result in accumulation of β-catenin which bypasses the growth-regulating effects of Wnt signaling resulting in important implications for cell differentiation, proliferation, and adhesion [5, 6]. GS is inherited as an autosomal dominant disorder with high penetrance and variable expressivity, though approximately 25 % of patients have de novo mutations and no family history [6]. The estimate of incidence of GS ranges from approximately 1 in 6,850 to 1 in 31,250 births [7–9].

A. Golant, M.D. (✉)
Department of Dermatology, The Mt. Sinai Hospital, New York, NY, USA
e-mail: alexandra.golant@mountsinai.org

J. A. Zeichner, M.D.
Department of Dermatology, Mt. Sinai School of Medicine, New York, NY, USA

J.A. Zeichner (ed.), *Acneiform Eruptions in Dermatology: A Differential Diagnosis*,
DOI 10.1007/978-1-4614-8344-1_29,

29.3 Clinical Features

In addition to the intestinal manifestations of FAP, patients with GS have characteristic extraintestinal manifestations—both cutaneous and extracutaneous.

29.3.1 Cutaneous Findings

Cutaneous lesions and bony abnormalities in GS often appear during childhood and adolescence, frequently before polyposis develops. Epidermoid cysts are the most common cutaneous finding in GS, affecting approximately one-third of patients [10]. Epidermoid cysts are firm, well-circumscribed dermal nodules that contain soft keratin secretions. They may be present at birth but often occur at puberty, occur in multiplicity in more than 50 % of patients, and tend to occur in unusual locations such as the face, scalp, and extremities [10]. Cysts in GS typically occur earlier than ordinary cysts, as seen in patient with acne. Though the majority of cysts are asymptomatic, they can be pruritic, inflamed, or ruptured [10]. Cutaneous cysts showing unusual histological features—namely, a mixture of epidermoid, trichilemmal, and/or pilomatricoma-like features—are considered a hallmark of GS [6].

Desmoid tumors are benign fibrous mesenchymal neoplasms that result from the proliferation of well-differentiated fibroblasts seen in 3–30 % of patients with GS [2, 6, 11], with average onset around age 30 and a marked female predominance (70–85 %) [6, 11, 12]. Desmoid tumors in GS are associated with mutations occurring downstream of codon 1400 of the APC gene [6, 12] and can be located in the abdominal region (intra-abdominally or within the abdominal wall) or extra-abdominally in the shoulder girdle, chest well, and inguinal regions [12, 13]. Physical exam may reveal a well-circumscribed, firm, flesh-colored tumor [13]. These tumors may occur spontaneously or at incision sites, commonly developing after colectomy which is a leading cause of morbidity in GS [12]. Although cytologically benign and non-metastatic, desmoid tumors are locally aggressive and can be invasive, recur after excision, and even lead to death [11].

Fibromas are another feature of GS and may occur in the skin, subcutaneous tissues, mesentery, or even retroperitoneum [11]. Nuchal fibromas classically present with diffuse swelling and induration of the back of the neck [2, 6]. "Gardner fibromas" arise in the first decade of life, favor the trunk or paraspinal region, and can serve as a desmoid precursor [11]. Lipomas, leiomyomas, trichoepitheliomas, and neurofibromas are other skin findings less commonly observed in GS [2, 6, 11].

None of the cutaneous lesions in GS have been reported to progress to malignancy.

29.3.2 Extracutaneous Findings

Osteomas occur in approximately 20 % of patients with GS and favor the mandible and maxilla. Less frequently, they can develop in long bones or the skull and are commonly associated with cutaneous cysts [2, 6]. Osteomas can present as early as childhood and often predate intestinal polyposis. These tumors are benign and painless but may be multiple or grow to reach significant enough size to be detected on physical exam [11]. Other skeletal abnormalities in GS include exostoses, endostoses, and cortical thickening of the long bones [11].

Dental anomalies are well described in GS and are seen in approximately 20 % of patients. These include odontomas and odontogenic cysts; absent, supernumerary, or rudimentary teeth; and multiple dental caries [2, 6].

Congenital hypertrophy of the retinal pigment epithelium (CHRPE) affects approximately two-thirds of patients with GS and can be an early sign of the syndrome [14]. CHRPE is a patch of darkly pigmented retinal epithelium that can be detected on ophthalmologic exam at birth [13]. While unilateral solitary CHRPE is not specific for FAP, multiple or bilateral lesions are considered highly specific for FAP [2, 6, 15]. In GS, CHRPE is associated with mutations between codons 767 and 1513 [16].

Importantly, patients with GS are at increased risk for the development of several extracolonic malignancies. These include duodenal cancer, papillary thyroid carcinoma (mostly in females), brain tumors (glioblastoma, astrocytoma, medulloblastoma), hepatoblastoma (mostly in children), pancreatic and biliary tract carcinomas, adrenal adenoma, and various sarcomas (including fibrosarcoma and osteosarcoma) [2, 5, 6, 11, 17].

29.3.3 Gastrointestinal Manifestations

FAP is characterized by the development of hundreds of adenomatous polyps of the colorectum that typically appear in the second decade [2]. These polyps invariably undergo malignant transformation resulting in colorectal carcinoma (CRC) at a mean age of 39 years if undetected or untreated [18]. Polyps occur primarily in the colon (typically bilaterally, but may initially be right sided) [13], but can also be found in the small intestine and stomach in over 50 % of patients [6]. Consideration of FAP or GS is often made when a patient presents with GI symptoms including bleeding, anemia, abdominal pain, diarrhea, constipation, or weight loss.

29.4 Work-Up

Patients suspected of having FAP/GS should be managed by a multidisciplinary medial team, including dermatologists, gastroenterologists, geneticists, and surgeons. The diagnosis of FAP should be suspected in any patient found to have multiple colorectal adenomas with any of the manifestations described above or in first-degree relatives of affected family members. In a patient who has cysts with an atypical histology, along with a history of jaw cysts, the diagnosis of GS should be considered. These may present prior to gastrointestinal signs in some patients.

Genetic testing for APC mutations is required for a definitive diagnosis of FAP. Molecular testing for *APC* mutations is commercially available and recommended for all patients suspected of having FAP/GS and their first-degree relatives.

Cutaneous cysts in patients with GS usually demonstrate the same microscopic changes as ordinary epidermoid cysts (lining of keratinizing epithelium including a granular layer containing loose lamellar keratin within the cyst) but also classically demonstrate cysts with pilomatrical differentiation (containing areas of ghost cell keratinization) [19]. "Gardner fibromas" appear as sheets of thick, haphazardly arranged collagen bundles with interspersed bland fibroblasts [20]. Intestinal polyps of GS show adenomatous hyperplasia of the mucosa [21].

29.5 Treatment

Management of the extraintestinal and intestinal manifestations of GS necessitates involvement of a multidisciplinary medical team. Symptomatic epidermoid cysts can be managed by intralesional steroid injection or surgical excision [1]. Desmoid tumors can be managed by surgical excision, though there is a high rate of recurrence and recurring tumors may be more aggressive [6]. If wide surgical excision of desmoid tumors fails, hormonal therapy (e.g., tamoxifen, raloxifene), and/or anthracycline-containing chemotherapy can be tried [22]. Some osteomas in GS may be amenable to surgical intervention [6, 11]. Medications that affect prostaglandin metabolism, such as nonsteroidal anti-inflammatory drugs, have been reported to reduce the risk of colorectal cancer and desmoids tumors [23].

Because of the significant risk of malignancy, strict screening regimens are crucial for patients with FAP/GS. Due to the inevitability of developing CRC, patients with FAP/GS should undergo annual sigmoidoscopy starting at age 10–15 and prophylactic colectomy is typically recommended when polyps are identified or by the end of the 2nd or 3rd decade [5, 6, 18]. Chemoprevention with cyclooxygenase inhibitors (i.e., celecoxib) has been associated with some level of polyp regression, but is not adequate to control the cancer risk [24].

Other recommended screening includes upper GI endoscopy every 1–3 years (depending on polyp burden) along with annual thyroid exam due to risk of malignancy [18, 25]. Annual abdominal ultrasounds and monitoring of serum α-fetoprotein levels during the first 5 years of life are recommended due to risk of hepatoblastoma in this age group [1]. Ophthalmologic exam should be performed upon consideration of the diagnosis of FAP/GS to evaluate for the presence of CHRPE. Panoramic dental radiographs can detect osteomas, odontomas, and supernumerary teeth, and long-bone x-rays can be used to detect osteomas [2]. No consensus exists for routine screening for the detection of desmoid tumors, but palpable masses or symptoms should be explored using computerized tomography [1].

Genetic counseling is an extremely important consideration and all family members should be offered genetic testing and be evaluated for evidence of GS.

29.6 Conclusion

Gardner syndrome affects multiple body systems, including the skin, soft tissue, bone, gastrointestinal system, as well as other solid organs. Recognition of cutaneous signs may provide an early diagnosis and can be lifesaving with proper management.

References

1. Juhn E, Khachemoune A. Gardner syndrome: skin manifestations, differential diagnosis and management. Am J Clin Dermatol. 2010;11(2):117–22.
2. Ponti G, Pellacani G, Seidenari S, Pollio A, Muscatello U, Tomasi A. Cancer-associated genodermatoses: skin neoplasms as clues to hereditary tumor syndromes. Crit Rev Oncol Hematol. 2012;85(3):239–56.
3. Nieuwenhuis MH, Vasen HF. Correlations between mutation site in APC and phenotype of familial adenomatous polyposis (FAP): a review of the literature. Crit Rev Oncol Hematol. 2007;61(2):153–61.
4. Wallis YL, Morton DG, McKeown CM, Macdonald F. Molecular analysis of the APC gene in 205 families: extended genotype-phenotype correlations in FAP and evidence for the role of APC amino acid changes in colorectal cancer predisposition. J Med Genet. 1999; 36(1): 14–20.
5. Doxey BW, Kuwada SK, Burt RW. Inherited polyposis syndromes: molecular mechanisms, clinicopathology, and genetic testing. Clin Gastroenterol Hepatol. 2005;3(7):633–64.
6. Kanitakis J. Adnexal tumours of the skin as markers of cancer-prone syndromes. J Eur Acad Dermatol Venereol. 2010;24(4):379–87.
7. Bussey HJR. Familial polyposis coli: Family studies, histopathology, differential diagnosis, and results of treatment. Baltimore: Johns Hopkins University Press; 1975
8. Järvinen HJ. Epidemiology of familial adenomatous polyposis in Finland: impact of family screening on the colorectal cancer rate and survival. Gut. 1992;33(3):357–60.
9. Bülow S, Faurschou Nielsen T, Bülow C, Bisgaard ML, Karlsen L, Moesgaard F. The incidence rate of familial adenomatous polyposis. Results from the Danish Polyposis Register. Int J Colorectal Dis. 1996;11(2):88–91.
10. Shen Z, Hoffman JD, Hao F, Pier E. More than just skin deep: faciocutaneous clues to genetic syndromes with malignancies. Oncologist. 2012;17(7):930–6.
11. Bayliss SJ, Berk DR, Burton BK, Cohen BA, Bree AF, Sybert VP. Other genodermatoses. In: Bolognia JL, Jorizzo JL, Schaffer JV, editors. Dermatology. St. Louis, MO: Mosby/Elsevier; 2012.
12. Leal RF, Silva PV, Ayrizono Mde L, Fagundes JJ, Amstalden EM, Coy CS. Desmoid tumor in patients with familial adenomatous polyposis. Arq Gastroenterol. 2010;47(4):373–8.
13. Shah KR, Boland CR, Patel M, Thrash B, Menter A. Cutaneous manifestations of gastrointestinal disease: part I. J Am Acad Dermatol. 2013;68(2):189.e1–189.e21.
14. Shields JA, Shields CL, Shah PG, et al. Lack of association among typical congenital hypertrophy of the retinal pigment epithelium, adenomatous polyposis and Gardner syndrome. Ophthalmology. 1992;99(11):1709–13.
15. Baker RH, Heinemann MH, Miller HH, DeCosse JJ. Hyperpigmented lesions of the retinal pigment epithelium in familial adenomatous polyposis. Am J Med Genet. 1988;31(2): 427–35.
16. Bisgaard ML, Bülow S. Familial adenomatous polyposis (FAP): genotype correlation to FAP phenotype with osteomas and sebaceous cysts. Am J Med Genet A. 2006;140(3):200–4.

17. Tsao H. Update on familial cancer syndromes and the skin. J Am Acad Dermatol. 2000; 42(6):939–69.
18. Jasperson KW, Tuohy TM, Neklason DW, Burt RW. Hereditary and familial colon cancer. Gastroenterology. 2010;138(6):2044–58.
19. Pujol RM, Casanova JM, Egido R, Pujol J, de Moragas JM. Multiple familial pilomatricomas: a cutaneous marker for Gardner syndrome? Pediatr Dermatol. 1995;12(4):331–5.
20. Coffin CM, Hornick JL, Zhou H, Fletcher CD. Gardner fibroma: a clinicopathologic and immunohistochemical analysis of 45 patients with 57 fibromas. Am J Surg Pathol. 2007; 31(3):410–6.
21. Naylor EW, Lebenthal E. Early detection of adenomatous polyposis coli in the Gardner's syndrome. Pediatrics. 1979;63(2):222–7.
22. de Camargo VP, et al. Clinical outcomes of systemic therapy for patients with deep fibromatosis (desmoid tumor). Cancer. 2010;116(9):2258–65.
23. Hughes-Fulford M, Boman B. Growth regulation of Gardner's syndrome colorectal cancer cells by NSAIDs. Adv Exp Med Biol. 1997;407:433–41.
24. Boardman LA. Heritable colorectal cancer syndromes: recognition and preventive management. Gastroenterol Clin North Am. 2002;31(4):1107–31.
25. Gallagher MC, Phillips RK, Bulow S. Surveillance and management of upper gastrointestinal disease in familial adenomatous polyposis. Fam Cancer. 2006;5(3):263–73.

Chapter 30
Gorlin Syndrome

Madelaine Haddican and James Spencer

30.1 Introduction

Basal cell nevus syndrome (BCNS) is an autosomal dominantly inherited condition first described in 1960 by Dr. Gorlin and Dr. Goltz [1]. BCNS is known by several other names including nevoid basal cell carcinoma syndrome, basal cell carcinoma nevus syndrome, Gorlin syndrome, and Gorlin-Goltz syndrome. Although BCNS demonstrates a high degree of penetrance, the diagnosis can be challenging due to its variable expressivity even within families [2, 3] and the age-dependent appearance of certain traits associated with this disorder. Some of the more frequent and characteristic features of BCNS include multiple basal cell carcinomas (BCCs), odontogenic keratocysts, skeletal abnormalities, palmar and/or plantar pits, calcified falx cerebri, and facial dysmorphism [1]. Other clinical features found in association with BCNS include neoplasms such as medulloblastoma, ovarian fibroma, and cardiac fibromas [4–7].

30.2 Background

BCNS results from mutations in the PTCH1 tumor suppressor gene which is found on chromosome 9q22.3-q31 [8]. The product of the PTCH1 gene normally represses gene transcription in the Hedgehog signaling pathway by acting as a transmembrane receptor for the Sonic Hedgehog (SHH) ligand [9]. The Hedgehog signaling pathway was first described as a developmental pathway during research on the fruit fly, *Drosophila melanogaster* [10]. Post-developmentally in humans, the Hedgehog signaling pathway is typically only active in hair follicles and skin cells [11].

M. Haddican, M.D. (✉) • J. Spencer, M.D.
Department of Dermatology, Mount Sinai School of Medicine, New York, NY, USA
e-mail: madelaine.haddican@mountsinai.org

J.A. Zeichner (ed.), *Acneiform Eruptions in Dermatology: A Differential Diagnosis*,
DOI 10.1007/978-1-4614-8344-1_30, © Springer Science+Business Media New York 2014

The neoplasms of the syndrome require two hits to the PTCH1 gene, with a mutation in the second normal allele [12]. However, some clinical features of BCNS, such as palmar pits, bifid rib, and macrocephaly, only require the inherited defective allele [3].

Women and men appear to be equally affected by BCNS. However, the prevalence of BCNS ranges from 1/57,000 to 1/256,000 depending on the studied population [13, 14]. It should be noted that certain clinical manifestations of BCNS, mainly BCCs, are less prevalent in darker skin individuals [15].

30.3 Clinical Presentation

More than 100 different clinical features have been found in association with BCNS [16]. The most frequent and characteristic features of BCNS have been listed chronologically by age of presentation.

Facial Dysmorphism: Most individuals with BCNS have one or more of the following "coarse" facial features: macrocephaly, frontal bossing, broad nasal bridge, prognathism, high arched eyebrows and/or palate, and cleft lip/palate [4, 17]. Patients with BCNS sometimes have a history of being delivered by cesarean section due to macrocephaly which is the most common facial dysmorphism associated with BCNS [18].

Skeletal Abnormalities: In addition to abnormal skull findings, other skeletal abnormalities typically present at birth include bifid ribs, vertebral abnormalities, Sprengel shoulder, pectus deformity, short 4th metacarpal, and syndactyly of the digits [7].

Ocular Abnormalities: Other congenital abnormalities associated with BCNS include severe eye defects such as strabismus, hypertelorism, telecanthus, cataracts, glaucoma, microphthalmia, orbital cyst, and coloboma [6, 14, 17].

Cardiac Fibromas: Less than 5 % of patients with BCNS develop cardiac fibromas which typically appear in the first year of life [6]. The detection of this benign tumor qualifies as one of the minor criteria for the diagnosis. In general, cardiac fibromas are asymptomatic, but they can cause conduction defects (arrhythmias) and ventricular outflow obstruction [19].

Medulloblastoma: Less than 5 % of patients with BCNS also present with medulloblastomas. Compared to sporadic medulloblastomas which usually occur between the ages of 6 and 10, medulloblastomas in association with BCNS are more common in male patients and typically present by 2 years of age [13, 20].

Odontogenic (Jaw) Keratocysts: Approximately 90 % of patients with BCNS develop multiple jaw keratocysts which occur mostly in the mandible [14]. These keratocysts have been reported as early as 4 years old, but typically occur during

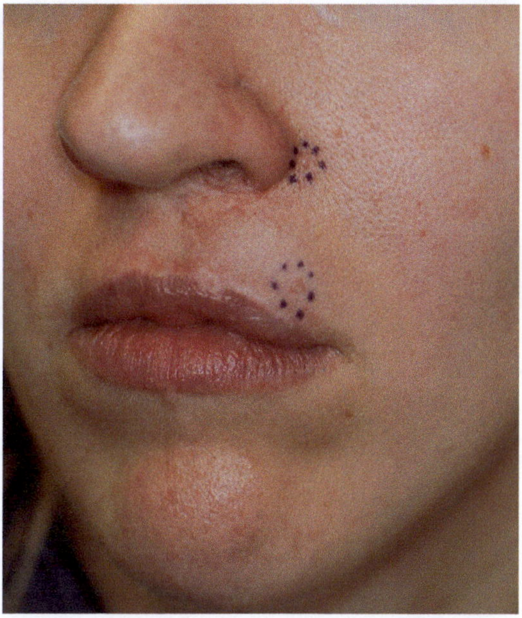

Fig. 30.1 2 mm pearly papules on the face. Biopsies revealed these lesions to be basal cell carcinomas (Photo credit: Joshua A. Zeichner, M.D.)

the second and third decade of life [21]. The presentation of these keratocysts ranges from asymptomatic to painless jaw swelling, tooth disruption, and rarely jaw fracture [22].

BCCs: BCCs in patients with BCNS occur in more than 75 % of Caucasians (Fig. 30.1) but less often in African American and Asian patients [15, 23]. BCCS in BCNS has been reported as early as 3 years of age, but the peak incidence occurs at 20 years of age [6]. They typically occur in sun-exposed area. While only a small percentage are locally invasive, they are challenging to treat and surgical management is potentially disfiguring [17].

Palmoplantar Pitting: Approximately 80 % of patients with BCNS develop palmoplantar pitting typically beginning in the second decade of life [24] (Fig. 30.2).

Intracranial Calcification: In a study of 105 individuals with BCNS (mean age of 32.5 years), approximately 65 % of these patients had intracranial calcification, particularly of the falx cerebri [4].

Ovarian Fibromas: Approximately 15–25 % of female patients with BCNS have ovarian fibroma which is often bilateral and calcified [4, 6]. Most are asymptomatic and are usually discovered incidentally, but some can undergo torsion [3].

Lymphomesenteric Cysts: The exact incidence and age of presentation for lymphomesenteric cysts is unknown. They are also usually asymptomatic [23].

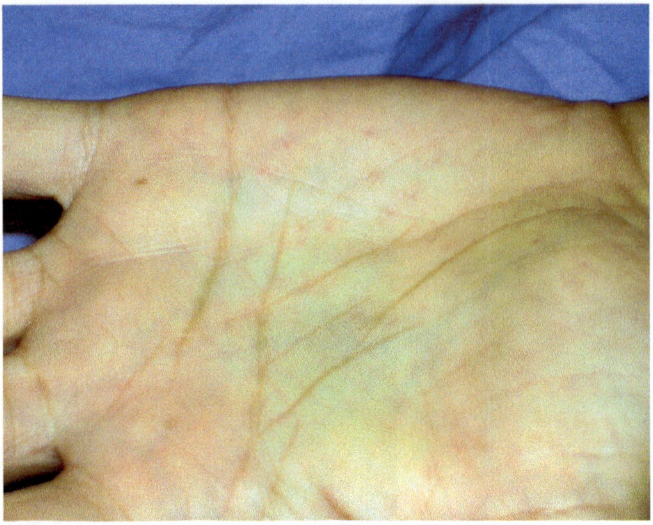

Fig. 30.2 1–2 mm depressed papules on the palms (Photo credit: Joshua A. Zeichner, M.D.)

30.4 Work-Up

The diagnosis of BCNS is typically based on the constellation of clinical manifestations [25]. Depending on the age of the patient, the following criteria can be used to establish the diagnosis:

- Physical examination for facial dysmorphism [26].
- X-rays to detect skeletal abnormalities [7].
- Ophthalmologic evaluation [3].
- Measurement of head circumference to evaluate for macrocephaly [25].
- Echocardiography to evaluate for the presence of a cardiac fibroma [25].
- Brain MRI for the detection of a medulloblastoma [25].
- Panoramic jaw X-rays to evaluate for odontogenic keratocysts [27]
- Skin examination (including biopsies of suspected lesions) for BCCs [25].
- Pelvic ultrasound examination to evaluate for ovarian fibromas in females [25].

There have been no formal studies to help clarify the best combination of clinical features which most accurately leads to a diagnosis of BCNS. The diagnostic criteria for BCNS generally include either two major criteria or one major and two minor criteria. The major criteria include BCC before 20 years old or excessive numbers of BCCs, odontogenic (jaw) keratocyst before 20 years old, palmar and/or plantar pitting, calcification of the falx cerebri, medulloblastoma, and family history of BCNS. The minor criteria include rib abnormalities, other skeletal malformations, macrocephaly, cleft/lip palate, ovarian/cardiac fibroma, lymphomesenteric cysts, and ocular abnormalities [25].

30.5 Treatment

There is no cure for BCNS and patients are managed based on syndrome-related findings [3]. The different clinical manifestations are treated similarly in patients without the disorder. However, surveillance guidelines for the detection of different tumors and odontogenic cysts are important; and thus, patients with BCNS need to be treated under the care of several specialists including medical geneticists, dermatologists, oral surgeons, and plastic surgeons [25]. Fortunately, the life span of patient with BCNS is not significantly different from the average [3], but exposure to ionizing and UV radiation should be minimized to reduce the total number of BCCs [28].

For the management of BCCs, a regular complete skin examination by a dermatologist every 2–4 months is recommended for patients with BCNS [3, 25]. Due to the increased number of BCCs typically present during a lifetime, there is a tendency to reserve surgical treatment for aggressive or invasive tumors in order to prevent disfigurement [3, 29]. Although the majority of BCCs are nodular in BCNS, topical application of 0.1 % tretinoin cream, 5-fluorouracil cream, and imiquimod 5 % cream is effective for treating superficial BCCs and has been used for these BCCs as well [3, 29, 30]. One of the more novel therapeutic approaches for BCC involves photodynamic therapy (PDT) which is the topical application of an agent, such as 5-aminolevulinic acid (ALA, Levulan®, DUSA Pharmaceuticals, Inc., Wilmington, MA, USA) or methyl ester form, methyl 5-aminolevulinate (MAL, Metvixia TM, Galderma, Princeton, NJ, USA) [31, 32]. Both ALA and MAL are converted to a photosensitizer protoporphyrin IX in tumor cells. MAL-PDT is unique in not only demonstrating a high efficacy in the treatment of superficial BCC; it has also been shown to be effective in the treatment of nodular BCC [33]. Vismodegib, an oral Hedgehog pathway inhibitor, has also been shown to be an important option in the treatment of BCCs. However, the side effects of oral vismodegib, including muscle spasms, hair loss, altered taste sensation, weight loss, fatigue, nausea, decreased appetite, and diarrhea, may not be well tolerated in some patients [34, 35]. Additionally, a topical inhibitor of the Hedgehog pathway has shown promising results in a randomized trial for patients with BCNS [36].

While great care is taken to treat BCC's, prophylactic therapy may be used to prevent growth of new cancers. Given these patients' high risk for continually developing BCCs, therapy to prevent them can save disfiguring treatments. Acitretin has been shown to reduce the size of clinically apparent skin cancers and may been used as chemoprevention [37]. While the efficacy of acitretin has been described for squamous cell carcinomas (SCCs), the drug may be used for patients with BCNS. Nonsteroidal anti-inflammatory drugs (NSAIDs) are also used as chemoprevention for SCCs. Oral celecoxib has been shown to be effective in suppression BCCs in both mice and humans with PTCH1 gene mutations [38].

For the detection of odontogenic keratocysts, annual dental panoramic X-rays are recommended beginning at the age of eight [27]. These cysts are typically removed by wide excision/enucleation with curettage but have a high rate of recurrence [23,

39]. There is some evidence that oral vismodegib is also an important treatment option for keratocysts; however, more studies are needed in patients with BCNS [40].

Notably in pediatric patients, surveillance for the development of medulloblastoma and cardiac fibroma is important. An annual cranial MRI is recommended until 8 years of age for the detection of a medulloblastoma [25]. For the treatment of a medulloblastoma, radiation therapy should be avoided because it causes multiple BCCs to develop in the field of radiation [28]. To monitor for the presence of a cardiac fibroma, an echocardiogram should be completed in the first year of life. Asymptomatic patients with a cardiac fibroma should be closely followed by a pediatric cardiologist [25].

30.6 Conclusion

Gorlin syndrome is an autosomal dominant condition characterized by countless number of basal cell carcinomas, in combination with various other findings such as odontogenic (jaw) keratocysts and palmar and/or palmar pits, and medulloblastoma. Treatment requires a multidisciplinary approach to monitor the various organ systems involved. Dermatologists play a crucial role not only in treating skin cancers but also in preventing the onset of new malignancies.

References

1. Gorlin RJ, Goltz RW. Multiple nevoid basal-cell epithelioma, jaw cysts, and bifid rib. A syndrome. N Engl J Med. 1960;262:908.
2. Anderson D, Taylor W, Falls H, Davidson R. The nevoid basal cell carcinoma syndrome. Am J Hum Genet. 1967;19:12–22.
3. Lo Muzio L. Nevoid basal cell carcinoma syndrome (Gorlin syndrome). Orphanet J Rare Dis. 2008;3:32.
4. Kimonis VE, et al. Clinical manifestations in 105 persons with nevoid basal cell carcinoma syndrome. Am J Med Gen. 1997;69:300.
5. Shanley S, et al. Nevoid basal cell carcinoma syndrome: review of 118 affected individuals. Am J Med Genet. 1994;50:282.
6. Evans DG, Ladusans EJ, Rimmer S, Burnell LD, Thakker N, Farndon PA. Complications of the naevoid basal cell carcinoma syndrome: results of a population based study. J Med Genet. 1993;30:460–4.
7. Ratcliffe JF, Shanley S, Chenevix-Trench G. The prevalence of cervical and thoracic congenital skeletal abnormalities in basal cell naevus syndrome; a review of cervical and chest radiographs in 80 patients with BCNS. Br J Radiol. 1995;68:596–9.
8. Farndon PA, Del Mastro RG, Evans DG, Kilpatrick MW. Location of gene for Gorlin syndrome. Lancet. 1992;339:581–2.
9. Booth DR. The hedgehog signaling pathway and its role in basal cell carcinoma. Cancer Metastasis Rev. 1999;18:261.
10. Hahn H, Wicking C, Zaphiropoulous PG, Gailani MR, Shanley S, Chidambaram A, Vorechovsky I, Holmberg E, Unden AB, Gillies S, et al. Mutations of the human homolog of Drosophila patched in the nevoid basal cell carcinoma syndrome. Cell. 1996;85:841–51.

11. Gailani M, Bale A. Developmental genes and cancer: role of patched in basal cell carcinoma of the skin. J Natl Cancer Inst. 1997;89:1103.
12. Levanat S, Gorlin R, Fallet S, et al. A two-hit model for developmental defects in Gorlin syndrome. Nat Genet. 1996;12:85.
13. Evans DG, Farndon PA, Burnell LD, Gattamaneni HR, Birch JM. The incidence of Gorlin syndrome in 173 consecutive cases of medulloblastoma. Br J Cancer. 1991;64:959–61.
14. Lo Muzio L, Nocini PF, Savoia A, Consolo U, Procaccini M, Zelante L, Pannone G, Bucci P, Dolci M, Bambini F, et al. Nevoid basal cell carcinoma syndrome. Clinical findings in 37 Italian affected individuals. Clin Genet. 1999;55:34–40.
15. Goldstein AM, Pastakia B, DiGiovanna JJ, Poliak S, Santucci S, Kase R, Bale AE, Bale SJ. Clinical findings in two African-American families with the nevoid basal cell carcinoma syndrome (NBCC). Am J Med Genet. 1994;50:272–81.
16. Farndon PA. Gorlin (naevoid basal cell carcinoma) syndrome. In: Eeles R, Easton DF, Ponder BAJ, Eng C, editors. Genetic predisposition to cancer. London: Hodder Arnold; 2004. p. 193–213.
17. Gorlin RJ. Nevoid basal-cell carcinoma syndrome. Medicine (Baltimore). 1987;66:98.
18. Hogge WA, Blank C, Roochvarg LB, Hogge JS, Wulfsberg EA, Raffel LJ. Gorlin syndrome (naevoid basal cell carcinoma syndrome): prenatal detection in a fetus with macrocephaly and ventriculomegaly. Prenat Diagn. 1994;14:725–7.
19. Jones KL, Wolf PL, Jensen P, et al. The Gorlin syndrome: a genetically determined disorder associated with cardiac tumor. Am Heart J. 1986;111:1013.
20. Lacombe D, Chateil JF, Fontan D, Battin J. Medulloblastoma in the nevoid basal-cell carcinoma syndrome: case reports and review of the literature. Genet Couns. 1990;1:273.
21. Woolgar JA, Rippin JW, Browne RM. The odontogenic keratocyst and its occurrence in the nevoid basal cell carcinoma syndrome. Oral Surg Oral Med Oral Pathol. 1987;64:727–30.
22. Myoung H, Hong SP, Hong SD, et al. Odontogenic keratocyst: review of 256 cases for recurrence and clinicopathologic parameters. Oral Surg Oral Med Oral Pathol Oral Radiol Endon. 2001;91:328.
23. Gorlin RJ. Nevoid basal cell carcinoma syndrome. Dermatol Clin. 1995;13:113–25.
24. Gutierrez MM, Mora RG. Nevoid basal cell carcinoma syndrome. A review and case report of a patient with unilateral basal cell nevus syndrome. J Am Acad Dermatol. 1986;15:1023–30.
25. Bree AF, Shah MR, BCNS Colloquium Group. Consensus statement from the first international colloquium on basal cell nevus syndrome. Am J Med Genet A. 2011;155:2091–7.
26. Soekarman D, Fryns JP, Casaer P, Berghe H. Van Den: increased head circumference and facial cleft as presenting signs of the nevoid basal-cell carcinoma syndrome. Genet Couns. 1991;2:157–62.
27. Lo Muzio L, Nocini P, Bucci P, Pannone G, Consolo U, Procaccini M. Early diagnosis of nevoid basal cell carcinoma syndrome. J Am Dent Assoc. 1999;130:669–74.
28. Frentz G, Munch-Petersen B, Wulf HC, et al. The nevoid basal cell carcinoma syndrome: sensitivity to ultraviolet and X-ray irradiation. J Am Acad Dermatol. 1987;17:637.
29. Van der Geer S, et al. Treatment of basal cell carcinomas in patients with nevoid basal cell carcinoma syndrome. J Eur Acad Dermatol Venereol. 2008;23:308.
30. Gollnick H, Barona CG, Frank RG, et al. Recurrence rate of superficial basal cell carcinoma following treatment with imiquimod 5 % cream: conclusion of a 5-year long-term follow-up study in Europe. Eur J Dermatol. 2008;18:677–82.
31. Hsi RA, Rosenthal DI, Glatstein E. Photodynamic therapy in the treatment of cancer:current state of the art. Drugs. 1999;57:725–34.
32. Morton CA, MacKie RM, Whitehurst C, Moore JV, McColl JH. Photodynamic therapy for basal cell carcinoma: effect of tumor thickness and duration of photosensitizer application on response. Arch Dermatol. 1998;134:248–9.
33. Horn M, Wolf P, Wulf HC, et al. Topical methyl aminolaevulinate photodynamic therapy in patients with basal cell carcinoma prone to complications and poor cosmetic outcome with conventional treatment. Br J Dermatol. 2003;149:1242–9.

34. LoRusso PM, Rudin CM, Reddy JC, Tibes R, Weiss GJ, Borad MJ, Hann CL, Brahmer JR, Chang I, Darbonne WC, Graham RA, Zerivitz KL, Low JA, Von Hoff DD. Phase I trial of hedgehog pathway inhibitor vismodegib (GDC-0449) in patients with refractory, locally advanced or metastatic solid tumors. Clin Cancer Res. 2011;17:2502–11.
35. http://www.roche.com/media/media_releases/med-cor-2011-06-20.html
36. Skvara H, Kalthoff F, Meingassner JG, et al. Topical treatment of Basal cell carcinomas in nevoid basal cell carcinoma syndrome with a smoothened inhibitor. J Invest Dermatol. 2011; 131:1735.
37. Lebwohl M, Tannis C, Carrasco D. Acitretin suppression of squamous cell carcinoma: case report and literature review. J Dermatolog Treat. 2003;14 Suppl 2:3–6. Review.
38. Tang JY, Aszterbaum M, Athar M, et al. Basal cell carcinoma chemoprevention with nonsteroidal anti-inflammatory drugs in genetically predisposed PTCH1+/– humans and mice. Cancer Prev Res (Phila). 2010 Jan;3(1):25–34.
39. Dominguez FV, Keszler A. Comparative study of keratocysts, associated and non-associated with nevoid basal cell carcinoma syndrome. J Oral Pathol. 1988;17:39–42.
40. Goldberg LH, Landau JM, Moody MN, et al. Resolution of odontogenic keratocysts of the jaw in basal cell nevus syndrome with GDC-0449. Arch Dermatol. 2011;147:839.

Chapter 31
Muir-Torre Syndrome

Adam J. Luber and Joshua A. Zeichner

31.1 Introduction

Muir-Torre syndrome (MTS) is a rare, autosomal dominant genodermatosis characterized by sebaceous neoplasms, keratoacanthomas, and visceral malignancies [1, 2]. MTS is a phenotypic subset of hereditary nonpolyposis colorectal cancer (HNPCC) caused by mutations in mismatch repair genes associated with microsatellite instability [3]. Due to the increased risk in developing visceral malignancies, it is important that the proper diagnosis to be made as early as possible and family members be evaluated for MTS and its associated cancers.

MTS was first described separately by Muir [4] and Torre [5] in 1967 and 1968, respectively. Muir first reported a patient with a sebaceous adenoma, multiple keratoacanthomas of the face, and multiple carcinomas of the gastrointestinal tract [4]. Torre described a case of multiple sebaceous neoplasms in a patient with a history of two gastrointestinal malignancies [5]. The combined name of the syndrome was created in 1982 when Fahmy et al. reported 20 cases with a similar constellation of findings [6].

31.2 Background

MTS is inherited as an autosomal dominant disorder with variable penetrance and expressivity [3]. The syndrome has a slight male predilection, with a male to female ratio of 3:2 and a mean age of 53 (ranging from the 30s to 80s) at the time of diagnosis [7, 8]. A 2004 study reported that more than 200 cases of MTS have been described in the literature since 1982 [3]. There is limited data on an ethnic or ancestral predisposition to MTS; however, the majority of cases are reported in

A.J. Luber, B.A. (✉)
Department of Dermatology, Mt Sinai Hospital, New York, NY, USA

J.A. Zeichner, M.D.
Department of Dermatology, Mt. Sinai School of Medicine, New York, NY, USA

J.A. Zeichner (ed.), *Acneiform Eruptions in Dermatology: A Differential Diagnosis*,
DOI 10.1007/978-1-4614-8344-1_31,

Caucasian patients residing in the developed world [2]. MTS is observed in 28 % of families and 9 % of individuals with HNPCC [9]. The two disorders share similar genetic mechanisms—both are caused by mutations in mismatch repair genes, which produce enzymes involved in maintaining accurate DNA replication in cells [10].

MTS is caused by heterozygous germline mutations in one of the following mismatch repair genes: MutS homolog 2 (MSH2), MutL homolog 1 (MLH1), or MutS homolog 6 (MSH6). The mismatch repair mechanism prevents errors in the short, repeat sequences of DNA, called microsatellites. Ninety percent of mutations in MTS occur in MSH2 on chromosome 2 [11, 12]. Mismatch repair deficiency results from an inherited germline mutation combined with a somatic loss-of-function mutation in the contralateral wild-type allele. Ensuing errors in DNA replication at multiple loci begin to accumulate and are termed microsatellite instability (MSI), which promote tumor formation [13].

In HNPCC, approximately 75 % of germline mutations are seen in either MSH2 or MLH1, with the remainder of mutations in MSH6 and postmeiotic segregation increased 2 (PMS2) [3, 9]. Mutations in MSH2 disrupt the MSH2-MSH6 heterodimer, ultimately causing a lack of expression of the MSH6 protein in both MTS and HNPCC [14].

31.3 Clinical Presentation

A diagnosis of MTS is made by the presence of at least one sebaceous gland neoplasm and at least one visceral malignancy, in the absence of any known predisposing factors [15]. While sebaceous adenomas are the most common sebaceous neoplasms found in MTS (68 %), sebaceous carcinomas (30 %), sebaceous epitheliomas (sebaceoma), keratoacanthomas with sebaceous differentiation (seboacanthoma), or basal cell carcinomas with sebaceous differentiation are included in the diagnostic criteria (sebaceous hyperplasia and nevus sebaceous of Jadassohn are excluded) [13]. Alternatively, when no sebaceous tumor is present, a patient can be diagnosed with MTS based on a personal history of multiple keratoacanthomas and visceral malignancies in the setting of a family history of MTS [1, 10, 16].

Sebaceous neoplasms are yellow papules or nodules that are typically found on the head, neck, or trunk; sporadic cases are almost exclusively on the head and neck [10, 16, 17]. Keratoacanthomas are rapidly appearing, erythematous papules or nodules that are seen in 25 % of patients with MTS [15]. While some patients with MTS present with a solitary sebaceous neoplasm, it is more common to see several and sometimes hundreds of tumors [1]. Excluding sebaceous carcinomas, the sebaceous neoplasms associated with MTS have low malignant potential and rarely metastasize. Sebaceous carcinomas, particularly when located in periocular regions, are aggressive tumors that invade angiolymphatic space [7].

Cutaneous manifestations can present prior to (30 % of cases), concurrently with (10 %), or after (60 %) the diagnosis of internal malignancy [15]. Reports have documented skin lesions preceding internal malignancy by 25 years or developing 37 years after [8]. Sixty-one percent of internal malignancies associated with MTS arise from the alimentary system, with colorectal carcinoma being the most common [3, 18]. MTS-associated colorectal carcinoma usually develops proximal to the splenic flexure and typically appears by age 50. In contrast, colorectal carcinoma in the general population is diagnosed, on average, 10 years later (age range 55–65) and is commonly located in the distal colon [7, 13]. Other visceral malignancies linked to MTS include genitourinary, breast, hematologic, head and neck, small intestine, and stomach [19].

While MTS-associated malignancies are usually less aggressive than their sporadic counterparts, approximately 60 % of patients affected by the syndrome will develop metastatic disease [20]. Few studies have examined survival rates among individuals with MTS, however, MTS-associated neoplasms may be more surgically responsive compared to sporadic carcinomas [2].

31.4 Work-Up

Laboratory evaluation for MTS can be conducted by peripheral blood samples to detect germline mutations at commercial laboratories. Many pathologists suggest that any sebaceous neoplasm that is difficult to classify should be investigated as a MTS lesion [13]. In general, histopathological examination of sebaceous neoplasms in MTS reveals the equivalent findings as the same lesion in non-MTS individuals [10, 16].

Immunohistochemical (IHC) analysis of the tumor specimens has become a popular method to differentiate MTS-associated neoplasms. The IHC assays are highly sensitive and specific since the antibodies target the DNA mismatch repair enzymes known to be linked to MTS—MLH1, MSH2, and MSH6. The absence of these enzymes on IHC analysis (i.e., loss of expression) is consistent with a MTS-associated neoplasm [10]. Polymerase chain reaction (PCR) assays can detect MSI in tissue specimens of MTS-associated malignancies [14].

MTS is diagnosed based on specific criteria, including the presence of multiple sebaceous neoplasms, skin lesions located outside of the head and neck region, and sebaceous neoplasms with high specificity for MTS (such as seboacanthoma). In addition, a personal or family history of colorectal cancer before the age of 50 or other HNPCC-related malignancy (small bowel, gastric, endometrial, bladder, ureteral, renal, biliary, pancreatic, or glioblastoma) increases the probability of MTS [15].

31.5 Treatment

Benign sebaceous neoplasms can be treated with cryotherapy, curettage, or simple excision depending on the size and location of the lesion. Wide, local excision with 5–6 mm margins or Mohs micrographic surgery is the recommended treatments for sebaceous carcinomas [1, 7]. Radiotherapy has been successful in treating surgically difficult sebaceous carcinomas located on the orbit or ocular adnexa [21, 22].

Oral isotretinoin, alone or in combination with interferon-alpha, is used to limit the growth of existing sebaceous tumors and to prevent new tumor development.

Additionally, topical fluorouracil and imiquimod are employed as chemoprophylaxis therapies in reducing the burden of keratoacanthomas and basal cell carcinomas that may be associated with MTS [7, 23, 24]. Lymphadenopathy warrants fine needle aspiration for further inspection, followed by regional lymphadenectomy if lymph node involvement is present [2]. Patients with a visceral malignancy require proper oncologic management beyond the scope of this chapter.

Managing patients and families affected by MTS requires a multidisciplinary approach including primary care physicians, dermatologists, gastroenterologists, oncologists, surgeons, and geneticists [2, 25]. Because of the syndrome's inheritance pattern, family members who acquire the DNA mismatch repair defect have a considerably increased risk of developing visceral malignancies and should commit to routine cancer surveillance [13].

Patients with MTS, as well as asymptomatic carriers of mutations, require annual physical examinations by a primary care physician and dermatologist. Beginning at ages 25–30, individuals should undergo colonoscopy or evaluation with barium enema every 3–5 years. Regular chest radiographs and serial renal ultrasounds are also useful screening tests. Females should have annual breast exams, mammograms, and Pap smears. Annual laboratory studies include urinalysis, complete blood count, carcinoembryonic antigen, and erythrocyte sedimentation rate [2, 15, 25].

31.6 Conclusion

Muir-Torre Syndrome is a disease characterized by both cutaneous and systemic changes. Patients diagnosed with sebaceous gland tumors, especially multiple tumors, should be offered genetic tests to detect mutations in mismatch repair genes associated with MTS [2, 3, 25]. These skin lesions often serve as a herald sign to a potentially life-threatening internal malignancy. Regular and strict dermatology follow-up is critical for affected individuals and their family members.

References

1. Schwartz RA, Torre DP. The Muir-Torre syndrome: a 25-year retrospect. J Am Acad Dermatol. 1995;33(1):90–104.
2. Ponti G, Ponz de Leon M. Muir-Torre syndrome. Lancet Oncol. 2005;6(12):980–7.
3. Curry ML, Eng W, Lund K, Paek D, Cockerell CJ. Muir-Torre syndrome: role of the dermatopathologist in diagnosis. Am J Dermatopathol. 2004;26(3):217–21.
4. Muir EG, Bell AJ, Barlow KA. Multiple primary carcinomata of the colon, duodenum, and larynx associated with kerato-acanthomata of the face. Br J Surg. 1967;54(3):191–5.
5. Torre D. Multiple sebaceous tumors. Arch Dermatol. 1968;98(5):549–51.
6. Fahmy A, Burgdorf WH, Schosser RH, Pitha J. Muir-Torre syndrome: report of a case and reevaluation of the dermatopathologic features. Cancer. 1982;49(9):1898–903.
7. Higgins HJ, Voutsalath M, Holland JM. Muir-Torre syndrome: a case report. J Clin Aesthet Dermatol. 2009;2(8):30–2.

8. Cohen PR, Kohn SR, Kurzrock R. Association of sebaceous gland tumors and internal malignancy: the Muir-Torre syndrome. Am J Med. 1991;90(5):606–13.
9. South CD, Hampel H, Comeras I, Westman JA, Frankel WL, De la Chapelle A. The frequency of Muir-Torre syndrome among Lynch syndrome families. J Natl Cancer Inst. 2008; 100(4):277–81.
10. Eisen DB, Michael DJ. Sebaceous lesions and their associated syndromes: part II. J Am Acad Dermatol. 2009;61(4):563–80.
11. Mangold E, Rahner N, Friedrichs N, et al. MSH6 mutation in Muir-Torre syndrome: could this be a rare finding? Br J Dermatol. 2007;156(1):158–62.
12. Lynch HT, Fusaro RM. The Muir-Torre syndrome in kindreds with hereditary nonpolyposis colorectal cancer (Lynch syndrome): a classic obligation in preventive medicine. J Am Acad Dermatol. 1999;41(5):797–9.
13. Hare HH, Mahendraker N, Sarwate S, Tangella K. Muir-Torre syndrome: a rare but important disorder. Cutis. 2008;82(4):252–6.
14. Marazza G, Masouyé I, Taylor S, et al. An illustrative case of Muir-Torre syndrome: contribution of immunohistochemical analysis in identifying indicator sebaceous lesions. Arch Dermatol. 2006;142(8):1039–42.
15. Bayliss SJ, Berk DR. Muir-Torre syndrome. In: Bolognia JL, Jorizzo JL, Schaffer JV, editors. Dermatology. 3rd ed. St. Louis, MO: Elsevier; 2012.
16. Eisen DB, Michael DJ. Sebaceous lesions and their associated syndromes: part I. J Am Acad Dermatol. 2009;61(4):549–62.
17. Dores GM, Curtis RE, Toro JR, Devesa SS, Fraumeni Jr JF. Incidence of cutaneous sebaceous carcinoma and risk of associated neoplasms: insight into Muir-Torre syndrome. Cancer. 2008;113(12):3372–81.
18. Akhtar S, Oza KK, Khan SA, Wright J. Muir-Torre syndrome: case report of a patient with concurrent jejunal and ureteral cancer and a review of the literature. J Am Acad Dermatol. 1999;41(5):681–6.
19. Cohen PR. Muir-Torre syndrome in patients with hematologic malignancies. Am J Hematol. 1992;40(1):64–5.
20. Poleksic S. Keratoacanthoma and multiple carcinomas. Br J Dermatol. 1974;91(4):461–3.
21. Pardo FS, Wang CC, Albert D, Stracher MA. Sebaceous carcinoma of the ocular adnexa: radiotherapeutic management. Int J Radiat Oncol Biol Phys. 1989;17(3):643–7.
22. Hata M, Koike I, Omura M, Maegawa J, Ogino I, Inoue T. Noninvasive and curative radiation therapy for sebaceous carcinoma of the eyelid. Int J Radiat Oncol Biol Phys. 2012;82(2): 605–11.
23. Spielvogel RL, DeVillez RL, Roberts LC. Oral isotretinoin therapy for familial Muir-Torre syndrome. J Am Acad Dermatol. 1985;12(3):475–80.
24. Pettey AA, Walsh JS. Muir-Torre syndrome: a case report and review of the literature. Cutis. 2005;75(3):149–55.
25. Cohen PR, Kohn SR, Davis DA, Kurzrock R. Muir-Torre syndrome. Dermatol Clin. 1995; 13(1):79–89.

Chapter 32
Reed's Syndrome

Kristen Pacific and Jason Emer

32.1 Introduction

Multiple cutaneous and uterine leiomyomatosis (MCUL), also known as Reed's syndrome, is an autosomal dominant genetic condition. Affected individuals have an increased predisposition to develop benign smooth muscle tumors (leiomyomas) in the skin and uterus. Affected females frequently develop uterine leiomyomas (fibroids) that are larger and more numerous and emerge earlier than those in the general population. Subsets of these patients are at risk for renal cell carcinoma (RCC) and have been determined to have mutations in the fumarate hydratase (FH) gene. In individuals or families without RCC, the syndrome may be referred to as multiple cutaneous leiomyomatosis (MCL) or MCUL. The term hereditary leiomyomatosis and RCC (HLRCC) refers to families with an increased prevalence of smooth muscle tumors and RCC as a result of the FH genetic defect. Since cutaneous leiomyomas are not exceptionally common, their presence—whether single or in multiplicity—should raise suspicion of underlying uterine leiomyomas and the possibility of real disease. Increased clinical awareness is important due to the association between coexisting cutaneous and systemic diseases.

32.2 Background

The coexistence of benign smooth muscle growths in the skin and in the uterus is known as Reed's syndrome [1]. In 1973, Reed et al reported on two families in which members of successive generations demonstrated cutaneous leiomyomas,

K. Pacific, B.A. • J. Emer, M.D. (✉)
Department of Dermatology, Mount Sinai School of Medicine, New York, NY, USA
e-mail: pacifick@dickinson.edu; Jason.emermd@gmail.com

J.A. Zeichner (ed.), *Acneiform Eruptions in Dermatology: A Differential Diagnosis*,
DOI 10.1007/978-1-4614-8344-1_32, © Springer Science+Business Media New York 2014

uterine leiomyomas, and/or leiomyosarcomas, establishing an autosomal dominant pattern of inheritance [2, 3].

Cutaneous leiomyomas are benign tumors composed of smooth muscle fibers that arise from either the arrector pili muscles surrounding the hair follicles; the dartos muscle of genital, nipple, or areola skin or the smooth muscle of the vasculature [4, 5]. In Reed's syndrome, they appear to be of the type originating from the arrector pili of the hair follicle [6–8]. Affected individuals with Reed's syndrome develop leiomyomas that are larger, more numerous, and emerge earlier than those in the general population. In addition, affected females develop uterine disease. Since its first reports, Reed's syndrome has been reported in only about 100 families across the globe, making it rare in the general population [1]. Although HLRCC has been observed in patients of many ethnic backgrounds, the incidence is reportedly higher among those of Eastern European descent [9]. The association of MCUL with papillary type 2 RCC is known [10, 11]. The disease predisposing gene has been identified as fumarate hydrase (FH), a gene encoding an enzyme that operates in the mitochondrial citric acid cycle (Krebs cycle) and is intimately involved in cellular energy metabolism [12, 13].

Familial studies have localized the predisposition for Reed's syndrome to chromosome 1q42.3–43, namely, the MCUL1 locus of the gene encoding FH [5, 14–16]. The discovery occurred shortly after researchers reported that some individuals with MCL were also at risk of developing an aggressive form of RCC. After significant genetic research, germline and somatic mutations along with loss of heterozygosity in FH of tumor tissue was identified. Mutations of the missense, nonsense, frameshift, insertion, and splice-site types have been discovered in the FH gene [13]. Mutation analysis of 21 North American families with HLRCC identified germline mutations of the FH gene in 100 % (21/21) [9]. Of families with HLRCC, 62 % (13/21) had RCC and 76 % (16/21) had cutaneous leiomyomas. Of female FH mutation carriers, 100 % (22/22) had uterine fibroids. Other reports have identified FH mutations in approximately 75 % of MCUL cases [17].

FH alterations are believed to correlate with tumor formation in families with HLRCC; however, the pathological mechanism for this relationship is not entirely clear. A cell that lacks functional FH has a subsequent metabolic derangement due to its defective Krebs cycle [18]. It has been suggested that pseudohypoxia due to defective enzymatic metabolism may drive cellular transformation and tumorigenesis [19]. Additionally, recent genetic analysis suggests that FH may act as a tumor suppressor gene, but the consequence thereof has yet to be determined.

32.3 Clinical Presentation

Clinical characteristics of HLRCC may include cutaneous leiomyomas, uterine leiomyomas, and/or renal tumors. Cutaneous leiomyomas are rare in the general population, but are observed in 76–87 % of HLRCC prognoses thus are cutaneous marker of systemic disease [20].

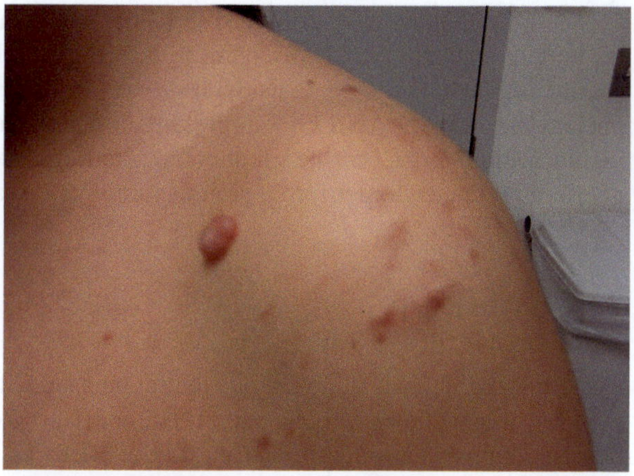

Fig. 32.1 Multiple red-brown papules and nodules in a cluster on the left shoulder

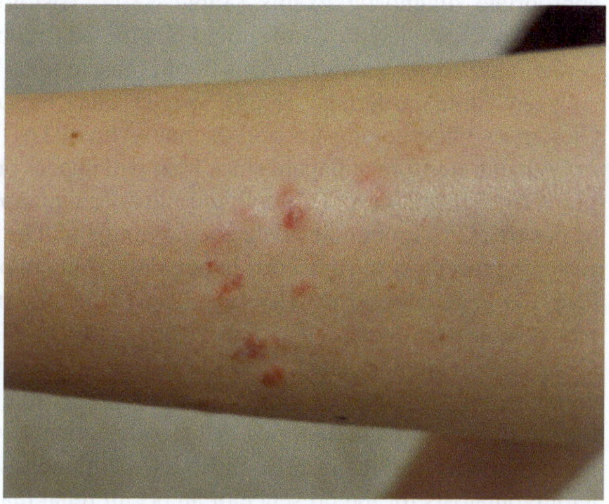

Fig. 32.2 Multiple erythematous papules on the leg of an adult woman. She frequently complained that the lesions would become tender (Photo credit: Joshua A. Zeichner, M.D.)

Reed's syndrome manifests during the second to fourth decade of life, with solitary or multiple cutaneous leiomyomas, which appear as firm skin-colored or pink-brown papules or nodules ranging from 0.2 to 2 cm in diameter [5, 7, 11] (Figs. 32.1 and 32.2). A pseudo-Darier sign may be present, which is a transient piloerection or elevation of a lesion induced by rubbing. The clinical presentation of multiple lesions has been described in various patterns or distributions, such as bilateral and symmetric, clustered, linear, zosteriform, dermatomal like, or disseminated [4, 21]. Although commonly distributed over the trunk, the face may also be affected.

It is important to consider a leiomyoma in any indolent nodular or papular growth associated with pain. In 89–92 % of cases, patients experience localized photosensitivity and pain upon contact, injury or exposure to change in temperature [20]. An acute increase in size and/or number of lesions and/or an increase in pain should be suggestive of worsening disease or the rare possibility of malignant degeneration.

Accurate diagnosis is critical due to the potential for concealed malignancy. As leiomyomas are classically painful, the complete list of painful papulonodules should all be taken into consideration on initial evaluation [22]. The popular pneumonic "LEND AN EGG" represents a list of painful tumors of the skin that includes leiomyoma, eccrine spiradenoma, neuroma, dermatofibroma, angiolipoma, neurilemmoma, endometrioma, glomus tumor, and granular cell tumor [23].

32.4 Work-Up

The clinical diagnosis of cutaneous leiomyomas may be challenging and ultimately requires histopathological analysis. It is important to differentiate a case of simple benign cutaneous leiomyomas from that of HLRCC. A high index of suspicion is required in order to ensure that patients are properly screened and receives the appropriate diagnostic exams (Table 32.1). Histological analyses exhibit very distinctive characteristics and should be utilized for confirmation of diagnosis.

On microscopic examination, smooth muscle fiber bundles are interspersed with collagen within the dermis [24, 25]. Special stains, including Masson's trichrome, Van Gieson, or phosphotungstic acid–hematoxylin (PTAH), can be used to distinguish smooth muscle from collagen, since both will appear pink-red on hematoxylin–eosin stain [26]. The markers of smooth muscle differentiation (desmin and actin) will also be positive [27]. Immunohistochemical staining will be negative for estrogen and progesterone receptors in cutaneous leiomyomas, but are positive in uterine leiomyomas [28]. FH gene enzyme activity in cultured skin fibroblasts or lymphoblastoid cells may demonstrate decreased activity (≤60 %) [29].

Any individual presenting with cutaneous leiomyomas should be given a complete physical examination with a comprehensive history, including a focus on the family and surgical histories. All female patients with MCL should be evaluated for uterine disease. Currently, the NIH recommends evaluating all patients with leiomyomatosis for the presence of an occult renal malignancy [29, 30]. Referral to genetics for further work-up may also be prudent.

Table 32.1 Screening recommendations in a patient with multiple cutaneous leiomyomatosis

Complete history with focus on family and surgical histories
Complete physical examination including pelvic examination
Skin biopsy with special stains such as Masson–Trichrome, Van Gieson, Desmin, and Actin
Pelvic ultrasound
Renal ultrasound
Complete blood count
Complete metabolic panel
Urinalysis
Genetic analysis for fumarate hydratase mutation
Referral to gynecology
Referral to nephrology
Referral to genetic counseling if fumarate hydratase mutation suspected and/or confirmed

32.5 Treatment

Treatment of cutaneous leiomyomas is dictated by the number of lesions and the degree of discomfort or cosmetic nuisance. Camouflage cosmetics (makeup) and avoidance of painful triggers, such as cold and/or pressure, may be all that is needed. When only a few lesions are present, surgical excision is the gold standard for complete removal, but may have a high rate of recurrence and possibly require skin grafting for larger lesions [4]. Recurrences have been reported to occur from 6 weeks to more than 15 years following excision [31]. Destructive methods, such as electrodessication or cryotherapy, may be employed for small, individual, or few lesions, but little benefit over excision has been demonstrated and unwanted scarring and recurrence may occur as a consequence [32].

Medical management plays a limited role in hastening the formation of new lesions and facilitating the resolution of current ones, but can be utilized for symptomatic pain relief. Medications known to affect smooth muscle contraction, such as nitroglycerine, nifedipine, phenoxybenzamine, and doxazosin, can provide effective pain relief [4]. The theory behind this method of treatment is that muscle contraction and subsequent nerve stimulation is responsible for the characteristic stabbing, shocking, and/or striking pain described by a majority of patients found to have these tumors [33–35]. Medications that target the activity of nerves are of special interest because of an increased nerve density within and around leiomyomas [36]. Gabapentin or pregabalin and/or topical analgesics, such as lidocaine or capsaicin, may be successful in patients with temperature-induced tenderness [37].

Recent studies show promising results from novel therapies such as botulinum toxin injection and carbon dioxide laser ablation for pain control [38–40]. Botulinum toxin type A is used in various pain syndromes as it is believed to work by inhibiting the release of neuropeptides, including substance P and glutamate, thus reducing central pain signals [41, 42]. Carbon dioxide laser ablation provides an alternative to invasive surgical techniques, facilitates myolysis, and offers pain relief [40, 43].

References

1. Hereditary leiomyomatosis and renal cell cancer. Available at http://ghr.nlm.nih.gov/condition=hereditaryleiomyomatosisandrenalcellcancer. Accessed 18 Sep 2012
2. Reed WB, Walker R, Horowitz R. Cutaneous leiomyomata with uterine leiomyomata. Acta Derm Venereol. 1973;53(5):409–16.
3. Kloepfer HW, Krafchuk J, Derbes V, Burks J. Hereditary multiple leiomyoma of the skin. Am J Hum Genet. 1958;10(1):48–52.
4. Holst VA, Junkins-Hopkins JM, Elenitsas R. Cutaneous smooth muscle neoplasms: clinical features, histologic findings, and treatment options. J Am Acad Dermatol. 2002;46(4): 477–90.
5. Costella TM, Romiti N, Almeida JR, et al. Do you know this syndrome? An Bras Dermatol. 2011;86(4):815–24.
6. Orellana Diaz O, Hernandez PE. Leiomyoma cutis and leiomyosarcoma: a 10-year study and a short review. J Dermatol Surg Oncol. 1983;9(4):283–7.

7. Badeloe S, Frank J. Clinical and molecular genetic aspects of hereditary multiple cutaneous leiomyomatosis. Eur J Dermatol. 2009;19(6):545–51.
8. Malhotra P, Walia H, Singh A, Ramesh V. Leiomyoma cutis: a clinicopathological series of 37 cases. Indian J Dermatol. 2010;55(4):337–41.
9. Wei MH, Toure O, Glenn GM, et al. Novel mutations in FH and expansion of the spectrum of phenotypes expressed in families with hereditary leiomyomatosis and renal cell cancer. J Med Genet. 2006;43(1):18–27.
10. Kiuru M, Launonen V. Hereditary leiomyomatosis and renal cell cancer (HLRCC). Curr Mol Med. 2004;4(8):869–75.
11. García Muret MP, Pujol RM, Alomar A, et al. Familial leiomyomatosis cutis et uteri (Reed's syndrome). Arch Dermatol Res. 1988;280:S29–32.
12. Toro JR, Nickerson ML, Wei MH, et al. Mutations in the fumarate hydratase gene cause hereditary leiomyomatosis and renal cell cancer in families in North America. Am J Hum Genet. 2003;73(1):95–106.
13. Alam NA, Olpin S, Leigh IM. Fumarate hydratase mutations and predisposition to cutaneous leiomyomas, uterine leiomyomas and renal cancer. Br J Dermatol. 2005;153(1):11–7.
14. Tomlinson IP, Alam NA, Rowan AJ, et al. Germline mutations in FH predispose to dominantly inherited uterine fibroids, skin leiomyomata and papillary renal cell cancer. Nat Genet. 2002;30(4):406–10.
15. Kiuru M, Launonen V, Hietala M, et al. Familial cutaneous leiomyomatosis is a two-hit condition associated with renal cell cancer of characteristic histopathology. Am J Pathol. 2001; 159(3):825–9.
16. Alam NA, Bevan S, Churchman M, et al. Localization of a gene (MCUL1) for multiple cutaneous leiomyomata and uterine fibroids to chromosome 1q42.3–q43. Am J Hum Genet. 2001;68(5):1264–9.
17. Alam NA, Rowan AJ, Wortham NC, et al. Genetic and functional analyses of FH mutations in multiple cutaneous and uterine leiomyomatosis, hereditary leiomyomatosis and renal cancer, and fumarate hydratase deficiency. Hum Mol Genet. 2003;12(11):1241–52.
18. Badeloe S, van Geel M, van Steensel MA, et al. Diffuse and segmental variants of cutaneous leiomyomatosis: novel mutations in the fumarate hydratase gene and review of the literature. Exp Dermatol. 2006;15(9):735–41.
19. Sudarshan S, Pinto PA, Neckers L, Linehan WM. Mechanisms of disease: hereditary leiomyomatosis and renal cell cancer—a distinct form of hereditary kidney cancer. Nat Clin Pract Urol. 2007;4(2):104–10.
20. Mitchum MD, Adams EG, Holcomb KZ. JAAD Grand Rounds quiz. A 46-year-old man with agminated papules on the buttock. Reed syndrome. J Am Acad Dermatol. 2012;66(2):337–9.
21. Smith CG, Glaser DA, Leonardi C. Zosteriform multiple leiomyomas. J Am Acad Dermatol. 1998;38(2 Pt 1):272–3.
22. Naverson DN, Trask DM, Watson FH, Burket JM. Painful tumors of the skin: "LEND AN EGG". J Am Acad Dermatol. 1993;28(2 Pt 2):298–300.
23. Apatenko AK, Turusov VS. The painful tumours of the skin. Neoplasma. 1968;15(2): 187–202.
24. Lehtonen HJ. Hereditary leiomyomatosis and renal cell cancer: update on clinical and molecular characteristics. Fam Cancer. 2011;10(2):397–411.
25. Kilpatrick SE, Mentzel T, Fletcher CD. Leiomyoma of deep soft tissue. Clinicopathologic analysis of a series. Am J Surg Pathol. 1994;18(6):576–82.
26. Spencer JM, Amonette RA. Tumors with smooth muscle differentiation. Dermatol Surg. 1996;22(9):761–8.
27. Miettinen M, Lehto VP, Virtanen I. Antibodies to intermediate filament proteins. The differential diagnosis of cutaneous tumors. Arch Dermatol. 1985;121(6):736–41.
28. McGinley KM, Bryant S, Kattine AA, et al. Cutaneous leiomyomas lack estrogen and progesterone receptor immunoreactivity. J Cutan Pathol. 1997;24(4):241–5.

29. Pithukpakorn M, Toro JR. Hereditary leiomyomatosis and renal cell cancer. In: Pagon RA, Bird TD, Dolan CR, Stephens K, editors. Genereviews. Seattle, Washington: University of Washington; 1993–2006.
30. Rongioletti F, Fausti V, Ferrando B, et al. A novel missense mutation in fumarate hydratase in an Italian patient with a diffuse variant of cutaneous leiomyomatosis (Reed's syndrome). Dermatology. 2010;221(4):378–80.
31. Fisher WC, Helwig EB. Leiomyomas of the skin. Arch Dermatol. 1963;88:510–20.
32. Montgomery H, Winkelmann RK. Smooth-muscle tumors of the skin. AMA Arch Derm. 1959;79(1):32–40.
33. George S, Pulimood S, Jacob M, Chandi SM. Pain in multiple leiomyomas alleviated by nifedipine. Pain. 1997;73(1):101–2.
34. Thompson JA. Jr Therapy for painful cutaneous leiomyomas. J Am Acad Dermatol. 1985; 13(5 Pt 2):865–7.
35. Batchelor RJ, Lyon CC, Highet AS. Successful treatment of pain in two patients with cutaneous leiomyomata with the oral alpha-1 adrenoceptor antagonist, doxazosin. Br J Dermatol. 2004;150(4):775–6.
36. Thyresson HN, Su WP. Familial cutaneous leiomyomatosis. J Am Acad Dermatol. 1981; 4(4):430–4.
37. Haugen RN, Tharp MD. The use of gabapentin for recurrent painful attacks with multiple piloleiomyomas. J Drugs Dermatol. 2008;7(4):401–2.
38. Sifaki MK, Krueger-Krasagakis S, Koutsopoulos A, et al. Botulinum toxin type A-treatment of a patient with multiple cutaneous piloleiomyomas. Dermatology. 2009;218(1):44–7.
39. Onder M, Adien E. A new indication of botulinum toxin: leiomyoma-related pain. J Am Acad Dermatol. 2009;60(2):325–8.
40. Christenson LJ, Smith K, Arpey CJ. Treatment of multiple cutaneous leiomyomas with CO2 laser ablation. Dermatol Surg. 2000;26(4):319–22.
41. Aoki KR. Review of a proposed mechanism for the antinociceptive action of botulinum toxin type A. Neurotoxicology. 2005;26(5):785–93.
42. Aoki KR. Pharmacology and immunology of botulinum toxin type A. Clin Dermatol. 2003; 21(6):476–80.
43. Hindley JT, Law PA, Hickey M, et al. Clinical outcomes following percutaneous magnetic resonance image guided laser ablation of symptomatic uterine fibroids. Hum Reprod. 2002; 17(10):2737–41.

Chapter 33
Tuberous Sclerosis

Omar Pacha and Adelaide Hebert

33.1 Introduction

Tuberous sclerosis or tuberous sclerosis complex (TSC) is a genetic disorder that classically causes skin changes, intellectual disability, and seizures. This relatively common condition often involves the face with angiofibromas (adenoma sebaceum) that in the earliest stages may be misinterpreted as acne lesions. Variable expressivity complicates the diagnosis and epidemiology of this autosomal dominant disorder. Current treatment focuses on mechanical removal of the angiofibromas. Recently, topical or systemic IL-2 inhibitors like rapamycin have also shown promise as a therapy [1].

33.2 Background

TSC is caused by a mutation in either the *TSC1* or *TSC2* genes with resultant loss of cell growth control. While TSC is an autosomal dominant disorder, the majority of cases are not inherited. Instead, 65–85 % arise from spontaneous mutations [2]. The two genes are distinct in location and function but produce nearly indistinguishable clinical presentation. Mutations in *TSC2* are found in more than half of the total number of patients. In about one fifth of patients, no mutation is identified in either of the *TSC1* or *TSC2* genes [3]. The range of prevalence estimates vary widely from 1 in 5,800 to 1 in 25,000 in the Caucasian population [4, 5].

The biological roles of hamartin (the protein product of *TSC1*) and tuberin (the protein product of *TSC2*) have been fairly well defined. They form a multimeric

O. Pacha (✉) • A. Hebert
Department of Dermatology, University of Texas Health Science Center, Houston, Houston, TX, USA
e-mail: omar.pacha@uth.tmc.edu; Adelaide.a.hebert@uth.tmc.edu

J.A. Zeichner (ed.), *Acneiform Eruptions in Dermatology: A Differential Diagnosis*, DOI 10.1007/978-1-4614-8344-1_33, © Springer Science+Business Media New York 2014

complex that functions in the mTOR pathway. The mTOR pathway plays an important role in cell growth and proliferation hence its effect on cell growth. The loss of function of either gene leads to increased activation of this pathway. The TSC complex interacts with Rheb, a member of the RAS subfamily, and stimulates conversion of Rheb to its inactive form. Loss of function TSC complex mutation leads to an increase in active Rheb, which in turn increases downstream mTOR expression.

33.3 Clinical Presentation

Presentation for TSC in the skin varies widely from a few subtle angiofibromas to diffuse angiofibromatosis with shagreen patches and ash-leaf macules, with clinical manifestations depending largely on the genetic expression in a given patient. Ash-leaf macules and shagreen patches are more likely to be present either at birth or shortly thereafter. Angiofibromas, however, may appear at any time but most often appear in late childhood or early adolescence frequently appearing much like the papules of acne vulgaris. Angiofibromas are several millimeter in diameter, fleshy pink to red papules. These can occur singly or in clusters of hundreds often in a malar distribution (Fig. 33.1). Koenen tumors are subungual fibromas that are pathognomonic for TSC (Fig. 33.2). Ash-leaf macules are hypopigmented macules that generally have a single broad side that tapers into a narrow tip, while shagreen patches are hamartomas of connective tissue that are typically raised, irregularly shaped, and firmer than surrounding tissue.

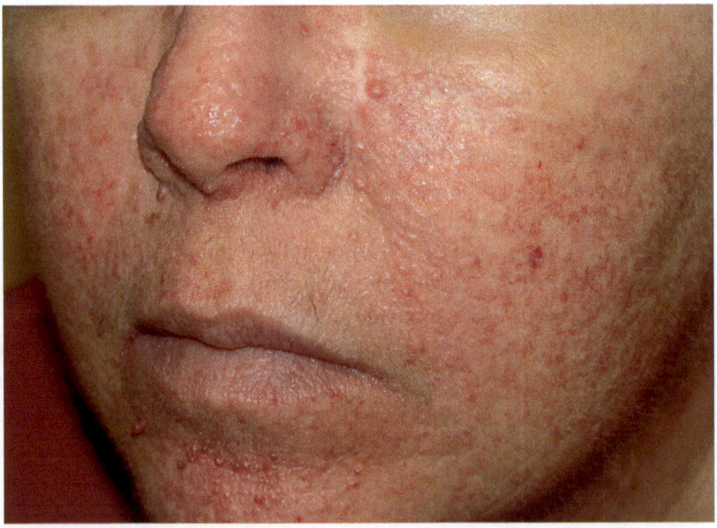

Fig. 33.1 Thousands of angiofibromas cover the face of a patient with Tuberous Sclerosis (Photo credit: Joshua A. Zeichner, M.D.)

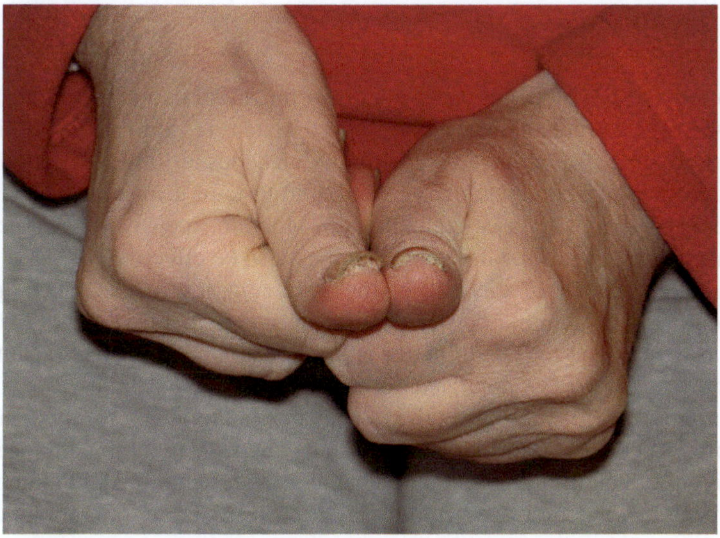

Fig. 33.2 Reddish to flesh-colored, smooth, firm subungual papules. Koenen tumors may also appear in a periungual distribution, emerging along the nail folds (Photo credit: Joshua A. Zeichner, M.D.)

In addition to the multiple skin findings, TSC also has effects on internal organ systems as well. The presence of skin changes should prompt a more thorough work-up to examine for possible renal lesions, neurologic findings, and pulmonary manifestations. Sequelae from internal organ involvement can cause serious morbidity and mortality [6].

33.4 Work-Up

Diagnosis of TSC is based upon diagnostic criteria and therefore cannot simply be made upon any one clinical finding such as the presence of angiofibromas. Diagnosis of TSC requires associated lesions of two or more organ systems or at least two different lesions in the same organ to confirm diagnosis [7]. In fact, some of the so-called pathognomonic features such as intellectual disability and epilepsy are so common in the general population that they are not specific enough to contribute to diagnosis [8]. For this reason a list of criteria was set forth to establish consensus as to a reliable and consistent method of diagnosis [9]. Complete diagnosis and the evaluation of TSC go beyond the scope of this text; however, one or more angiofibromas, without other appropriate findings, do not suffice for diagnosis nor does it imply a work-up for TSC is warranted. Angiofibromas occur in over 90 % of individuals with TSC. However, a variant of angiofibromas occur commonly in the general population and are known as fibrous papules of the nose or simply fibrous papules. These may occur singly or multiply but only rarely in as high numbers or as diffusely as is manifest in the angiofibromas of TSC [10].

33.5 Treatment

The treatment of TSC depends on the patient's clinical status and radiologic findings. Diagnosis and treatment should include appropriate referral to a TSC clinic if possible with adequate follow-up and screening. Cutaneous lesions can be monitored or treated depending on patient preference and overall status using mechanical removal or Argon and /or CO2 laser technologies. More inexpensively, radiofrequency ablation, chemical peel, and dermabrasion may also be effective [11, 12].

With the discovery of the role of the TSC complex in the mTOR pathway, utilization of mTOR inhibitors was identified as a potential treatment of all tumors in TSC patients. One mTOR inhibitor is sirolimus, also known as rapamycin, an immunosuppressant FDA-approved for use in transplant patients. Sirolimus has shown promise in clinical trials both systemically and topically for the treatment of angiofibromas [13, 14]. This therapeutic strategy appears to inhibit angiogenesis by decreasing production of vascular endothelial growth factor [15]. Ongoing clinical trials are underway to study sirolimus as an effective and safe for mainstream treatment.

References

1. Hofbauer GFL, Marcollo-Pini A, Corsenca A, et al. The mTOR inhibitor rapamycin significantly improves facial angiofibroma lesions in a patient with tuberous sclerosis. Br J Dermatol. 2008;159:473–5.
2. Osborne JP, Fryer A, Webb D. Epidemiology of tuberous sclerosis. Ann N Y Acad Sci. 1991; 615:125–7.
3. Sancak O, Nellist M, Goedbloed M, et al. Mutational analysis of the TSC1 and TSC2 genes in a diagnostic setting: genotype–phenotype correlations and comparison of diagnostic DNA techniques in tuberous sclerosis complex. Eur J Hum Genet. 2005;13:731–41.
4. Morrison PJ. Tuberous sclerosis: epidemiology, genetics and progress towards treatment. Neuroepidemiology. 2009;33:342–3.
5. OSBORNE JP, FRYER A, WEBB D. Epidemiology of tuberous sclerosis. Ann N Y Acad Sci. 1991;615:125–7. doi:10.1111/j.1749-6632.1991.tb37754.x.
6. Weiner DM, Ewalt DH, Roach ES, Hensle TW. The tuberous sclerosis complex: a comprehensive review. J Am Coll Surg. 1998;187:548–61.
7. Roach ES, Sparagana SP. Diagnosis of tuberous sclerosis complex. J Child Neurol. 2004; 19:643.
8. Józwiak S, Schwartz RA, Janniger CK, Michałowicz R, Chmielik J. Skin lesions in children with tuberous sclerosis complex: their prevalence, natural course, and diagnostic significance. Int J Dermatol. 1998;37:911–7. doi:10.1046/j.1365-4362.1998.00495.x.
9. Roach ES, Gomez MR, Northrup H. Tuberous sclerosis complex consensus conference: revised clinical diagnostic criteria. J Child Neurol. 1998;13:624–8.
10. Sand M, Sand D, Thrandorf C, Paech V, Altmeyer P, Bechara FG. Review Cutaneous lesions of the nose 2010. Head Face Med. 2010;6:7.
11. Swaroop MR, Nischal KC, Rajesh Gowda CM, Umashankar NU, Basavaraj HB, Sathyanarayana BD. Radiofrequency ablation of adenoma sebaceum. J Cutan Aesthet Surg. 2008;1:89.

12. Kaufman AJ, Grekin RC, Geisse JK, Frieden IJ. Treatment of adenoma sebaceum with the copper vapor laser. J Am Acad Dermatol. 1995;33:770–4.
13. Salido R, Garnacho-Saucedo G, Cuevas-Asencio I, Ruano J, Galán-Gutierrez M, Vélez A, Moreno-Giménez J. Sustained clinical effectiveness and favorable safety profile of topical sirolimus for tuberous sclerosis—associated facial angiofibroma. J Eur Acad Dermatol Venereol. 2011. doi:10.1111/j.1468-3083.2011.04212.x.
14. Kaufman ME, Curtis AR, Fleischer AB. Successful treatment of angiofibromata of tuberous sclerosis complex with rapamycin. J Dermatol Treat. 2012;23(1):46–8.
15. Guba M, Von Breitenbuch P, Steinbauer M, et al. Rapamycin inhibits primary and metastatic tumor growth by antiangiogenesis: involvement of vascular endothelial growth factor. Nat Med. 2002;8:128–35.

Part V
Other Mimickers of Acne Vulgaris

Chapter 34
Acne Scarring

Neal Bhatia, Consuelo Veronica David, Salar Hazany, and Aman Samrao

34.1 Introduction

The inflammatory lesions caused by acne such as papules, pustules, nodules, and cysts can result in two types of changes to the skin—temporary pigment changes and true scarring. These lesions are common and can be just as must a source of psychologically distress to patients as active acne lesions. While pigment changes are temporary and resolve on their own over months to years, true scars are permanent. The appearance of true scars may be improved with various modalities including intralesional cortisone injections and laser therapies. Pigmentary alteration will be covered in another chapter, and in the following we will review true scars.

34.2 Background

True scars result from permanent changes to the epidermis, dermis, and subcutaneous tissue. Following the initial injury, tissue undergoes three stages of wound healing: inflammation, granulation, and tissue remodeling [1]. During tissue remodeling, keratinocytes and fibroblasts produce enzymes that dictate the proportion of matrix metalloproteinases (MMPs) to MMP inhibitors. Exuberance of the wound healing response, as well as a predominance of either MMPs or MMP inhibitors, determines how a scar will heal [1]. Acne scars are classified as atrophic or hypertrophic, and a summary of their clinical appearances is summarized (Table 34.1). Although research supports a genetic predisposition for the development of keloids, such a predisposition has not been suggested for atrophic scars.

N. Bhatia, M.D. (✉) • C.V. David, M.D. • S. Hazany, M.D. • A. Samrao, M.D.
Division of Dermatology, Harbor-UCLA Medical Center, 1000 W. Carson Street,
Box 259, Torrence, CA 90502, USA
e-mail: bhatiaharbor@gmail.com

J.A. Zeichner (ed.), *Acneiform Eruptions in Dermatology: A Differential Diagnosis*,
DOI 10.1007/978-1-4614-8344-1_34, © Springer Science+Business Media New York 2014

Table 34.1 Morphologies of acne scars

Morphology	Description	Shape
Atrophic		
Ice pick	<2 mm orifice; tapers as it extends to dermis or subcutaneous tissue	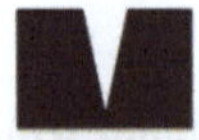
Boxcar (shallow)	<0.5 mm, shallow flat-bottomed scars with sharply demarcated vertical walls	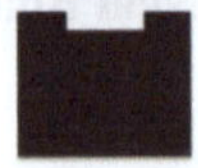
Boxcar (deep)	>0.5 mm, flat-bottomed scar with sharply demarcated vertical walls	
Rolling	4–5 mm with sloped borders	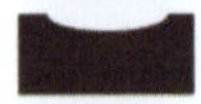
Sinus tract	Contiguous connections in the dermis and/or subcutaneous tissue. Sometimes epithelialized	
Hypertrophic		
Hypertrophic	Papules and plaques that are elevated above the skin surface to a greater degree than normal, but remain within the boundaries of the original area of damage	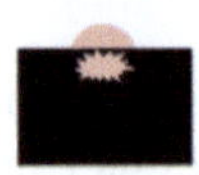
Keloid	Smooth papules and plaques that are elevated above the skin surface to a greater degree than normal extend beyond the boundaries of the original area of involvement. Can by symptomatic	

[a]Most of the atrophic scars are based on the Jacob's classification scheme [4]

In general, patients with darker skin types more commonly develop keloids than patients of other skin types, although the exact prevalence is not known. It is widely accepted that keloids develop as a result of a genetic predisposition with an environmental influence. It is unclear whether the predisposition to keloids results in single Mendelian or polygenetic disorder. Both autosomal dominant with incomplete penetrance and autosomal recessive modes have been reported [2, 3]. Chromosomes 2q23 and 7p11 mutations and HLA-DRB1*15, HLA-DQA1*0104, DQ-B1*0501, and DQB1*0503 all may play a role [2].

34.3 Clinical Appearance

34.3.1 Atrophic Scars

Atrophic scars are depressions caused by loss of substance in epidermis, dermis, or subcutis. They may appear pigmented due to increased visibility of vasculature and how they reflect light [1, 4]. The appearance of these scars may be described as

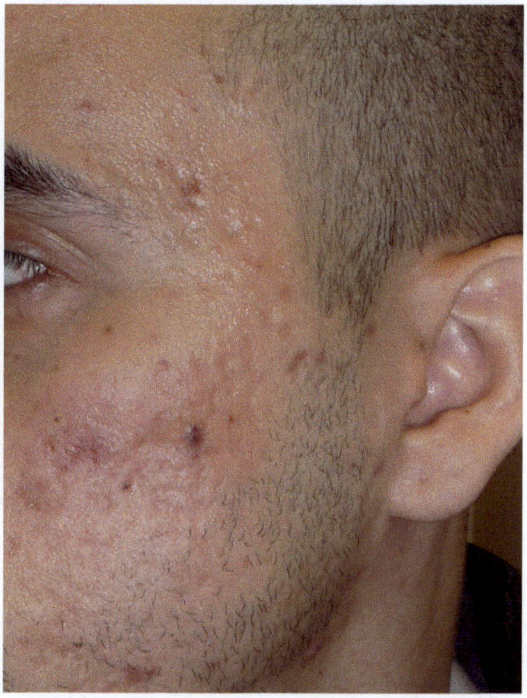

Fig. 34.1 Atrophic acne scarring in a man in his twenties. Boxcar scars with well-defined borders are evident on the temples, while smoother, rolling scars are present on the cheeks (Photo credits: Joshua A. Zeichner, M.D.)

flat-bottomed, narrow, wrinkled, ice pick, depressed, crater-like, atrophic, narrow, wide, or deep (Fig. 34.1). In 2001, Jacobs et al. proposed a classification system that unifies the terminology to describe atrophic scars [5]. In this scheme, atrophic scars are classified as ice pick, rolling, or boxcar. These subtypes are categorized based on depth, width, and architecture of the lesions. Accurate categorization can provide guidance to clinicians when determining treatment options.

Ice pick scars are narrow (<2 mm), well-defined, epithelialized tracts that extend to the deep dermis and even subcutaneous tissue. The scar orifice starts out wide and tapers at the base. They are frequently seen on the cheeks [5].

Rolling scars are wider than ice pick scars (4–5 mm or larger), but shallow. They have gently sloped surfaces that create a soft, undulating, uneven appearance of the skin. Rolling scars result from scarring and tethering of the dermis to the subcutaneous tissue [5].

Boxcar scars, like rolling scars, can be shallow, round, square. or oval depressions. However, they are sharply demarcated and have vertical walls. The base of boxcar scars is flat and is frequently the same size as the opening at the surface. Boxcar scars can be divided into shallow (<0.5 mm) and deep (>0.5 mm) [5].

A final form of atrophic scarring that is not included in the Jacob classification is the sinus tract. Sinus tracts are contiguous connections in the dermis and subcutaneous tissue which may have more than one epidermal orifice; they can result in significant morbidity.

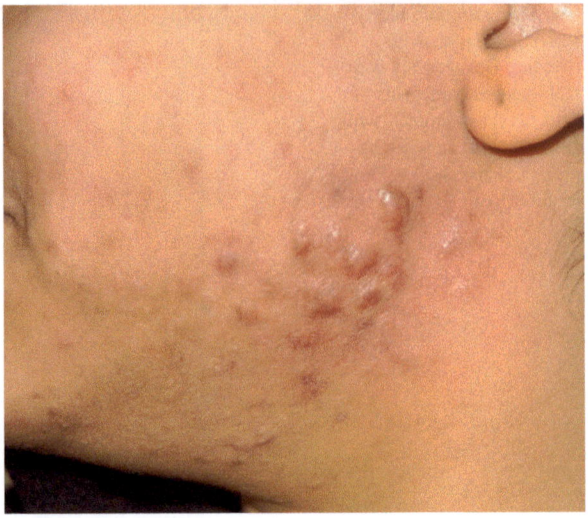

Fig. 34.2 Both hypertrophic and keloidal scars are present on the jawline of this woman. Keloidal scars grow beyond the border of the original area of skin damage (Photo credits: Joshua A. Zeichner, M.D.)

34.3.2 Hypertrophic Scars

Hypertrophic scars and keloids are two types of scars resulting from over-exuberant wound healing responses with excess collagen deposition and decreased collagenase activity [1]. Hypertrophic scars are lesions that elevate above the skin surface, but remain within the boundaries of the original area of damage [6]. These lesions may spontaneously involute. Keloids on the other hand are lesions with collagen deposition beyond the border of the original wound (Fig. 34.2). Histologically, keloids are characterized by thick, hyalinized collagen bundles [6, 7]. Keloids can be painful, itchy, and burn. Importantly, keloids due to acne should not be confused with acne keloidalis nuchae, a primary cicatricial alopecia that has no association with acne vulgaris [8].

34.4 Work-Up

The diagnosis of acne scarring is based on clinical appearance, and little work-up is necessary. Patients should be educated on the difference between post-inflammatory erythema or pigmentation and true acne scarring. It is important to set realistic expectations on outcomes, treatment options, and the time course for improvement. Psychosocial issues should also be addressed, as acne scars can have a large impact on self esteem and be a source of depression [9].

Scars have distinct histologic appearances. The various atrophic scar subtypes are similar, with an atrophic epidermis and effacement of the rete ridges. Collagen fibers are arranged parallel to the epidermis, while blood vessels are oriented perpendicular to the epidermis [5, 6, 10]. The epidermis of hypertrophic scars is similar to atrophic ones; however, they contain dense collagen bands and fibroblasts oriented parallel to the epidermis [8]. Abundant fibroblasts and pale mucinous stroma are present in newer scars while older scars have fewer fibroblasts [8]. Keloidal scars can be distinguished from hypertrophic scars by their unique hyalinized bundles of collagen. Moreover, keloids contain increased mucin and mast cells with less prominent blood vessels [8].

34.5 Treatment

Traditional treatments for atrophic acne scarring include surgical interventions, dermabrasion, and chemical peels. With advances in laser technology, the treatment armamentarium for scars has vastly expanded, providing patients with more options and improved outcomes. Hypertrophic scars on the other hand are largely treated with intralesional triamcinolone. While effective, risks include skin atrophy and hypopigmentation which improves over several months when it occurs. The risk of these adverse events increases with higher doses of triamcinolone.

Minor surgical procedures include punch excision, subcision, and punch grafting, which are performed under local anesthesia in the office. In a punch excision, the scar tissue is removed with a punch biopsy with or without a primary closure. A subcision is a lifting procedure, which attempts to raise the base of an atrophic scar upward towards the surface, making the skin smooth [11]. Using a large gauge needle probed parallel to the surface of the skin, scar tissue beneath the epidermis is broken apart [12, 13]. The lesion is left to heal so that new collagen is laid down in a more cosmetically elegant manner. Punch excision is very effective for ice pick scarring, whereas subcision is more effective for thick fibrotic scars. Punch grafting is a two-step method in which the scar is removed using a punch biopsy and replaced with harvested punched skin from an inconspicuous area [14, 15]. Punch excisions and grafts are especially helpful for deep, ice pick scars, which are not effectively treated with subcision, lasers, or similar modalities.

Dermal fillers such as collagen, hyaluronic acid, and calcium hydroxyapatite can be injected to lift depressed scars and achieve a smooth appearance at the skin's surface [11]. Optimal candidate lesions are broad, soft, and stretchable. Caution should be exercised not to inject hyaluronic acid too superficially in the skin, as to avoid a Tyndall effect. Lesions with underlying fibrosis are often subcised prior to placement of the filler.

Chemical peels have shown benefit to atrophic acne scars, even in patients with dark skin. Medium depth peels using 50 % trichloroacetic acid (TCA), Jessner's solution followed by 35 % TCA, or 70 % glycolic acid followed by 35 % TCA can produce a controlled wound to the level of the upper reticular dermis [16]. Deep chemical peels reach the mid-reticular dermis and can be useful to treat deep acne scars. Phenol peels have been the agent traditionally used, but must may cause cardiac arrhythmia so patients require cardiac monitoring during the procedure.

Laser resurfacing is especially useful in treating atrophic acne scars. Fractional photothermolysis (FP) was approved by the FDA in 2006 to treat acne scarring. This technology creates microscopic zones of thermal damage separated by areas of intact skin, allowing rapid reepithelialization and recovery. The photothermal injury produced in the dermis leads to collagen remodeling and improvement of the appearance of scares. Non-ablative fractional lasers leave the epidermis intact. They require less postoperative care, but often more treatment sessions needed compared to their ablative counterparts [17, 18].

While infrequently used since the advent of laser resurfacing, dermabrasion is an effective treatment for patients with atrophic acne scars. Mechanical dermabrasion using a diamond fraises or wire brushes causes injury to the dermis and induces dermal remodeling with fibroplasia, matrix formation, and collagen neogenesis [19, 20].

34.6 Conclusion

Acne is a significant source of morbidity when active as well as when it resolves with permanent scars. While the best treatment for acne scars is prevention with an early, effective treatment, several treatment modalities exist to improve the appearance of scars if they do develop. An understanding of the classification of acne scars is important to manage patient expectations and development a treatment regimen.

References

1. Thiboutot D, Gollnick H, Bettoli V, Dreno B, Kang S, Leyden JJ, et al. New insights into the management of acne: an update from the global alliance to improve outcomes in acne group. J Am Acad Dermatol. 2009;60:S1–50.
2. Shih B, Bayat A. Genetics of keloid scarring. Arch Dermatol Res. 2010;302:319–39.
3. Halim AS, Emami A, Salahshourifar I, Kannan TP. Keloid scarring: understanding the genetic basis, advances, and prospects. Arch Plast Surg. 2012;39:184–9.
4. Rivera AE. Acne scarring: a review and current treatment modalities. J Am Acad Dermatol. 2008;59:659–76.
5. Jacob CI, Dover JS, Kaminer MS. Acne scarring: a classification system and review of treatment options. J Am Acad Dermatol. 2001;45:109–17.
6. Rapini R. Practical dermatopathology. Houston: Elsevier-Mosby; 2012.
7. Verhaegen PD, van Zuijlen PP, Pennings NM, van Marle J, Niessen FB, van der Horst CM, et al. Differences in collagen architecture between keloid, hypertrophic scar, normotrophic scar, and normal skin: an objective histopathological analysis. Wound Repair Regen. 2009; 17:649–56.
8. James W, Berger T, Elston D. Andrews' diseases of the skin clinical dermatology. Philadelphia: Elsevier-Saunders; 2011.
9. Levy LL, Zeichner JA. Management of acne scarring, part II: a comparative review of non-laser-based, minimally invasive approaches. Am J Clin Dermatol. 2012;13:331–40.
10. Fabbrocini G, Annunziata MC, D'Arco V, De Vita V, Lodi G, Mauriello MC, et al. Acne scars: pathogenesis, classification and treatment. Dermatol Res Pract. 2010;2010:893080.

11. Fife D. Practical evaluation and management of atrophic acne scars: tips for the general dermatologist. J Clin Aesthet Dermatol. 2011;4:50–7.
12. Orentreich D, Orentreich N. Acne scar revision update. Dermatol Clin. 1987;5:359–68.
13. Tsao SS, Dover JS, Arndt KA, Kaminer MS. Scar management: keloid, hypertrophic, atrophic, and acne scars. Semin Cutan Med Surg. 2002;21:46–75.
14. Johnson WC. Treatment of pitted scars: punch transplant technique. J Dermatol Surg Oncol. 1986;12:260–5.
15. Solotoff SA. Treatment for pitted acne scarring–postauricular punch grafts followed by dermabrasion. J Dermatol Surg Oncol. 1986;12:1079–84.
16. Al-Waiz MM, Al-Sharqi AI. Medium-depth chemical peels in the treatment of acne scars in dark-skinned individuals. Dermatol Surg. 2002;28:383–7.
17. Kim S, Cho KH. Clinical trial of dual treatment with an ablative fractional laser and a nonablative laser for the treatment of acne scars in Asian patients. Dermatol Surg. 2009;35:1089–98.
18. Ong MW, Bashir SJ. Fractional laser resurfacing for acne scars: a review. Br J Dermatol. 2012;166:1160–9.
19. Roenigk Jr HH. Dermabrasion for miscellaneous cutaneous lesions (exclusive of scarring from acne). J Dermatol Surg Oncol. 1977;3:322–8.
20. Yarborough Jr JM. Ablation of facial scars by programmed dermabrasion. J Dermatol Surg Oncol. 1988;14:292–4.

Chapter 35
Eosinophilic Pustular Folliculitis

Joy Makdisi and Adam Friedman

35.1 Introduction

First described in Japan by Ofuji in 1970 [1], eosinophilic pustular folliculitis (EPF) is a noninfectious inflammatory skin disease that manifests with coalescing papulopustular plaques. The disease is histologically characterized by eosinophilic infiltration of hair follicles. There are three known variants of EPF: classic (as originally described by Ofuji and predominantly affecting Japanese individuals), HIV-associated, and infantile.

35.2 Background

The majority of reported EPF cases are related to immunosuppression, while the classic and infantile EPF are far less common [2]. The classic variant of EPF is found predominantly in Japanese patients, though any race may be affected [3]. Males are more commonly affected than women, in a ratio generally reported as 4.8:1 [2, 4], though a study in Singapore found a ratio of 1.6:1 [5]. The incidence of classic EPF is concentrated in the third and fourth decades of life, with the average age of onset at 30 years [6].

The immunosuppression-related variant chiefly affects HIV-infected individuals, though cases have also been seen in intravenous drug abusers [7, 8]. There is also a tremendous male predominance; only six cases have been reported in female patients [9]. Most cases of HIV-related EPF have been seen in Caucasian patients, and the majority of cases reported are from the United States and Great Britain.

J. Makdisi, B.S. (✉) • A. Friedman, M.D.
Department of Medicine, Montefiore – Albert Einstein College of Medicine, 1300 Morris Park Ave Ullmann 107, Bronx, NY 10461, USA
e-mail: joy.makdisi@med.einstein.yu.edu

J.A. Zeichner (ed.), *Acneiform Eruptions in Dermatology: A Differential Diagnosis*, DOI 10.1007/978-1-4614-8344-1_35,

Patients tend to present to the doctors' offices later in the course of their disease, often once they have established acquired immunodeficiency syndrome [10].

The pathophysiology of EPF is largely unknown. Theories on its etiology take into account the prominent eosinophilic cellular infiltrate, the folliculocentric character of the lesions, and the distribution of the eruption. Hypersensitivity reactions to infection or medication, as well as an autoimmune etiology have been proposed as possible mechanisms of EPF [2]. For example, EPF can present similarly to a fungal folliculitis with respect to both its clinical and histological features; it is hypothesized that the folliculitis may be attributable to immune hyperreactivity to dermatophytes or other fungi [11]. This theory is supported by the positive therapeutic response in patients treated with antifungal agents [2]. Other possible antigenic sources investigated include mites (*Demodex folliculorum* and *Demodex brevis*) and bacteria (*Leptotrichia buccalis*) [2]. In addition, medications such as carbamazepine, minocycline, allopurinol, timepidium bromide [3, 12, 13], and silicone tissue injections [14] have been reported as possible causes of EPF skin reactions.

Given the high incidence of eosinophilic pustular reactions in the setting of coexisting immune dysfunction, it has been suggested that immune dysregulation may also be a contributing factor to EPF [15]. Furthermore, it has been proposed that the HIV-associated variant of EPF may also be an autoimmune disorder, with a component of sebum behaving as the target antigen [10, 16]. Of note, there are also cases of EPF in HIV-negative immunocompromised states, such as in lymphoma patients after autologous peripheral blood stem cell and allogeneic bone marrow transplantation [3, 17]. It is likely that this variant of EPF is a nonspecific manifestation that presents in the setting of a compromised immune system and may be provoked by various antigens [2]. Given these reported findings, it is critical to evaluate EPF patients for coexisting systemic disease [2]. Though many hypotheses have been proposed, more research is required to further elucidate the mechanism and conclusively determine the pathophysiology of EPF.

35.3 Clinical Presentation

Though HIV-related EPF and classic EPF (a.k.a. Ofuji's disease) appear similar histologically, they differ clinically. The classic form arises in healthy patients and generally presents with chronic, recurring, sterile, folliculocentric papules and pustules [10, 18]. These lesions usually develop into confluent annular plaques with central clearing [2]. The classic distribution includes seborrheic areas such as the face (85 %), back, and trunk (59 %), as well as non-hair-bearing areas such as the palms and soles (20 %) [2, 16, 18]. The lesions typically resolve without scarring, but may develop postinflammatory hyperpigmentation. Furthermore, pruritus affects <50 % of patients [10].

In HIV-associated EPF, immunocompromised patients universally present with a defining feature: chronic, severe, intractable pruritus [10]. Rather than confluent

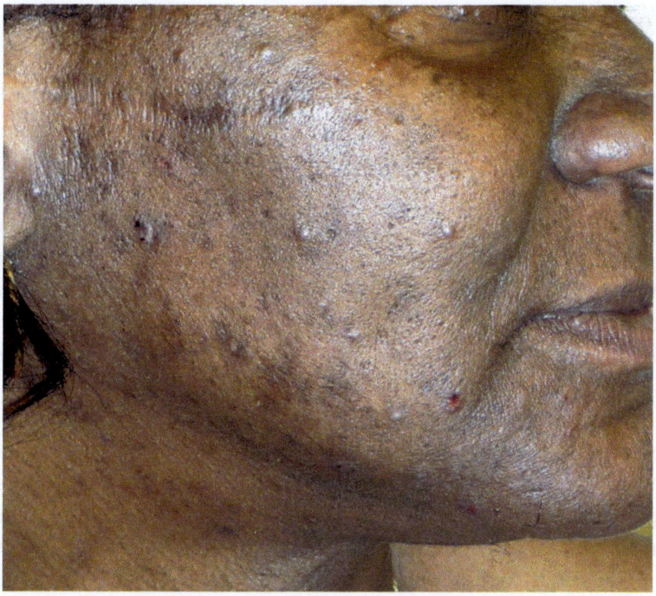

Fig. 35.1 Flesh colored and excoriated papules on face (Photo credits: Joshua A. Zeichner, M.D.)

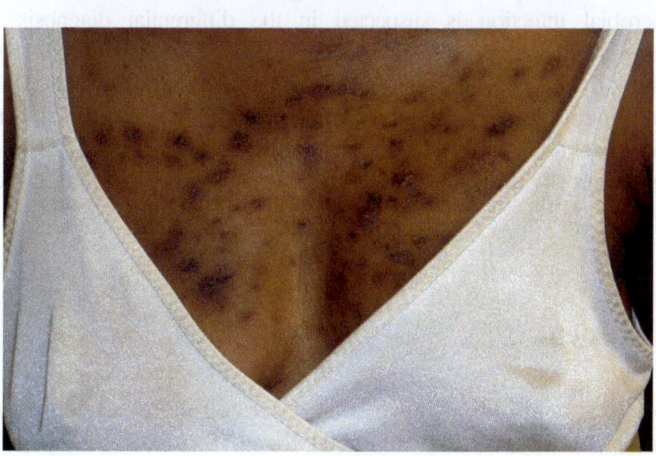

Fig. 35.2 Post-inflammatory pigmentation and excoriations on the chest. The patient complained of extreme itching, yet no primary lesions are visible. The patient is HIV positive (Photo credits: Joshua A. Zeichner, M.D.)

clusters, the lesions present as discrete, erythematous, perifollicular papules and pustules and are usually heavily excoriated (see Figs. 35.1 and 35.2) [6, 10, 19]. There are more rare presentations with confluent erythematous, plaques [20]. The distribution of HIV-associated EPF is predominantly on the trunk, though a significant number of patients also have head and neck lesions [8, 20–22]. Acral involvement is uncommon [10], in contrast to classic EPF [18].

35.4 Work-Up

Patients with suspected EPF should have a complete blood count with differential, as peripheral eosinophilia has been found in up to 35 % of classic EPF patients [1, 6] and 50 % of HIV-associated EPF patients [8, 10, 21, 22]. In the classic form, a mild to moderate leukocytosis may be present, whereas a leukopenia may be present in the HIV-associated variant [18]. Serum IgE levels have also been reported to be elevated significantly in a large number of HIV-associated EPF patients, as compared to levels in HIV controls [21, 23]. Patients tend to have a CD4 count less than 250–300 cells/ml [21].

The EPF variants share common findings on histopathologic analysis: noninfectious infiltration of eosinophils. Eosinophilic spongiosis and pustulosis are seen on pathology, particularly in the infundibulum of the hair follicle [18]. The infiltrate often extends to the adjacent sebaceous gland and duct [18]. In addition, there is a perivascular and perifollicular infiltrate consisting of lymphocytes [18]. When taking the biopsy, it is necessary o acquire an entire papule or pustule with a contiguous follicle for adequate histopathological diagnosis. In addition, because EPF is folliculocentric, serial sections may be necessary to visualize the inflamed follicle and confirm the diagnosis [2, 10]. Routine hematoxylin and eosin stain should be performed, as well as specific stains for fungi and bacteria.

If a microbial infection is suspected in the differential diagnosis, skin swabs for microscopy and culture and scrapings for mycologic examination should be performed.

It is clinically difficult to distinguish between the different HIV-associated folliculitides, including EPF and infective folliculitis. However, routine bacterial and fungal cultures are usually negative in HIV-associated EPF [21, 24]. Furthermore, histology is diagnostic and can be used to differentiate between infective folliculitis and EPF [10].

35.5 Treatment

A myriad of treatment options have been described with variable results. Topical corticosteroids are the first-line treatment for all forms of EPF [6]. The dose is modified depending on the age of the patient: mild to moderate potency for children and moderate to high potency for adults [2, 6]. Topical tacrolimus also appears to be an effective first-line agent [6, 25].

Classic EPF is often treated with nonsteroidal anti-inflammatory drug derivatives, most commonly oral indomethacin [3, 5, 6, 10]. Throughout the many years of use by Japanese dermatologists, it appears to be the most effective treatment for the classic form of the disease. One case series of 25 patients found indomethacin to be effective in 92 % of patients [26].

If topical corticosteroids and oral indomethacin are unsuccessful in treating HIV-associated EPF, a variety of other treatment options can be utilized. These include itraconazole, metronidazole, and 5 % permethrin cream [3, 6, 10]. In addition, antihistamines, including cetirizine and cyproheptadine, are often utilized in the treatment of HIV-associated EPF because of the severe pruritus that is characteristic of the disease [6, 10, 27].

HIV-associated EPF can develop 3–6 months after beginning highly active antiretroviral therapy, but interestingly, it also responds quite well to the therapy [6, 28, 29]. It is best to reassure patients that as the immune system is strengthened and the CD4 count rises above 250, the disease shows improvement and often complete resolution [2].

If the topical and oral agents discussed above prove ineffective, phototherapy with ultraviolet B (UVB) is considered the "gold standard" treatment and can often be curative [6].

There are several other EPF treatments that demonstrate some efficacy but it is less certain if the benefit of these treatments outweighs their risk. These include psoralen plus UVA (PUVA) photochemotherapy, which has been utilized with some therapeutic success [10, 30]. However, ultraviolet treatments cease to be efficacious once they are withdrawn [2]. Systemic corticosteroids have also been used with success, but caution must be taken to avoid the many well-known potential adverse effects of prolonged systemic steroid use [2]. Other treatments in this category include synthetic retinoids, oral cyclosporine, interferon-α, and interferon-γ [6]. In addition, twice daily dapsone has also shown some therapeutic success [31]. Finally, in chronic EPF that is unresponsive to the treatments discussed above, ionizing radiation has proven to be effective [6].

Whereas HIV-associated EPF tends to resolve with highly active antiretroviral therapy and the subsequent rising CD4 counts, classic EPF tends to follow a chronic and relapsing course for many years. Because of this, the prognosis is generally considered poor [2]. More recently, patients have achieved complete remission with indomethacin and tacrolimus [2].

35.6 Conclusion

EPF is a noninfectious papulopustular disease characterized by an eosinophilic infiltrate concentrated perifollicularly. It exists in three distinct variants, and though it can occur in persons with normal immune status, it is a possible sign of immunosuppression. Though the etiology is unclear, several hypotheses suggest that it is likely multifactorial; hypersensitivity to various antigenic stimuli in combination with immune dysregulation are both discussed in the literature. A variety of treatment options are available, though a definitive successful treatment strategy is not obvious. Because the pathophysiology remains unclear, EPF treatment must be tailored to individual patients according to their subtype. Often patients go through several courses of treatment and medication changes before achieving successful results. Due to the chronic relapsing course, most EPF patients need maintenance treatment [5]. It is hoped that with continued research and increased awareness of the disease, earlier diagnosis and more effective treatment can be realized.

References

1. Ofuji S. Eosinophilic pustular folliculitis. Dermatologica. 1987;174(2):53.
2. Nervi SJ, Schwartz RA, Dmochowski M. Eosinophilic pustular folliculitis: a 40 year retrospect. J Am Acad Dermatol. 2006;55(2):285–9.
3. Dmochowski M SR. Eosinophilic pustular folliculitis. eMedicine Dermatology [journal serial online]. 2006. Available at: http://emedicine.com/derm/topic120.htm. Accessed 15 Dec 2012.
4. Takematsu H, Nakamura K, Igarashi M, Tagami H. Eosinophilic pustular folliculitis. Report of two cases with a review of the Japanese literature. Arch Dermatol. 1985;121(7):917.
5. Tang MBY, Tan E, Chua SH. Eosinophilic pustular folliculitis (Ofuji's disease) in Singapore: a review of 23 adult cases. Australas J Dermatol. 2003;44(1):44–7.
6. Ellis E, Scheinfeld N. Eosinophilic pustular folliculitis: a comprehensive review of treatment options. Am J Clin Dermatol. 2004;5(3):189–97.
7. Ferrandiz CRM, Barranco JC, Clotet B, Lorenzo JC. Eosinophilic pustular folliculitis in patients with acquired immunodeficiency syndrome. Int J Dermatol. 1992;31(3):193–5.
8. Basarab T, Jones RR. HIV-associated eosinophilic folliculitis: case report and review of the literature. Br J Dermatol. 1996;134(3):499–503.
9. Hayes BB, Hille RC, Goldberg LJ. Eosinophilic folliculitis in 2 HIV-positive women. Arch Dermatol. 2004;140(4):463.
10. Fearfield L, Rowe A, Francis N, Bunker C, Staughton R. Itchy folliculitis and human immunodeficiency virus infection: clinicopathological and immunological features, pathogenesis and treatment. Br J Dermatol. 1999;141(1):3.
11. Haupt HM, Stern JB, Weber CB. Eosinophilic pustular folliculitis: fungal folliculitis? J Am Acad Dermatol. 1990;23(5):1012–4.
12. Kimura K, Ezoe K, Yokozeki H, Katayama I, Nishioka K. A case of eosinophilic pustular folliculitis (Ofuji's disease) induced by patch and challenge tests with indeloxazine hydrochloride. J Dermatol. 1996;23(7):479.
13. Maejima H, Mukai H, Hikaru E. Eosinophilic pustular folliculitis induced by allopurinol and timepidium bromide. Acta Derm Venereol. 2002;82(4):316–7.
14. Wong TW, Tsai YM, Lee J, Hsu ST, Sheu HM. Eosinophilic pustular folliculitis (Ofuji's disease) in a patient with silicone tissue augmentation. J Dermatol. 2004;31(9):727.
15. Magro CM, Crowson AN. Eosinophilic pustular follicular reaction: a paradigm of immune dysregulation. Int J Dermatol. 1994;33(3):172–8.
16. Takematsu H, Tagami H. Eosinophilic pustular folliculitis. Studies on possible chemotactic factors involved in the formation of pustules. Br J Dermatol. 2006;114(2):209–15.
17. Keida T, Hayashi N, Kawashima M. Eosinophilic pustular folliculitis following autologous peripheral blood stem-cell transplantation. J Dermatol. 2004;31(1):21.
18. Johnston R. Chapter 15: Diseases of cutaneous appendages. In: Weedon D, editor. Weedon's skin pathology essentials. 3rd ed. London: Churchill Livingstone Elsevier; 2012. p. 302.
19. Buchness MR, Lim HW, Soter NA. AIDS-related eosinophilic pustular folliculitis. J Am Acad Dermatol. 1991;25(5 Pt 1):866.
20. Soeprono FF, Schinella RA. Eosinophilic pustular folliculitis in patients with acquired immunodeficiency syndrome: report of three cases. J Am Acad Dermatol. 1986;14(6):1020–2.
21. Rosenthal D, LeBoit PE, Klumpp L, Berger TG. Human immunodeficiency virus-associated eosinophilic folliculitis: a unique dermatosis associated with advanced human immunodeficiency virus infection. Arch Dermatol. 1991;127(2):206.
22. Frentz G, Niordson AM, Thomsen K. Eosinophilic pustular dermatosis: an early skin marker of infection with human immunodeficiency virus? Br J Dermatol. 1989;121(2):271–4.
23. Maurer T, Berger T. Serum IgE levels in eosinophilic folliculitis—an inflammatory disease of HIV infection. J Invest Dermatol. 1994;102:619.
24. McCalmont TH, Altemus D, Maurer T, Berger TG. Eosinophilic folliculitis. The histologic spectrum. Am J Dermatopathol. 1995;17(5):439.

25. Kabashima K, Sakurai T, Miyachi Y. Treatment of eosinophilic pustular folliculitis (Ofuji's disease) with tacrolimus ointment. Br J Dermatol. 2004;151(4):949–50.
26. Ota T, Hata Y, Tanikawa A, Amagai M, Tanaka M, Nishikawa T. Eosinophilic pustular folliculitis (Ofuji's disease): indomethacin as a first choice of treatment. Clin Exp Dermatol. 2001; 26(2):179–81.
27. Harris D, Ostlere L, Buckley C, Johnson M, Rustin M. Eosinophilic pustular folliculitis in an HIV-positive man: response to cetirizine. Br J Dermatol. 1992;126(4):392–4.
28. Moyle M, Woolley IJ, Thevarajan I, Korman TM. Eosinophilic folliculitis: an example of 'immune reconstitution folliculitis'? AIDS. 2004;18(17):2350–2.
29. Rajendran PM, Dolev JC, Heaphy Jr MR, Maurer T. Eosinophilic folliculitis: before and after the introduction of antiretroviral therapy. Arch Dermatol. 2005;141(10):1227.
30. Buchness MR, Lim HW, Hatcher VA, Sanchez M, Soter NA. Eosinophilic pustular folliculitis in the acquired immunodeficiency syndrome. N Engl J Med. 1988;318(18):1183–6.
31. Steffen C. Eosinophilic pustular folliculitis (Ofuji's disease) with response to dapsone therapy. Arch Dermatol. 1985;121:921–3.

Chapter 36
Favre-Racouchot Syndrome

Silvina Pugliese, Andrea Smith, Rachel Epstein, and Abel Torres

36.1 Introduction

Favre-Racouchot syndrome (nodular elastosis with cysts and comedones) is a distinct variant of solar elastosis most frequently found in elderly Caucasian men. The estimated prevalence is 1.5–6 % in the general population. This syndrome is characterized by yellow nodules and plaques accentuated by enlarged, open comedones and dilated cysts, often accompanied by other cutaneous findings of actinic damage.

36.2 Background

The prevalence of Favre-Racouchot syndrome in the 40–60 year-old population is estimated at 6 %, while a more recent study of 25–74 year-olds identified a prevalence of 1.4 % [1, 2]. A study of agricultural workers found a 2.5 % prevalence [3]. Favre-Racouchot is more common in elderly, Caucasian males. Many of the affected individuals have a chronic history of excessive ultraviolet (UV) radiation from occupational and recreational exposures.

A number of theories have been postulated regarding the etiology of Favre-Racouchot. Extensive UV damage has been strongly associated with the development of this disorder, with actinic damage believed to cause degeneration of elastin, and structural loss leading to the abnormal enlargement of comedones [4]. Hedelund confirmed this association by finding that both UV-A1 and UV-B exposure provoked comedonal and cystic formation in a patient with Favre-Racouchot, with UV-B radiation leading to more extensive skin changes [5]. This relationship is so well established

S. Pugliese, M.D. (✉) • A. Smith, M.D. • R. Epstein, D.O. • A. Torres, M.D.
Department of Dermatology, Loma Linda University, 11370 Anderson Street Suite 2600, Loma Linda, CA 92354, USA
e-mail: spugliese@llu.edu

J.A. Zeichner (ed.), *Acneiform Eruptions in Dermatology: A Differential Diagnosis*, DOI 10.1007/978-1-4614-8344-1_36, © Springer Science+Business Media New York 2014

that Lim et al. have recently identified Favre-Racouchot as a consequence of UV exposure [6]. It should be noted that host predisposition plays a modulating role, as many individuals with chronic UV exposure do not develop Favre-Racouchot.

Multiple case reports have linked radiation therapy to the development of Favre-Racouchot, including Breit et al., who reported a case that developed a mere 2 weeks after cessation of radiation therapy to the nasopharynx and neck [7].

Smoking is associated with a higher incidence of developing Favre-Racouchot syndrome. This relationship is believed to be dose-dependent, as smokers with Favre-Racouchot were found to have a significantly greater pack-year smoking history than smokers without Favre-Racouchot [8]. For years, smoking has been implicated in photoaging and has been found to particularly affect the development of comedones [9].

Lastly, systemic and topical steroids have been postulated to play a contributing role in the development of Favre-Racouchot [5]. UV damage, smoking, radiation therapy, and corticosteroids stimulate the associated clinical features of Favre-Racouchot disease via atrophy of the skin, loss of normal elastic fibers, keratinization of the pilosebaceous follicle, and increased comedone formation [10].

36.3 Clinical Presentation

Favre-Racouchot develops in areas of extensive sun exposure, and is classically found periorbitally, with predilection for the skin adjacent to the lateral canthi, as well as the malar eminences. Early changes include yellow plaques accentuated by enlarged, open, black comedones. These plaques later develop into distinct nodules. In addition to comedones, later lesions also show cystic dilations filled with retained keratin. Furrows are often present. Inflammatory lesions are not associated with Favre-Racouchot [10, 11]. These findings are usually bilateral, although they can be unilateral (Fig. 36.1).

Given its association with UV exposure, other skin findings linked to actinic damage often coexist (e.g., actinic keratoses, cutis rhomboidalis nuchae, and skin cancer). To date, this syndrome is not directly associated with any systemic symptoms or internal malignancies. The differential diagnosis for this disorder includes chloracne, cutis rhomboidalis nuchae, colloid milium, and actinic granuloma [12].

36.4 Work-Up

When evaluating a patient for Favre-Racouchot syndrome, a pertinent history should be taken with special attention to smoking habits, history of UV light exposure, radiation exposure, topical or systemic corticosteroid use, and routine use of comedogenic cosmetics.

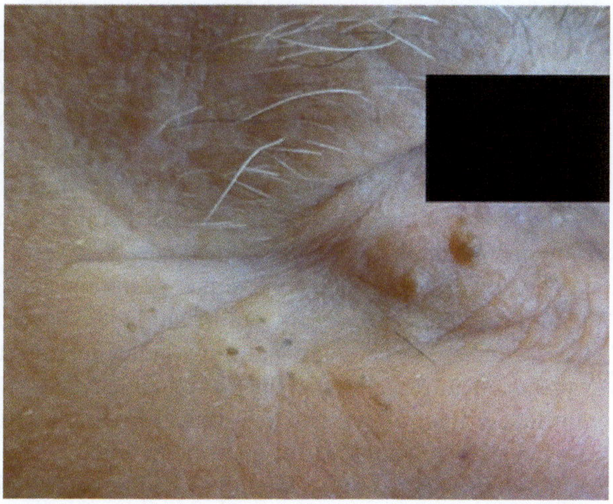

Fig. 36.1 Periorbital cystic nodules and enlarged open comedones on a background of chronic actinic damage

A differential diagnosis, as noted above, should be entertained given any pertinent historical findings. An important differential diagnosis is chloracne from toxin exposures such as aromatic hydrocarbons. Recognizing this diagnosis may have clinical, therapeutic, and even financial implications for the patient especially if there was an occupational exposure.

The time course of development of lesions may help point to the etiology. For example, Patterson et al. report a woman with rapid development of Favre-Racouchot comedones after radiation therapy [10]. Generally, affected patients will report a long gradual development of lesions in sun-exposed areas.

36.5 Treatment

Treatment for Favre-Racouchot has traditionally been difficult as it is often invasive and the unsightly lesions recur. The condition largely has aesthetic implications. No increase in skin cancers, ulcerations, or infections has been reported to our knowledge. Therefore, the features that most concern the patient should guide formation of treatment goals.

Prior therapies should be elucidated from the patient. Any contributing factors, if found, should be discontinued such as smoking or application of topical steroid formulations. Consistent and appropriate sun protection and avoidance should be emphasized.

Two main components need to be addressed when discussing therapeutic options: the presence of large disfiguring open comedones and the photodamaged surrounding skin.

Historically, chemical peels in conjunction with manual abrasion techniques were treatment standards. However, currently, the mainstay of therapy for Favre-Racouchot remains the topical retinoids [13]. The topical retinoids are first-line treatment for several reasons including their ability to address both the comedonal and photoaging aspects of Favre-Racouchot [7]. This therapy is non-invasive and can be applied in the comfort of the patient's home.

The disadvantage of topical retinoid therapy is that it is not very effective in resolving the larger and deeper comedones. Kaya et al. propose that topical retinoids are only effective on small comedones <1 mm in size [14]. Another adverse effect is their potential to cause significant irritation. However, these patients with thickened skin secondary to photodamage may better tolerate topical retinoid therapy [13]. A precursor to retinoic acid called retinaldehyde has been reported to be effective with less irritant effect than the topical retinoids [10]. Retinaldehyde is commercially available in a variety of over-the-counter retinol-containing products.

Oral retinoids have also been reported to be effective in the treatment of Favre-Racouchot. Low dose isotretinoin is the most frequently reported regimen with dosing ranging from 0.05 to 0.1 mg/kg for 4–6 months [10]. Oral isotretinoin is generally used in conjunction with topical retinoids. Disadvantages to this approach include but are not limited to serious side effects such as transaminitis, hyperlipidemia, a possible association with inflammatory bowel disease, and severe xerosis.

Comedonal extraction is still an important component of treatment for the large open comedones characteristic of Favre-Racouchot. Most often a traditional comedone extractor is used to do this. Kaya et al. also proposed a more efficient method for extracting these large open comedones on loose, thin skin using a standard dissecting forceps [14]. Mavilia et al. have also reported using forceps for extraction with CO_2 laser [15]. Comedone extraction is an effective therapeutic tool especially when combined with other treatment modalities including topical retinoids, dermabrasion, and even superficial CO_2 laser.

Comedone extraction can easily and quickly be performed in the office setting and allows for immediate improvement in appearance. Unfortunately, the comedones frequently recur after extraction, as the epithelial lining of the cyst is still present. In addition, extraction may result in superficial skin infections and inflammation. To prevent this, topical antibacterial ointments, such as mupirocin, are recommended for 5–14 days following extractions [14, 15].

Finally, in more severe cases, surgical interventions can be considered. Simple excisions can be used to excise large plaques and nodules. If necessary, excisions can be staged allowing for decreased tension on wounds during healing. Surgical therapies are particularly challenging for Favre-Racouchot, as the skin is by definition thin with damaged elastic fibers and altered collagen rendering it very friable. This makes it difficult to close any defects with ideal cosmesis. Sharkey et al. reported a case where incisional wound healing was poor and required both a staged excision and dermabrasion to obtain an acceptable cosmetic result [16].

Overall, the most efficacious treatments are those that combine therapeutic modalities. Since there is no cure for this condition, successive treatments are often necessary. Patients with this syndrome need to be treated with individually tailored regimens. Avoidance of risk factors such as excessive sun exposure, long term steroid use, and tobacco should be discussed. The importance of proper sun protection should also be addressed to help limit the potential actinic damage. When considering therapeutic options, physicians must take into consideration their patient's skin type, predominant lesion, likelihood of recurrence, and willingness to undergo high-risk procedures. Even though this condition is not life threatening, it can result in significant psychological, emotional, and social distress. Quality of life must therefore be taken into consideration when treating this relatively benign skin condition.

References

1. Aguis JRG. Grouped periorbital comedones. Br J Dermatol. 1964;76:158–64.
2. Schäfer T, Merkl J, Klemm E, Wichmann HE, Ring J, KORA Study Group. The epidemiology of nevi and signs of skin aging in the adult general population: results of the KORA-survey 2000. J Invest Dermatol. 2006;126(7):1490–6.
3. Cellini A, Offidani A. An epidemiological study on cutaneous diseases of agricultural workers authorized to use pesticides. Dermatology. 1994;189(2):129–32.
4. Sams Jr WM. Sun-induced aging. Dermatol Clin. 1986;4:509–16.
5. Hedelund L, Wulf HC. Favre-Racouchot disease provoked by UV-A1 and UV-B exposure. Arch Dermatol. 2004;140(1):129–31.
6. Lim HW, James WD, Rigel DS, Maloney ME, Spencer JM, Bhushan R. Adverse effects of ultraviolet radiation from the use of indoor tanning equipment: time to ban the tan. J Am Acad Dermatol. 2011;64(5):893–902.
7. Breit S, Flaig MJ, Wolff H, Plewig G. Favre-Racouchot-like disease after radiation therapy. J Am Acad Dermatol. 2003;49(1):117–9.
8. Keough GC, Laws RA, Elston DM. Favre-Racouchot syndrome: a case for smokers' comedones. Arch Dermatol. 1997;133(6):796–7.
9. Green AC, Hughes MC, McBride P, Fourtanier A. Factors associated with premature skin aging (photoaging) before the age of 55: a population-based study. Dermatology. 2011; 222(1):74–80.
10. Patterson WM, Fox MD, Schwartz RA. Favre-Racouchot disease. Int J Dermatol. 2004; 43(3):167–9.
11. Calderone DC, Fenske NA. The clinical spectrum of solar elastosis. J Am Acad Dermatol. 1995;32:1016–24.
12. Lewis KG, Bercovitch L, Dill SW, Robinson-Bostom L. Acquired disorders of elastic tissue: part I. Increased elastic tissue and solar elastotic syndromes. J Am Acad Dermatol. 2004; 51(1):1–21.
13. Rallis E, Karanikola E, Verros C. Successful treatment of Favre-Racouchot disease with 0.05% tazarotene gel. Arch Dermatol. 2007;143:810–2.
14. Kaya TI, Tursen AC, Yazici GI. A simple open comedone extraction technique for Favre-Racouchot disease. Photodermol Photoimmunol Photomed. 2005;21:275–7.
15. Mavilia L, Campolmi P, Santoro G, Lotti T. Combined treatment of Favre-Racouchot syndrome with a superpulsed carbon dioxide laser: report of 50 cases. Dermatol Ther. 2010;23:S4–6.
16. Sharkey MJ, Keller RA, Grabski WJ, McCollough ML. Favre-Racouchot syndrome: a combined therapeutic approach. Arch Dermatol. 1992;128:615–6.

Chapter 37
Hidradenitis Suppurativa

Deanna M. Sikorski and Kenneth J. Tomecki

37.1 Introduction

Hidradenitis suppurativa (HS), also known as acne inversa, is a chronic, debilitating inflammatory disease characterized by painful subcutaneous nodules and abscesses of intertriginous areas that contain both apocrine glands and terminal hairs.

37.2 Background

HS typically begins during the second and third decade of life, most often between the ages of 21 and 23, although cases of prepubertal HS and postmenopausal HS occasionally occur. The prevalence rate varies between 0.03 and 4 %, but true prevalence is probably 1 % in the general population [1, 2]. Women are more likely to be affected than men and disease distribution varies by gender. The groin and inframammary regions are more commonly affected in women, while the buttocks, perineum, and perianal area are more commonly affected in men.

The pathogenesis of HS is unclear and may include genetic, infectious, hormonal, behavioral, and even host defense factors. Once thought to be a disorder of the apocrine gland, HS actually represents follicular plugging as the primary event. As such, inflammation of the apocrine gland is not essential and apocrinitis is a secondary phenomenon.

Approximately 40 % of HS patients have familial HS, inherited as an autosomal dominant trait with 100 % penetrance. The likely defect may be a dysfunctional γ (gamma)-secretase-Notch pathway with mutations in Presenilin-1 (PSEN1), Presenilin

D.M. Sikorski, M.D. (✉) • K.J. Tomecki, M.D.
Department of Dermatology, The Cleveland Clinic Foundation, 9500 Euclid Avenue A61, Cleveland, OH 44195, USA
e-mail: sikorsd@ccf.org

J.A. Zeichner (ed.), *Acneiform Eruptions in Dermatology: A Differential Diagnosis*,
DOI 10.1007/978-1-4614-8344-1_37,

Enhancer-2 (PSENEN), and Nicastrin (NCSTN) genes, which encode proteins integral to γ (gamma)-secretase enzyme [3]. Gamma-secretase cleaves type 1 transmembrane proteins such as Notch, and mice without Notch-1 have occluded hair follicles, thought to be the initiating pathogenic event in HS.

HS is a component of the follicular occlusion tetrad which includes acne conglobata, dissecting cellulitis of the scalp, and pilonidal cysts. Known associations include acne vulgaris (30–70 %), obesity (51–75 %), smoking (70–89 %), and Crohn's disease. HS occasionally occurs with some genetic disorders, specifically keratosis-ichthyosis-deafness (KID) syndrome, Dowling-Degos Disease, SAPHO syndrome, PAPA syndrome, pachyonychia congenita, and Fox-Fordyce disease [1, 4].

37.3 Clinical Presentation

The onset of HS is usually insidious, typically affecting overweight or obese patients who develop tender, indurated papules, pustules, and subcutaneous nodules in the intertriginous areas (Figs. 37.1 and 37.2). Exact diagnosis may not be apparent initially, leading to incomplete evaluation and treatment. Disease may remit spontaneously within 7–10 days or persist for many months as non-tender nodules with subsequent recurrences. Disease distribution corresponds with the "milk line" location of apocrine-related mammary tissue in mammals, typically affecting the axillae most frequently (approximately 70 % of the time), followed by inguinal areas, inner thighs, perianal and perineal areas, mammary and inframammary area, buttocks, and less often the pubic region, scrotum, vulva, chest, scalp, and retroauricular region. Perianal and perineal disease is associated with more debilitation compared

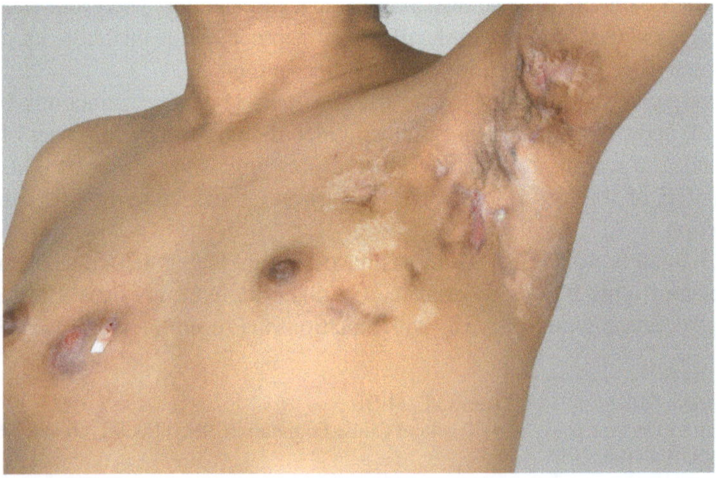

Fig. 37.1 Hidradenitis of the axillae and chest

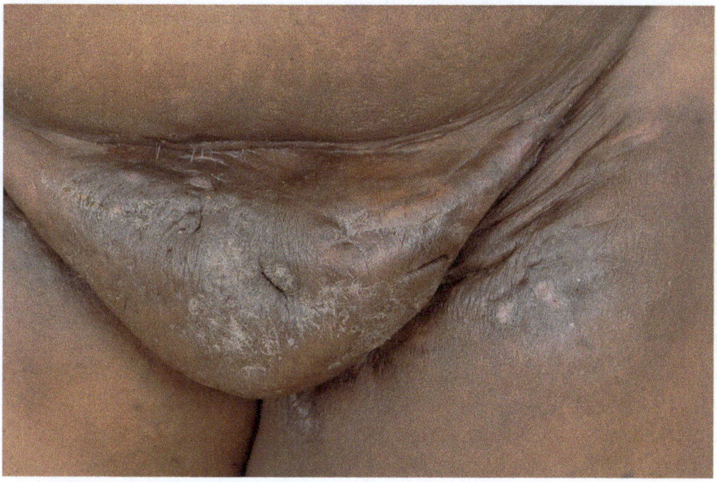

Fig. 37.2 Hidradenitis of the groin

to axillary disease; most patients with perianal and perineal involvement have recurrent disease and poorer quality of life [5].

During the course of the disease, additional nodules and plaques develop de novo or from extension of existing nodules, either on affected or adjacent skin or occasionally at distant sites. Fifty percent of patients experience a prodrome consisting of burning, stinging, pain, and pruritus, with or without hyperhidrosis, occurring 12–48 h before disease onset. The subcutaneous coalescence of neighboring cysts or the lateral extension of proliferating pilosebaceous material with rupture to the surface produces deep dermal abscesses and interlinked sinus tracts, which may lead to the formation of honeycombed fistulous tracts with chronic infection. Drainage from these tracts is common and may be serous, purulent, bloody, or a mixture and is often malodorous.

Ultimately, over time, disease becomes quiescent, invariably healing with scarring. Occasionally, indolent cysts may develop on the face, behind the ears, at the nape of the neck, on the trunk, and in the genital area. These cysts are more common in men. Sinus tracts can coalesce to form hypertrophic, fibrous fistulae, and subcutaneous sinus networks can form characteristic hypertrophic scars or dense, ropelike fibrotic bands. Fifty percent of patients develop the "tombstone comedone" of permanently dilated pores within an old "burned out" area of disease.

Most patients with chronic or untreated HS develop complications, e.g., anal, urethral, and rectal strictures, fistulae, and fecal incontinence from genitofemoral involvement or contractures and compromised mobility, especially in the axillae and thighs, from axillary or perianal disease. Other sequelae include spondyloarthropathy, pyogenic granuloma, lymphedema, lymphangiectasia [6], scrotal and vulvar edema, secondary infections including cellulitis and even septicemia, epidural abscesses, and sacral osteomyelitis. Metabolic sequelae are uncommon, but anemia, hypoproteinemia, and amyloidosis occasionally occur. Affected patients have a 4.6-fold increase in cutaneous SCC reported in HS patients with the mean time at diagnosis 25 years after the onset of HS. Most of the skin cancer (61 %) occurs in the perineum or on the buttocks, with men primarily affected (4:1). Skin cancer is often invasive and nearly half of affected patients die within 2 years of diagnosis. HS patients reportedly have a 50 % greater risk of malignancy, especially buccal cancer and primary hepatic cancer, though smoking and alcohol abuse are confounding variables that may explain this increase.

HS exhibits significant psychological and physiologic morbidity and social and economic hardships which contribute to a decreased quality of life. In one study, 144 HS patients, using the Dermatology Quality of Life Index (DQLI) questionnaire, had a mean score of 8.9, worse than mild to moderate psoriasis or alopecia. The high score was related to pain, malodorous discharge, genital disease or areas of intimacy, and lack of medical care related to patient hesitancy to disclose signs and symptoms. Another study of 61 hospitalized HS patients revealed similar results, with pain as the primary effect on quality of life. HS patients with severe disease are often unemployed, poor, and socially isolated. Employed patients with HS lose an average of 2–7 days of work per year, a number that tends to be greater in women.

37.4 Work-Up

The diagnosis is made clinically and biopsy is rarely necessary. The differential diagnosis includes infectious and inflammatory diseases such as acne, carbuncles, furuncles, inflamed cysts, fistulous abscess, granuloma inguinale, lymphogranuloma venereum, tuberculous abscess, noduloulcerative syphilis, actinomycosis, blastomycosis, nocardiosis, and cat scratch disease. HS can resemble Crohn's disease; if suggestive, GI and surgical evaluation may be necessary. Drainage warrants bacterial, fungal, and mycobacterial culture, which may reveal *Staphylococcus aureus* or Gram-negative organisms. Disease severity is variable and is quantified by the older Hurley scale or newer Sartorius scale.

37.5 Treatment

There is no uniformly successful therapy for HS. Standard treatment depends on the extent and severity of disease. Purely medical treatment is invariably prolonged since permanent cure is uncommon. Regardless of severity, all patients deserve information and education regarding preventative measures including the importance of good daily hygiene coupled with antimicrobial cleansers and reduction of heat, friction, and excessive sweating, including use of loose-fitting clothing. Adjunctive therapy should include smoking cessation, weight reduction, and support group referral.

Medical therapies include topical and systemic antibiotics, topical and systemic retinoids, systemic and intralesional corticosteroids, anti-androgens, dapsone, cyclosporine, and anti-TNF-alpha inhibitors. Mild HS is often treated with intralesional corticosteroids and/or short courses of topical or oral antibiotics, with selection based on sensitivities of cultured organisms, most commonly clindamycin or a tetracycline. Complete remission with antibiotic treatment is rare, but combination therapy with oral clindamycin and rifampicin [8] or with rifampicin, moxifloxacin, and metronidazole has produced remissions in patients with mild to moderate HS. Anti-androgen therapy with ethinylestradiol, cyproterone acetate, and finasteride has proven to be helpful in many patients. TNF-alpha inhibitors such as infliximab [9], etanercept [10], and adalimumab [11] have been effective in some patients with moderate to severe disease, but long-term results have been poor and the side effect profile of these drugs and their cost have limited their use. Despite successful use in acne, oral retinoids have not been shown to be effective in treating HS.

Surgical interventions with botulinum toxin, radiotherapy, carbon dioxide laser, long-pulsed neodymium: yttrium-aluminum-garnet (YAG) laser [12], and photodynamic [13] therapy have shown success in some patients. Incision and drainage has little benefit since recurrence is so common. Surgical excision remains one of the most successful therapies for recalcitrant HS, despite its appreciable morbidity and complications such as infection, scarring, graft failure, ischemic necrosis of myocutaneous flaps, and recurrence. A recent review of 72 surgical HS patients showed a recurrence rate of 54 % following excision to fascia with primary closure, but 19 % recurrence with myocutaneous flap and 13 % recurrence with split thickness skin graft [14].

References

1. Alikhan A, Lynch PJ, Eisen DB. Hidradenitis suppurativa: a comprehensive review. J Am Acad Dermatol. 2009;60:539–61.
2. Revuz JE, Canoui-poitrine F, Wolkenstein P, et al. Prevalence and factors associated with hidradenitis suppurativa: results from two case–control studies. J Am Acad Dermatol. 2008;59:596–601.
3. Wang B, Yang W, Wen W, et al. Gamma-secretase gene mutations in familial acne inversa. Science. 2010;330:1065.
4. Danby FW, Margesson LJ. Hidradenitis suppurativa. Dermatol Clin. 2010;28:779–93.
5. Matusiak L, Bieniek A, Szepietowski JC. Hidradenitis suppurativa markedly decreases quality of life and professional activity. J Am Acad Dermatol. 2010;62:706–8.
6. Moosbrugger EA, Mutasim DF. Hidradenitis suppurativa complicated by severe lymphedema and lymphangiectasias. J Am Acad Dermatol. 2011;64:1223–4.3.
7. Simonart T. Hidradenitis suppurativa and smoking. J Am Acad Dermatol. 2010;62:149–50.
8. Wall D, Kirby B. Rifampicin and clindamycin for hidradenitis. J Am Acad Dermatol. 2011; 64:790.
9. Grant A, Gonzalez T, Montgomery MO, Cardenas V, Kerdel FA. Infliximab therapy for patients with moderate to severe hidradenitis suppurativa: a randomized, double-blind, placebo-controlled crossover trial. J Am Acad Dermatol. 2010;62:205–17.
10. Lee RA, Dommasch E, Treat J, et al. A prospective clinical trial of open-label etanercept for the treatment of hidradenitis suppurativa. J Am Acad Dermatol. 2009;60:565–73.

11. Blanco R, Martínez-Taboada VM, Villa I, et al. Long-term successful adalimumab therapy in severe hidradenitis suppurativa. Arch Dermatol. 2010;145:580–84.
12. Mahmoud BH, Tierney E, Hexsel CL, Pui J, Ozog DM, Hamzavi IH. Prospective controlled clinical and histopathologic study of hidradenitis suppurativa treated with the long-pulsed neodymium:yttrium-aluminium-garnet laser. J Am Acad Dermatol. 2010;62:637–45.
13. Syed ZU, Hamzavi IH. Photomedicine and phototherapy considerations for patients with skin of color. Photodermatol Photoimmunol Photomed. 2011;27:10.
14. Rambhatla PV, Lim HW, Hamzavi I. A systematic review of treatments for hidradenitis suppurativa. Arch Dermatol. 2012;148:439–46.

Chapter 38
Perioral Dermatitis

Bryan Gammon and Bethanee J. Schlosser

38.1 Introduction

Perioral dermatitis (PD), a common acneiform facial eruption, was first described in the 1950s. The terms "light-sensitive seborrheid" and "steroid-induced rosacea-like dermatitis" were previously used to describe this condition [1, 2]. Given the now recognized periorbital, perinasal, and perioral distribution of lesions, the term periorificial dermatitis may be most appropriate [3].

38.2 Background

The exact etiology and pathogenesis of PD has not been elucidated. However, an association with the use/misuse of topical corticosteroids has been well established. Corticosteroid exposure through intranasal, inhaled, and systemic modes of delivery has also been reported to incite PD [4–8]. Not all cases of PD demonstrate a history of corticosteroid exposure [9].

Other specific environmental factors have not been identified, and patients do not exhibit photosensitivity. Suggestions of microbiologic pathogenesis due to *Candida* species, *Demodex folliculorum*, or fusiform bacteria have not been substantiated. Allergic contact dermatitis to constituents of dentifrices (i.e., fluoride) and cosmetics has been reported as a contributing factor in some cases although rechallenge with these same products after resolution of PD may not consistently incite recurrence of PD.

Although PD has been considered by some to be a variant of acne rosacea, the distribution of inflammatory lesions and absence of persistent background erythema and telangiectasia differentiate PD from acne rosacea.

PD affects both adults and children. Adult PD disproportionately affects females of reproductive age (25–40 years old). Pediatric PD affects both girls only slightly

B. Gammon, M.D. (✉) • B.J. Schlosser, M.D., Ph.D.
Department of Dermatology, Northwestern University, Chicago, IL, USA

J.A. Zeichner (ed.), *Acneiform Eruptions in Dermatology: A Differential Diagnosis*,
DOI 10.1007/978-1-4614-8344-1_38,

more often than boys with onset typically before 5 years old. Pediatric PD in children as young as 6 months has been reported [10]. There appears to be no racial predilection in pediatric or adult PD. PD has been shown to occur in siblings, but genetic predisposition has not been further elucidated [11].

38.3 Clinical Presentation

PD classically presents with erythematous papules, pustules, and occasionally vesicles on a background of variable erythema and fine scaling involving the perioral, periorbital, and perinasal skin (Figs. 38.1 and 38.2a). Inflammatory lesions may be singular or clustered with symmetric or unilateral distribution. Sparing of the skin immediately surrounding (within 5 mm) the vermilion border has been

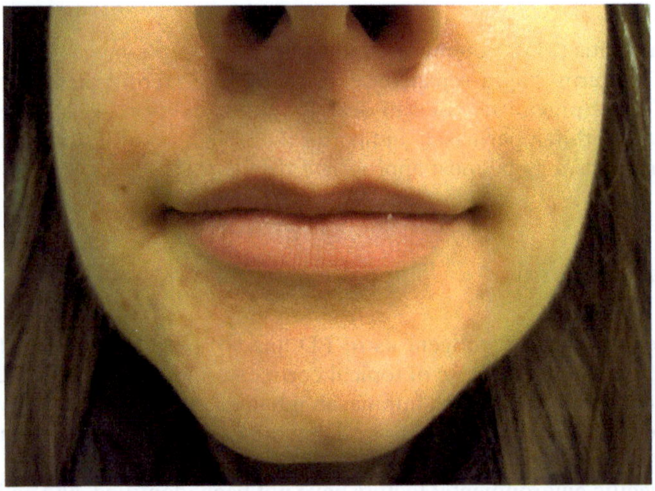

Fig. 38.1 Erythematous papules and pustules on a background of erythema and fine scaling involving the perioral and perinasal skin. Sparing of the skin immediately surrounding the vermilion border

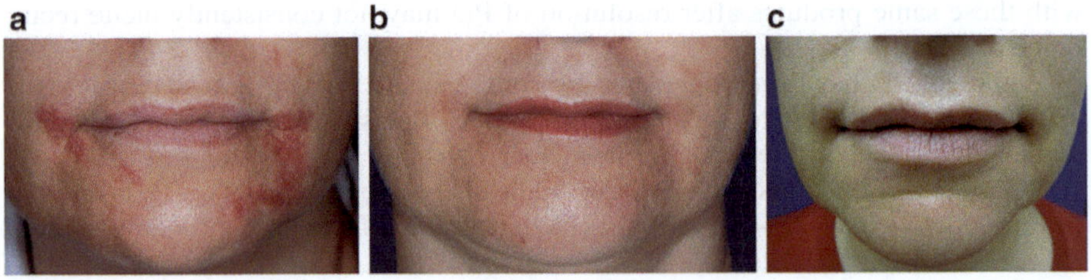

Fig. 38.2 (**a**) A patient at baseline before therapy for perioral dermatitis (**b**) 6 weeks after therapy with oral doxycycline and topical metronidazole for perioral dermatitis (**c**) 12 weeks after therapy with oral doxycycline and topical metronidazole for perioral dermatitis

Table 38.1 Clinical differential diagnosis of perioral dermatitis

Disorder	Distinguishing clinical features
Acne rosacea	Predilection for central face including the nose; background persistent erythema and telangiectasia
Acne vulgaris	Presence of comedones +/– nodulocystic lesions; possible truncal involvement
Allergic contact dermatitis	Rare pustules; potential exposure elicited through history
Cutaneous candidiasis	Concomitant angular cheilitis or intraoral candidiasis; immunocompromised host; +KOH microscopy, fungal culture
Demodex folliculorum infestation (dermatitis, demodicosis, folliculitis)	Associated pruritus; immunocompromised host; +KOH microscopy
Eosinophilic folliculitis	Pruritic papules and pustules; possible upper trunk involvement; immunocompromised (HIV+) host
Gram-negative folliculitis	Predominance of pustules in perioral distribution; history of antibiotic exposure
Impetigo	Pustules and erosions with honey-colored crust; +bacterial culture
Irritant contact dermatitis	Rare pustules; presence of fissures; potential exposure elicited through history
Lupus erythematosus	Malar erythema; absences of pustules; photo-exacerbation; non-facial eruption and systemic symptoms
Sarcoidosis	Firm erythematous to brown papules; +diascopy; multisystem involvement (pulmonary, ocular, musculoskeletal)
Seborrheic dermatitis	Predilection for nasolabial folds; greasy scale; possible scalp, brow and ear involvement
Tinea faciei, tinea incognito, Majocchi's granuloma	+KOH microscopy, fungal culture; possible scalp involvement

Definitions: KOH = potassium hydroxide

noted as a clinical hallmark (Fig. 38.1). Associated burning, stinging, or itching is commonly reported. Granulomatous PD manifests as skin-colored, erythematous, or yellow-brown papules. Exclusive perioral involvement is less common than multisite disease, and PD without perioral lesions (i.e., exclusive perinasal and/or periorbital lesions) is rare [10]. Extrafacial involvement is uncommon, and patients do not exhibit systemic symptoms.

PD is typically self-limited and resolves over several weeks to months. Recurrence is uncommon when corticosteroid exposure is avoided. Scarring is atypical.

The clinical differential diagnosis of PD includes both infectious and noninfectious inflammatory disorders (Table 38.1). A thorough history, clinical examination, review of systems, and simple diagnostic procedures (potassium hydroxide (KOH) microscopy) are usually sufficient to differentiate PD from its mimics. Patients who fail to respond to standard PD treatment or who exhibit an atypical clinical presentation should be reevaluated with additional diagnostic testing as needed.

38.4 Work-Up

The diagnosis of PD is typically rendered based on history and clinical presentation. Laboratory evaluation, biopsy, and microbiologic cultures are usually not performed. A thorough history often reveals preceding or current facial skin corticosteroid exposure, by topical or other routes; rebound exacerbation of the eruption upon cessation of corticosteroid use is characteristic.

Exposure to potential contactants should be investigated in order to differentiate PD from allergic and irritant contact dermatitis; cutaneous patch testing may be helpful [12, 13]. KOH microscopy of skin scrapings may be helpful in differentiating PD from demodicosis, perioral candidiasis, and tinea faciei [14, 15].

PD shows significant histopathologic overlap with acne rosacea. Biopsy of PD typically reveals mild spongiosis of the epidermis and follicular infundibulum with perivascular and perifollicular lymphohistiocytic inflammation in the papillary and superficial reticular dermis [16]. Papillary dermal edema can be seen. Perifollicular granulomas and multinucleate giant cells are sometimes evident, particularly in cases of granulomatous PD [17].

38.5 Treatment

There are no FDA-approved therapies for PD. While the therapeutic armamentarium for the treatment of PD is large, the level of evidence supporting many of the available agents is poor. Two systematic, evidence-based reviews of the literature suggest that some of the strongest evidence supports "zero therapy" for PD, i.e., withdrawal of any offending or exacerbating agents, such as topical or inhaled corticosteroids or cosmetics [18, 19]. Multiple trials have demonstrated that avoidance of topical corticosteroids and cosmetics results in improvement in 4 weeks and resolution within an average of 2–3 months. It is well recognized that continued use of topical corticosteroids and cosmetics prolongs PD regardless of treatment employed.

Cutaneous irritation and sensitivity may limit the utility of topical agents for PD though use of a gentle non-medicated cleanser and moisturizer may reduce this tendency. Topical metronidazole, as monotherapy or in combination with oral antibiotics, has demonstrated efficacy for PD (Fig. 38.2a–c). Use of topical metronidazole gel 0.75 % twice daily in children with PD demonstrated significant improvement after 8 weeks and resolution after 14 weeks [20]. A prospective, randomized, double-blind study comparing metronidazole cream 1 % twice daily with oral tetracycline 250 mg twice daily demonstrated significant reduction in papule number in the metronidazole group and complete resolution in the tetracycline group after 8 weeks [21].

Topical erythromycin may also provide benefit [22]. Topical erythromycin emulsion 2 % twice daily was superior to placebo in clearing papules with an average time to clearance of 7 weeks; topical erythromycin demonstrated similar efficacy to oral tetracycline [23]. A case series reported that 98 % of 700 patients cleared on topical erythromycin [24].

Pimecrolimus has been shown to expedite resolution of PD but may offer limited long-term benefit. Two randomized, placebo-controlled trials of adults with PD independently demonstrated that pimecrolimus cream 1 % twice daily significantly reduced erythema, scaling, and papule number after 2 weeks compared with vehicle. After 4 weeks, however, there was no significant difference between pimecrolimus and vehicle [25, 26].

Oral tetracycline remains the gold standard for the treatment of PD. Randomized controlled trials and large case series support the use of oral tetracycline as a first-line agent [27]. Oral tetracycline (250 mg twice daily) has been shown to be more effective for PD than topical metronidazole or topical erythromycin [21, 23]. Severe perioral dermatitis recalcitrant to erythromycin ointment 2 % has been shown to respond to oral tetracycline [24]. The use of doxycycline or minocycline in PD is supported by case reports and small series [7, 28, 29].

Additional therapeutic options for PD are supported by small, uncontrolled trials or case series which fail to assess whether an agent is more efficacious than zero therapy. Open-label studies of azelaic acid cream 20 % twice daily reported complete clearance within 5–6 weeks [30, 31]. A split-face study using photodynamic therapy (PDT) with 5-aminolevulinic acid showed greater lesion reduction with PDT than topical clindamycin gel 1 % at 1 month (92 % vs. 80 %); photosensitivity and post-inflammatory hyperpigmentation complicated PDT treatment [32]. A retrospective review of 25 patients treated with sodium sulfacetamide/sulfur 10/5 % reported clearance in 14 of 25 (56 %) after an average of 1.2 months of treatment [33]. Limited case reports detail the efficacy adapalene gel 0.1 % and isotretinoin [34, 35].

38.6 Conclusion

Perioral dermatitis is facial dermatosis of unclear etiology, but is frequently associated with preceding corticosteroid use. Patients typically present with erythematous papules around the mouth, nose, and eyes. Treatment should include withdrawal of offending agents including cosmetics and topical corticosteroids. Depending on severity, topical metronidazole or an oral tetracycline should be instituted for at least 8 weeks. Topical erythromycin applied twice daily provides greater benefit than zero therapy. Pimecrolimus cream may promote rapid clearance of PD papules but shows limited efficacy over the long term.

References

1. Frumess GM, Lewis HM. Light-sensitive seborrheid. AMA Arch Dermatol. 1957; 75(2):245–8.
2. Mihan R, Ayres Jr S. Perioral dermatitis. Arch Dermatol. 1964;89:803–5.
3. Kihiczak GG, Cruz MA, Schwartz RA. Periorificial dermatitis in children: an update and description of a child with striking features. Int J Dermatol. 2009;48(3):304–6.
4. Hafeez ZH. Perioral dermatitis: an update. Int J Dermatol. 2003;42(7):514–7.

5. Dubus JC, Marguet C, Deschildre A, et al. Local side-effects of inhaled corticosteroids in asthmatic children: influence of drug, dose, age, and device. Allergy. 2001;56(10):944–8.
6. Poulos GA, Brodell RT. Perioral dermatitis associated with an inhaled corticosteroid. Arch Dermatol. 2007;143(11):1460.
7. Adams SJ, Davison AM, Cunliffe WJ, Giles GR. Perioral dermatitis in renal transplant recipients maintained on corticosteroids and immunosuppressive therapy. Br J Dermatol. 1982;106(5):589–92.
8. Clementson B, Smidt AC. Periorificial dermatitis due to systemic corticosteroids in children: report of two cases. Pediatr Dermatol. 2012;29(3):331–2.
9. Wilkinson DS, Kirton V, Wilkinson JD. Perioral dermatitis: a 12-year review. Br J Dermatol. 1979;101(3):245–57.
10. Nguyen V, Eichenfield LF. Periorificial dermatitis in children and adolescents. J Am Acad Dermatol. 2006;55(5):781–5.
11. Weston WL, Morelli JG. Identical twins with perioral dermatitis. Pediatr Dermatol. 1998;15(2):144.
12. Nedorost ST. Medical pearl—the evaluation of perioral dermatitis: use of an extended patch test series. J Am Acad Dermatol. 2007;56(5 Suppl):S100–2.
13. Arutjunow V. Perioral dermatitis—an allergic disease? Hautarzt. 1978;29(2):89–91.
14. Bradford LG, Montes LF. Perioral dermatitis and *Candida albicans*. Arch Dermatol. 1972; 105(6):892–5.
15. Hsu CK, Hsu MM, Lee JY. Demodicosis: a clinicopathological study. J Am Acad Dermatol. 2009;60(3):453–62.
16. Hogan DJ. Perioral dermatitis. Curr Probl Dermatol. 1995;22:98–104.
17. Urbatsch AJ, Frieden I, Williams ML, Elewski BE, Mancini AJ, Paller AS. Extrafacial and generalized granulomatous periorificial dermatitis. Arch Dermatol. 2002;138(10):1354–8.
18. Hall CS, Reichenberg J. Evidence based review of perioral dermatitis therapy. G Ital Dermatol Venereol. 2010;145(4):433–44.
19. Weber K, Thurmayr R. Critical appraisal of reports on the treatment of perioral dermatitis. Dermatology. 2005;210(4):300–7.
20. Miller SR, Shalita AR. Topical metronidazole gel (0.75%) for the treatment of perioral dermatitis in children. J Am Acad Dermatol. 1994;31(5 Pt 2):847–8.
21. Veien NK, Munkvad JM, Nielsen AO, Niordson AM, Stahl D, Thormann J. Topical metronidazole in the treatment of perioral dermatitis. J Am Acad Dermatol. 1991;24(2 Pt 1):258–60.
22. Bikowski JB. Topical therapy for perioral dermatitis. Cutis. 1983;31(6):678–82.
23. Weber K, Thurmayr R, Meisinger A. A topical erythromycin preparation and oral tetracycline for the treatment of perioral dermatitis: a placebo-controlled trial. J Dermatol Treat. 1993; 4:57–9.
24. Weber K. How I, treat perioral dermatitis: non-compliance with the treatment guidelines. Dermatology. 2003;207(2):215.
25. Oppel T, Pavicic T, Kamann S, Brautigam M, Wollenberg A. Pimecrolimus cream (1%) efficacy in perioral dermatitis—results of a randomized, double-blind, vehicle-controlled study in 40 patients. J Eur Acad Dermatol Venereol. 2007;21(9):1175–80.
26. Schwarz T, Kreiselmaier I, Bieber T, et al. A randomized, double-blind, vehicle-controlled study of 1% pimecrolimus cream in adult patients with perioral dermatitis. J Am Acad Dermatol. 2008;59(1):34–40.
27. Macdonald A, Feiwel M. Perioral dermatitis: aetiology and treatment with tetracycline. Br J Dermatol. 1972;87(4):315–9.
28. Misago N, Nakafusa J, Narisawa Y. Childhood granulomatous periorificial dermatitis: lupus miliaris disseminatus faciei in children? J Eur Acad Dermatol Venereol. 2005;19(4):470–3.
29. Rosso JQ. Management of papulopustular rosacea and perioral dermatitis with emphasis on iatrogenic causation or exacerbation of inflammatory facial dermatoses: use of doxycycline-modified release 40mg capsule once daily in combination with properly selected skin care as an effective therapeutic approach. J Clin Aesthet Dermatol. 2011;4(8):20–30.

30. Jansen T. Azelaic acid as a new treatment for perioral dermatitis: results from an open study. Br J Dermatol. 2004;151(4):933–4.
31. Jansen T, Melnik BC, Schadendorf D. Steroid-induced periorificial dermatitis in children–clinical features and response to azelaic acid. Pediatr Dermatol. 2010;27(2):137–42.
32. Richey DF, Hopson B. Photodynamic therapy for perioral dermatitis. J Drugs Dermatol. 2006;5(2 Suppl):12–6.
33. Bendl BJ. Perioral dermatitis: etiology and treatment. Cutis. 1976;17(5):903–8.
34. Jansen T. Perioral dermatitis successfully treated with topical adapalene. J Eur Acad Dermatol Venereol. 2002;16(2):175–7.
35. Smith KW. Perioral dermatitis with histopathologic features of granulomatous rosacea: successful treatment with isotretinoin. Cutis. 1990;46(5):413–5.

Chapter 39
Photocontact Dermatitis

Nicholas Gulati and Emma Guttman-Yassky

39.1 Introduction

Photocontact dermatitis (PCD) belongs to the category of skin diseases known as photodermatoses, which are skin disorders caused or aggravated by ultraviolet (UV) radiation and/or visible light. PCD is divided into two categories: phototoxic and photoallergic. Phototoxic (photo-irritant) reactions are caused by direct damage to tissue resulting from light activation of the photosensitizing agent without an immunological basis. On the other hand, photoallergic reactions are cell-mediated immune responses in which the antigen is the light-activated photosensitizing agent and these reactions only occur after previous specific sensitization. PCD can be caused by either cutaneous contact or systemic uptake [1]. Chronic actinic dermatitis, a condition which is clinically similar to photodermatitis, can occur both as a sequelae of photoallergic reactions or de novo [2].

39.2 Background

The exact prevalence of PCD in the general population is not known. However, estimates of its frequency have ranged from 7 to 15 % for phototoxicity and 4 to 8 % for photoallergy [3–6].

Common phototoxic agents include coal-tar derivatives, dyes, antiarrhythmics, diuretics, non-steroidal anti-inflammatory drugs (NSAIDs), phenothiazines,

N. Gulati, B.A. (✉)
Laboratory for Investigative Dermatology, The Rockefeller University, 1230 York Ave, New York, NY 10065, USA
e-mail: ngulati@rockefeller.edu

E. Guttman-Yassky, M.D., Ph.D.
Department of Dermatology, Mount Sinai NY, New York, NY, USA

J.A. Zeichner (ed.), *Acneiform Eruptions in Dermatology: A Differential Diagnosis*, DOI 10.1007/978-1-4614-8344-1_39, © Springer Science+Business Media New York 2014

quinolones, tetracyclines, thiazides, sulfonamides, sulfonylureas, and, most commonly, plant-derived furocoumarins including psoralen. When phototoxicity results from exposure to a plant, vegetable, or fruit, the resulting dermatitis is called phytophotodermatitis. Examples of vegetables/fruits causing phytophotodermatitis include limes, figs, and parsley [7–9].

Photoallergic agents frequently encountered are sunscreens, fragrances, antibacterials, and NSAIDs [10]. UV filters used in sunscreens which commonly act as sensitizers include isopropyl dibenzoylmethane (now off the market), benzophenone-3, benzophenone-10, butyl methoxydibenzoyl-methane, oxybenzone, and *p*-aminobenzoic acid (PABA) [11, 12]. The UVB filter octyl methoxycinnamate, on the other hand, rarely produces photoallergic reactions [13]. Ketoprofen, an NSAID, although not commonly used topically, has been found to cause 82 % of contact photoallergies in a large retrospective study [14]. However, the relative potency of different agents to cause PCD is not well studied. This information is difficult to ascertain in the general population because most studies consider only the people who seek medical attention for preexisting skin conditions [15].

PCD is caused by compounds which absorb specific wavelengths of light (absorption spectrum). This spectrum usually approximates the wavelengths which lead to the clinical reaction (action spectrum). Most phototoxic sensitizers have action spectrums in the UV range but some are in the visible light range.

Phototoxic reactions are thought to be mediated through generation of oxygen free radicals, superoxide anions, hydroxyl radicals, and singlet oxygen, which in turn causes cytotoxic effects. Different phototoxic agents act at various cell sites such as the nucleus or cell membrane. There is also variety in the way different people handle drugs, thus potentially accounting for the range of susceptibilities to these reactions [16].

Although the exact mechanism of photoallergy is unknown, it is thought to involve an exogenous low molecular weight compound (hapten) combining with an endogenous protein only in the presence of UV or visible light in order to create an antigenic conjugate. This conjugate can then lead to a delayed-type hypersensitivity response in the skin and therefore the clinical appearance of dermatitis. In support of this theory, the photoallergen tetrachlorosalicylanilide has been shown to bind non-covalently to human serum albumin. However, upon irradiation with UV light, a covalently bound conjugate is formed [17]. Photoconjugates such as this are able to induce photoallergic responses when injected into guinea pigs [18].

The presumed initial step in the induction of delayed-type hypersensitivity is the uptake of applied hapten by antigen-presenting cells (APCs) such as Langerhans cells [19, 20]. Next, these APCs migrate to the local draining lymph nodes where they stimulate the proliferation of antigen-specific T cells [21, 22].

Uptake by APCs (in the context of photoallergy) is made easier by cell apoptosis, a process which could also explain the phototoxic capabilities of certain chemicals. To this end, several agents known to cause photoallergy and/or phototoxicity have been found to preferentially induce keratinocyte apoptosis upon irradiation with UVA light as compared to no irradiation [23].

39.3 Clinical Presentation

Phototoxic reactions are similar in appearance to a sunburn, exhibiting erythema, edema, stinging, and burning in areas exposed to the sun (Fig. 39.1). Sometimes, vesicles, bullae, and onycholysis are observed. Phototoxic agents might also occasionally cause delayed reactions with manifestations occurring after hours or several days. Symptoms resolve spontaneously with hyperpigmentation (due to stimulation of melanin synthesis) and desquamation over a time course of days to weeks; the eruption is rarely persistent [24].

Acute lesions of photoallergic reactions are limited to sun-exposed skin which has been in contact with the photoallergen. Patients usually present with pruritus and eczematous dermatitis with bullae and vesicles being rare. On repeated contact, lichenification occurs. In some cases, spreading to covered sites is possible as UVA-mediated reactions can occur under thin clothing [25].

PCD can present with variable severity depending on many factors such as the amount of the photosensitizer and the location, the nature of the activating radiation, thickness of the horny layer, degree of melanin pigmentation, and immunological status. Phototoxic and photoallergic reactions can be difficult to discriminate clinically, but there are several useful characteristics that can serve to distinguish the two. For example, phototoxic reactions can occur upon first exposure while photoallergic reactions require previous sensitization. Also, photoallergic reactions may "flare"

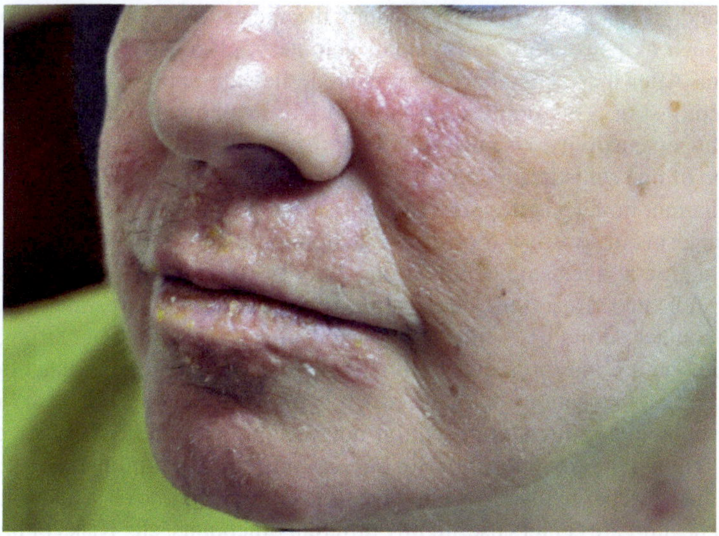

Fig. 39.1 Erythematous, tender plaques on the face that developed after application of a sunscreen and exposure to UV light outside. The robust photocontact dermatitis became secondarily infected, with the development of yellow crusted plaques (Photo credit: Joshua A. Zeichner, M.D.)

at distant previously involved sites while phototoxic reactions do not. Furthermore, the concentration of allergen required for a photoallergic reaction is often lower than that needed for a phototoxic reaction [26].

39.4 Work-Up

To diagnose PCD, it is necessary to question possible exposure to various photosensitizers such as medications, cosmetics, fragrances, and plant extracts. In order to distinguish PCD from the commoner allergic contact dermatitis, it is essential to validate a history of UV or visible light exposure. A valuable diagnostic clue is preferential involvement of photoexposed sites with relative sparing of shadow sites within the scalp, under the chin and nose, behind the ears, and around the eyes. Skin lesions usually develop in the spring or summer seasons due to high levels of sun exposure.

On histological examination, phototoxic reactions are characterized by sporadic necrotic keratinocytes with lymphocytic and neutrophilic dermal infiltrates. Despite causing a sunburn-like dermatitis, phototoxic reactions occur upon exposure to UV doses normally well-tolerated by the individual as opposed to the overdoses of UV radiation which lead to sunburn. The histological appearance of photoallergic reactions resembles an allergic contact dermatitis reaction. This includes parakeratosis, irregular acanthosis, and spongiosis as well as a lymphocytic infiltrate with some eosinophils in the dermis [27].

Key to the investigation of PCD is the photopatch test, a tool conceptually similar to the standard patch test. In this procedure, the agents to be tested are prepared in a vehicle such as petrolatum and a small volume is placed within plastic or metal chambers. After these chambers are prepared, they are applied in duplicate sets to the patient's skin. This duplication is important as photoallergens can also cause contact hypersensitivity. Usually after 48 h, the chambers are removed and the skin at the site of one set is irradiated with a light source. Then, usually at 24–72 h from the irradiation, both test sites are visually inspected and any observed reactions are graded in terms of severity. A positive reaction is defined as erythema, edema, and/or vesiculation at a test site. If this occurs only at the irradiated site, a diagnosis of PCD is indicated. Reactions equally positive at both sites are interpreted as an allergic contact dermatitis while reactions positive at both sites but stronger at the irradiated one are interpreted as both allergic and photoallergic contact dermatitis [28]. Having observations over several timepoints (i.e., 48 and 72 h) is useful because photoallergic reactions exhibit delayed onsets with courses increasing in severity while phototoxic reactions peak early on and then diminish.

The many steps involved in photopatch testing are not well standardized, and different health-care centers use slightly different timepoints, etc. Risks of photopatch testing include inadvertent sensitization to test materials, discomfort at test sites, "flares" at previously involved sites, and persistent hyperpigmentation at test sites.

39.5 Treatment

Individuals with acute PCD reactions including erythema and edema may find relief with ice-cold compresses of Burow's solution in a 1:10 dilution. For acute phototoxic reactions, aspirin or other NSAIDs can be used. Alternatively, for generalized cases, systemic corticosteroid therapy may provide prompt symptomatic relief.

The mainstay of treatment of PCD is avoidance of the offending agents as well as appropriate photoprotection. Protective clothing such as long-sleeved shirts and hats should be worn and sunscreens should be applied (provided they are not the offending agent) [29]. As needed, changes in lifestyle including avoidance of midday sun as well as alterations in leisure and occupational activities may be recommended. Special UV-absorbing plastic can be installed over windows and windscreens to improve photoprotection. For chronic cases that only respond to systemic corticosteroids and which have high morbidity, immunosuppressive agents such as azathioprine can be used [30].

39.6 Conclusion

Photocontact dermatitis is an inflammatory, facial dermatosis as a result of an immune-mediated or directly toxic reaction from an exogenous source. Correct diagnosis is important for proper management of the acute flare and prevention of future recurrences.

References

1. Lehmann P. Diagnostic approach to photodermatoses. J Dtsch Dermatol Ges. 2006;4(11):965–75.
2. Hawk JLM. Chronic actinic dermatitis. Photodermatol Photoimmunol Photomed. 2004;20(6):312–4.
3. Fotiades J, Soter NA, Lim HW. Results of evaluation of 203 patients for photosensitivity in a 7.3-year period. J Am Acad Dermatol. 1995;33(4):597–602.
4. Selvaag E. Clinical drug photosensitivity. A retrospective analysis of reports to the Norwegian Adverse Drug Reactions Committee from the years 1970–1994. Photodermatol Photoimmunol Photomed. 1997;13(1–2):21–3.
5. Crouch RB, Foley PA, Baker CS. Analysis of patients with suspected photosensitivity referred for investigation to an Australian photodermatology clinic. J Am Acad Dermatol. 2003;48(5):714–20.
6. Wong SN, Khoo LSW. Analysis of photodermatoses seen in a predominantly Asian population at a photodermatology clinic in Singapore. Photodermatol Photoimmunol Photomed. 2005;21(1):40–4.
7. Wagner AM, Wu JJ, Hansen RC, Nigg HN, Beiere RC. Bullous phytophotodermatitis associated with high natural concentrations of furanocoumarins in limes. Am J Contact Dermatitis. 2002;13(1):10–4.

8. Polat M, Oztas P, Dikilitas MC, Alli N. Phytophotodermatitis due to Ficus carica. Dermatol Online J. 2008;14(12):9.
9. Lagey K, Duinslaeger L, Vanderkelen A. Burns induced by plants. Burns. 1995;21(7):542–3.
10. Bylaite M, Grigaitiene J, Lapinskaite GS. Photodermatoses: classification, evaluation and management. Br J Dermatol. 2009;161 Suppl 3:61–8.
11. Schauder S, Ippen H. Contact and photocontact sensitivity to sunscreens. Review of a 15-year experience and of the literature. Contact Derm. 1997;37(5):221–32.
12. Szczurko C, Dompmartin A, Michel M, Moreau A, Leroy D. Photocontact allergy to oxybenzone: ten years of experience. Photodermatol Photoimmunol Photomed. 1994;10(4):144–7.
13. Darvay A, White IR, Rycroft RJ, et al. Photoallergic contact dermatitis is uncommon. Br J Dermatol. 2001;145(4):597–601.
14. Diaz RL, Gardeazabal J, Manrique P, et al. Greater allergenicity of topical ketoprofen in contact dermatitis confirmed by use. Contact Derm. 2006;54(5):239–43.
15. Agin PP, Ruble K, Hermansky SJ, McCarthy TJ. Rates of allergic sensitization and irritation to oxybenzone-containing sunscreen products: a quantitative meta-analysis of 64 exaggerated use studies. Photodermatol Photoimmunol Photomed. 2008;24(4):211–7.
16. Ferguson J. Photosensitivity due to drugs. Photodermatol Photoimmunol Photomed. 2002; 18(5):262–9.
17. Kochevar IE, Harber LC. Photoreactions of 3,3',4',5-tetrachlorosalicylanilide with proteins. J Invest Dermatol. 1977;68(3):151–6.
18. Pendlington RU, Barratt MD. Molecular basis of photocontact allergy. Int J Cosmet Sci. 1990;12(2):91–103.
19. Atarashi K, Kabashima K, Akiyama K, Tokura Y. Stimulation of Langerhans cells with ketoprofen plus UVA in murine photocontact dermatitis to ketoprofen. J Dermatol Sci. 2007; 47(2):151–9.
20. Miyachi Y, Takigawa M. Mechanisms of contact photosensitivity in mice: II. Langerhans cells are required for successful induction of contact photosensitivity to TCSA. J Invest Dermatol. 1982;78(5):363–5.
21. Gerberick GF, Ryan CA, Von Bargen EC, Stuard SB, Ridder GM. Examination of tetrachlorosalicylanilide (TCSA) photoallergy using in vitro photohapten-modified Langerhans cell-enriched epidermal cells. J Invest Dermatol. 1991;97(2):210–8.
22. Gerberick GF, Ryan CA, Fletcher ER, Howard AD, Robinson MK. Increased number of dendritic cells in draining lymph nodes accompanies the generation of contact photosensitivity. J Invest Dermatol. 1991;96(3):355–61.
23. Kurita M, Shimauchi T, Kobayashi M, et al. Induction of keratinocyte apoptosis by photosensitizing chemicals plus UVA. J Dermatol Sci. 2007;45(2):105–12.
24. Epstein JH. Phototoxicity and photoallergy. Semin Cutan Med Surg. 1999;18(4):274–84.
25. Lankerani L, Baron ED. Photosensitivity to exogenous agents. J Cutan Med Surg. 2004; 8(6):424–31.
26. Stein KR, Scheinfeld NS. Drug-induced photoallergic and phototoxic reactions. Expert Opin Drug Saf. 2007;6(4):431–43.
27. Hölzle E, Lehmann P, Neumann N. Phototoxic and photoallergic reactions. J Dtsch Dermatol Ges. 2009;7(7):643–9.
28. Anon X. Photopatch testing—methods and indications. British Photodermatology Group. Br J Dermatol. 1997;36(3):371–6.
29. Fourtanier A, Moyal D, Seité S. Sunscreens containing the broad-spectrum UVA absorber, Mexoryl SX, prevent the cutaneous detrimental effects of UV exposure: a review of clinical study results. Photodermatol Photoimmunol Photomed. 2008;24(4):164–74.
30. Yap LM, Foley P, Crouch R, Baker C. Chronic actinic dermatitis: a retrospective analysis of 44 cases referred to an Australian photobiology clinic. Australas J Dermatol. 2003; 44(4):256–62.

Chapter 40
Post-inflammatory Pigment Alteration

Rajiv I. Nijhawan and Andrew F. Alexis

40.1 Introduction

Post-inflammatory pigment alteration is a common sequela of acne vulgaris in darker skin types (Fitzpatrick skin phototypes IV–VI). Acne-associated dyschromia contributes considerably to the psychological and emotional distress experienced by acne patients and can often be of greater concern to the patient than the acne itself [1–3]. Post-inflammatory hyperpigmentation is seen much more frequently than post-inflammatory hypopigmentation; however, it is important to keep in mind that in addition to acne itself, various acne treatments can cause hyper- or hypopigmentation as a result of irritation.

40.2 Background

Post-inflammatory pigment alteration especially hyperpigmentation is a common presenting concern, especially in acne patients [4, 5]. In a hospital-based dermatology practice in New York City, dyschromia was the second most common presenting diagnosis second to acne in black patients [5]. Of note, in another study, 65.3 % of African-Americans, 52.7 % of Hispanics, and 47.4 % percent of Asians all had hyperpigmented macules secondary to acne [6]. While the multifactorial pathogenesis of acne appears to be the same in all skin types and ethnic populations [1], the innate qualities of each patient such as skin color and sensitivity to inflammation markedly individualizes this disease. The differences in skin color are attributed to the varying degrees of epidermal density and distribution of the melanin, activity of

R.I. Nijhawan, M.D. • A.F. Alexis, M.D., M.P.H. (✉)
Department of Dermatology, St. Luke's-Roosevelt Hospital Center, 1090 Amsterdam Avenue, Suite 11B, New York, NY 10025, USA
e-mail: alexisderm@yahoo.com

J.A. Zeichner (ed.), *Acneiform Eruptions in Dermatology: A Differential Diagnosis*,
DOI 10.1007/978-1-4614-8344-1_40, © Springer Science+Business Media New York 2014

the enzyme tyrosinase, variations in number, size, and groupings of the melanosomes, as well as the efficiency of melanosome transfer to keratinocyte [7–10].

A key characteristic in skin of color is the tendency for melanocytes to exhibit labile responses to inflammation and injury [11, 12], which contributes to the high prevalence of post-inflammatory hyperpigmentation in darker skin types. Inflammatory mediators, including prostaglandins and leukotrienes, can stimulate increased melanin synthesis, which can lead to increased pigment in the epidermis alone or also in the dermis [13]. When there is dermal involvement, there is disruption of the basal layer that leads to macrophages engulfing the melanin and the formation of melanophages. In addition, a study by Halder et al. examined biopsies in thirty black patients with acne vulgaris and found the presence of inflammation histologically even in clinically noninflammatory lesions such as comedones. In addition, papules and pustules displayed considerable inflammation histologically that extended significantly beyond the margins of each lesion [14]. While subclinical inflammation is likely a feature of acne vulgaris in all skin types, it may contribute to the tendency toward dyschromias in acne patients with skin of color [2].

40.3 Clinical Presentation

Post-inflammatory hyperpigmentation (PIH) from acneiform lesions appears as macules or patches of darker skin color in contrast to the patient's natural skin color (see Fig. 40.1). With dermal deposition of melanin, the duration of the hyperpigmentation

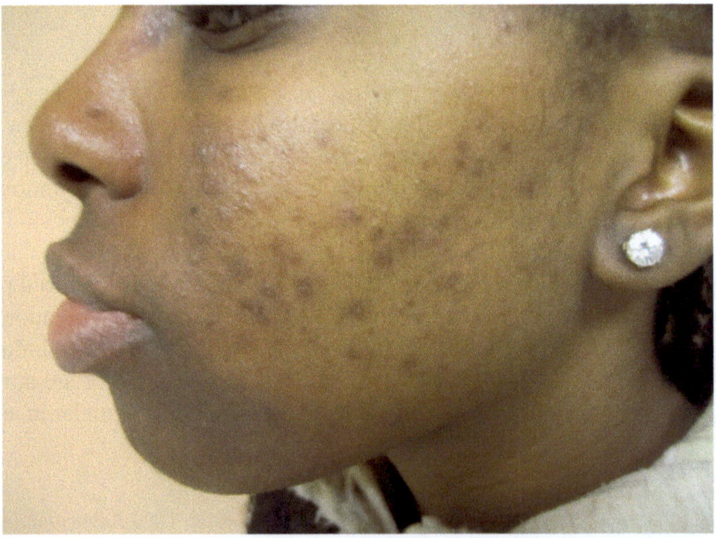

Fig. 40.1 An African-American woman with Fitzpatrick skin type VI and severe post-inflammatory hyperpigmentation associated with acne vulgaris

is prolonged and can last several months to years. Hypopigmentation can also be seen in acne patients as a sequela of irritant dermatitis from topical acne therapies. It can also be seen with the use of skin lightening agents to lighten PIH, typically presenting with perilesional halos of hypopigmentation.

40.4 Work-Up

Post-inflammatory pigment alteration from acne is generally a clinical diagnosis based on medical history and examination without need for laboratory tests, biopsies, or culture. Wood's lamp examination may assist the clinician in assessing the location of pigment involved as is used in melasma. Increased epidermal melanin usually enhances with Wood's lamp examination, whereas dermal pigment does not, though a mixed pattern can be noted [15]. It is important to be mindful of the potential for minocycline-induced pigmentation to mimic acne-associated PIH; however, the bluish gray pigment, the tendency to develop within preexisting scars, and frequent involvement of the mucous membranes and nail beds are distinguishing characteristics.

40.5 Treatment

One of the hallmarks of post-inflammatory hyperpigmentation management is sun protection with broad-spectrum sunscreens including physical blockers to prevent both ultraviolet and visible light induced melanogenesis [16] as well as wearing wide-brimmed hats and adhering to overall sun avoidance. Education regarding sunscreen use is especially important in patients with darker skin types (i.e., multiracial, Hispanic, black) since they are less likely to apply sunscreen when compared to non-Hispanic whites [17]. Cosmetic camouflage can be a useful adjunct. In regard to hyperpigmentation specific treatments, topical agents attempt to interfere with the enzymatic processes of melanin production, especially the rate-limiting enzyme tyrosinase. A combination of modalities is often needed for optimal management (see Table 40.1) [18].

Because of the often disfiguring nature of post-inflammatory hyperpigmentation, patients often attempt to self-treat these hyperpigmented areas with over-the-counter, herbal, and prescription fading, lightening, and bleaching agents from beauty supply stores and various pharmacies before even seeing a dermatologist. Hydroquinone (1,4 dihydroxybenzene), a tyrosinase inhibitor, is one of the most widely used bleaching agents. Branded and generic formulations are available in concentrations of 2–4 %, although higher concentrations can be compounded by specialty pharmacists [19]. The efficacy of hydroquinone, a first-line therapy for hyperpigmentation for close to 50 years [13], can be enhanced with consistent use broad-spectrum sun protection [20]. The most common side effects with use of

Table 40.1 Management options for post-inflammatory hyperpigmentation

Mainstay
• Broad-spectrum sunscreens
• Avoidance of intense sun exposure
• Early aggressive anti-inflammatory treatment of acne vulgaris to prevent development of dyschromias
• Tincture of time (spontaneous resolution of PIH with adequate control of primary inflammatory disorder)
Adjunctive therapies
• Cosmetic camouflage
• Topical skin lightening agents (hydroquinone, azelaic acid, cosmeceuticals)
• Topical retinoids
• Chemical peels (superficial)
• Microdermabrasion

hydroquinone are the risks of a "halo" of hypopigmentation on perilesional skin, irritant contact dermatitis (which must be monitored closely as this can potentiate post-inflammatory pigment alteration), and rarely exogenous ochronosis. The hypopigmented "halo" can be minimized by instructing patients to apply the bleaching agent using a cotton swab only to the darker areas to minimize the application on normal skin. When it does occur, hydroquinone application to the affected area(s) should be discontinued until repigmentation ensues, typically within several weeks.

Additional topical agents have also become mainstays of post-inflammatory hyperpigmentation management. Multiple studies have evidenced the efficacy of topical retinoids, not only for the management of acneiform eruptions themselves, but also for dyschromias [21–23]. Proposed mechanisms of topical retinoids for the improvement of hyperpigmentation include inhibition of tyrosinase induction in melanocytes, enhancement of desquamation that speed up sloughing of melanin in keratinocytes, inhibition of melanosome transfer from melanocytes to keratinocytes, allowing greater penetration of other active ingredients, and redistribution or dispersion of epidermal melanin [24, 25]. Clinicians must also be aware of the potential of topical retinoids to induce irritation that could also potentially potentiate post-inflammatory pigment alteration [22].

Studies of dual or triple agent combination therapies that may include a topical retinoid, hydroquinone, and a topical corticosteroid in comparison to single agents have shown to be more effective with a more rapid response in pigment disorders [26–31]. In a multicentered, investigator blinded, randomized study of 792 patients with post-inflammatory hyperpigmentation secondary to acne vulgaris that compared triple combination cream (fluocinolone acetonide 0.01 %, hydroquinone 4 %, and tretinoin 0.05 %) to each of its dyads, results indicated more patients treated with triple therapy for 8 weeks achieved clear or almost clear status than any of the dyad comparators [30]. Other therapeutic considerations for dyschromia include products containing azelaic acid, kojic acid, and glycolic acid [32–34].

Cosmeceuticals have become increasingly popular for consumers interested in hyperpigmentation remedies. Certain ingredients in these products have been subject to or are currently being evaluated in blinded controlled studies including soy, liquiritin (licorice extract), *N*-acetylglucosamine, niacinamide, mequinol (4-hydroxyanisole), vitamin C (ascorbic acid), oligopeptide, rucinol, tranexamic acid, and *N*-undecyl-10-enoyl-L-phenylalanine [19, 35–38]. Products that include soy or nicotinamide prevent melanosome transfer [39–41], while hydroquinone, arbutin, licorice, azelaic acid, and kojic acid inhibit tyrosinase [39]. Newer combination formulations such as emblica, kojic acid, and glycolic acid (Skinceuticals); lipo-hydoxy acid, glycolic acid, and kojic acid (La Roche-Posay); and kojic acid, licorice extract, and vitamin C (Neostrata) may also be useful adjuncts to the treatment of PIH. Potential emerging products for pigment disorders include grape seed extract, ellagic acid, linoleic acid, aleosin, green tea extracts, and lignin peroxidase [39, 42, 43]. While topical therapies are usually the initial approach to the treatment of post-inflammatory hyperpigmentation, physical therapies, such as chemical peels and microdermabrasion, may also be used as adjuncts to improve treatment outcomes.

Superficial chemical peels such as salicylic acid (20–30 %), glycolic acid (20–70 %), trichloroacetic acid [TCA] (10–25 %), and Jessner's solution as an adjunctive approach with topical agents may help improve hyperpigmentation by removing excess epidermal melanin and enhancing penetration of topical bleaching agents [39]. Various studies have reported that the addition of serial glycolic acid chemical peels to a topical regimen is beneficial for the treatment of hyperpigmentation from melasma with a trend toward more rapid and greater improvement [44–46], and this approach can similarly be applied to post-inflammatory hyperpigmentation. Burns et al. specifically studied this hyperpigmentation in nineteen patients with darker skin and found a trend toward more rapid and greater improvement when six serial glycolic acid peels were added to a topical regimen of 2 % hydroquinone/10 % glycolic acid gel twice daily as well as tretinoin 0.05 % cream at bedtime in comparison to those who only maintained the topical regimen without receiving the chemical peels [47].

In regard to serial salicylic acid peels, a study of 35 Korean patients receiving 30 % salicylic acid peels biweekly for 12 weeks found this to be a safe and effective therapy for acne in Asian patients [48]. However, there is limited evidence and some conflicting data regarding the efficacy of salicylic acid peels in the treatment of post-inflammatory hyperpigmentation [49–51], thus larger systemized studies are needed to better assess the utility of salicylic acid peels in post-inflammatory hyperpigmentation. When peels are performed on darker skin types, a conservative approach with slow titration of acid concentration is recommended to avoid adverse effects such as persistent redness, crusting, and pigmentary abnormalities. Discontinuation of topical retinoids 1 week prior to the chemical peel as well as application of sunscreen immediately following the chemical peel helps to minimize the risk of pigmentary complications following chemical peels.

While there is an increasing amount of literature on chemical peels for dyschromias, there is limited literature on photodynamic and other light-/laser-based therapies in the management of post-inflammatory hyperpigmentation [1, 19, 52]. Lasers are unpredictable in the treatment of hyperpigmentation and therefore are usually reserved for failures of combination topical therapy and chemical peels.

If considered, skin type should always be taken into account given the high risk of post-inflammatory hyperpigmentation [32]. While fractional nonablative lasers may be useful for hyperpigmentation, optimal treatment parameters for dyschromias in skin of color have not been well established and treatment outcomes are unpredictable; however, lower treatment levels and prophylactic use of hydroquinone both before and after laser treatment are recommended to minimize post-treatment hyperpigmentation [53–55].

Post-inflammatory hyperpigmentation secondary to acne vulgaris can be an extremely challenging process to manage, and thus the prevention of such lesions is paramount with early intervention and meticulous sun protection. Anti-inflammatory agents (including systemic therapies where appropriate) should be initiated as early as possible in patients prone to post-inflammatory hyperpigmentation [56]. Combination therapies with the addition of lightening agents have shown to be beneficial, and chemical peels can be considered as second-line approaches. New therapeutic agents, however, are needed including alternatives to hydroquinone and improved strategies for the treatment of resistant dermal pigmentation.

References

1. Davis EC, Callender VD. A review of acne in ethnic skin: pathogenesis, clinical manifestations, and management strategies. J Clin Aesthet Dermatol. 2010;3(4):24–38. PubMed PMID: 20725545. Pubmed Central PMCID: 2921746. Epub 2010/08/21. eng.
2. Alexis AF. Acne in patients with skin of color. J Drugs Dermatol. 2011;10(6):s13–6. PubMed PMID: 21780341. Epub 2011/07/26. eng.
3. Shah SK, Alexis AF. Acne in skin of color: practical approaches to treatment. J Dermatolog Treat. 2010;21(3):206–11. PubMed PMID: 20132053. Epub 2010/02/06. eng.
4. Halder RM. Hair and scalp disorders in blacks. Cutis. 1983;32(4):378–80. PubMed PMID: 6226494. Epub 1983/10/01. eng.
5. Alexis AF, Sergay AB, Taylor SC. Common dermatologic disorders in skin of color: a comparative practice survey. Cutis. 2007;80(5):387–94. PubMed PMID: 18189024. Epub 2008/01/15. eng.
6. Taylor SC, Cook-Bolden F, Rahman Z, Strachan D. Acne vulgaris in skin of color. J Am Acad Dermatol. 2002;46(2 Suppl Understanding):S98–106. PubMed PMID: 11807471. Epub 2002/01/25. eng.
7. Iozumi K, Hoganson GE, Pennella R, Everett MA, Fuller BB. Role of tyrosinase as the determinant of pigmentation in cultured human melanocytes. J Invest Dermatol. 1993;100(6):806–11. PubMed PMID: 8496620. Epub 1993/06/01. eng.
8. Staricco RJ, Pinkus H. Quantitative and qualitative data on the pigment cells of adult human epidermis. J Invest Dermatol. 1957;28(1):33–45. PubMed PMID: 13416674. Epub 1957/01/01. eng.
9. Seiji M, Shimao K, Birbeck MS, Fitzpatrick TB. Subcellular localization of melanin biosynthesis. Ann N Y Acad Sci. 1963;100:497–533. PubMed PMID: 13992624. Epub 1963/02/15. eng.
10. Jimbow K, Quevedo Jr WC, Fitzpatrick TB, Szabo G. Some aspects of melanin biology: 1950–1975. J Invest Dermatol. 1976;67(1):72–89. PubMed PMID: 819593. Epub 1976/07/01. eng.
11. Ruiz-Maldonado R, Orozco-Covarrubias ML. Postinflammatory hypopigmentation and hyperpigmentation. Semin Cutan Med Surg. 1997;16(1):36–43. PubMed PMID: 9125764. Epub 1997/03/01. eng.

12. Grimes PE, Stockton T. Pigmentary disorders in blacks. Dermatol Clin. 1988;6(2):271–81. PubMed PMID: 3378372. Epub 1988/04/01. eng.
13. Grimes PE. Management of hyperpigmentation in darker racial ethnic groups. Semin Cutan Med Surg. 2009;28(2):77–85. PubMed PMID: 19608057. Epub 2009/07/18. eng.
14. Halder R, Holmes Y, Bridgeman-Shah S, Kligman A. A clinical pathological study of acne vulgaris in black females. J Invest Dermatol. 1996;106(4):888.
15. Gilchrest BA, Fitzpatrick TB, Anderson RR, Parrish JA. Localization of malanin pigmentation in the skin with Wood's lamp. Br J Dermatol. 1977;96(3):245–8. PubMed PMID: 857837. Epub 1977/03/01. eng.
16. Pathak MA, Riley FC, Fitzpatrick TB. Melanogenesis in human skin following exposure to long-wave ultraviolet and visible light. J Invest Dermatol. 1962;39:435–43. PubMed PMID: 13941837. Epub 1962/11/01. eng.
17. Summers P, Bena J, Arrigain S, Alexis AF, Cooper K, Bordeaux JS. Sunscreen use: Non-Hispanic Blacks compared with other racial and/or ethnic groups. Arch Dermatol. 2011;147(7):863–4. PubMed PMID: 21768492. Epub 2011/07/20. eng.
18. Alexis AF, Lamb A. Concomitant therapy for acne in patients with skin of color: a case-based approach. Dermatol Nurs. 2009;1:33–6. PubMed PMID: 19283960. Epub 2009/03/17. eng.
19. Sheth VM, Pandya AG. Melasma: a comprehensive update Part II. J Am Acad Dermatol. 2011;65(4):699–714. PubMed PMID: 21920242. Epub 2011/09/17. eng.
20. Vazquez M, Sanchez JL. The efficacy of a broad-spectrum sunscreen in the treatment of melasma. Cutis. 1983;32(1):92, 95–6. PubMed PMID: 6349944. Epub 1983/07/01. eng.
21. Bulengo-Ransby SM, Griffiths CE, Kimbrough-Green CK, Finkel LJ, Hamilton TA, Ellis CN, et al. Topical tretinoin (retinoic acid) therapy for hyperpigmented lesions caused by inflammation of the skin in black patients. N Engl J Med. 1993;328(20):1438–43. PubMed PMID: 8479462. Epub 1993/05/20. eng.
22. Grimes P, Callender V. Tazarotene cream for postinflammatory hyperpigmentation and acne vulgaris in darker skin: a double-blind, randomized, vehicle-controlled study. Cutis. 2006;77(1):45–50. PubMed PMID: 16475496. Epub 2006/02/16. eng.
23. Dogra S, Kanwar AJ, Parsad D. Adapalene in the treatment of melasma: a preliminary report. J Dermatol. 2002;29(8):539–40. PubMed PMID: 12227492. Epub 2002/09/14. eng.
24. Romero C, Aberdam E, Larnier C, Ortonne JP. Retinoic acid as modulator of UVB-induced melanocyte differentiation. Involvement of the melanogenic enzymes expression. J Cell Sci. 1994;107(Pt 4):1095–103. PubMed PMID: 8056833. Epub 1994/04/01. eng.
25. Ortonne JP. Retinoid therapy of pigmentary disorders. Dermatol Ther. 2006;19(5):280–8. PubMed PMID: 17014483. Epub 2006/10/04. eng.
26. Taylor SC, Torok H, Jones T, Lowe N, Rich P, Tschen E, et al. Efficacy and safety of a new triple-combination agent for the treatment of facial melasma. Cutis. 2003;72(1):67–72. PubMed PMID: 12889718. Epub 2003/08/02. eng.
27. Grimes PE. A microsponge formulation of hydroquinone 4% and retinol 0.15% in the treatment of melasma and postinflammatory hyperpigmentation. Cutis. 2004;74(6):362–8.
28. Kligman AM, Willis I. A new formula for depigmenting human skin. Arch Dermatol. 1975;111(1):40–8. PubMed PMID: 1119822. Epub 1975/01/01. eng.
29. Lynde CB, Kraft JN, Lynde CW. Topical treatments for melasma and postinflammatory hyperpigmentation. Skin Therapy Lett. 2006;11(9):1–6. PubMed PMID: 17075653. Epub 2006/11/01. eng.
30. Baumann L, Grimes P, Pandya AG, et al. Triple combination cream is an effective treatment for post-inflammatory hyperpigmentation. Presented at the 65th Annual American Academy of Dermatology Conference, Washington, DC, 3–5 Feb 2007
31. Guevara IL, Pandya AG. Melasma treated with hydroquinone, tretinoin, and a fluorinated steroid. Int J Dermatol. 2001;40(3):212–5. PubMed PMID: 11422530.
32. Rendon M, Berneburg M, Arellano I, Picardo M. Treatment of melasma. J Am Acad Dermatol. 2006;54(5 Suppl 2):S272–81. PubMed PMID: 16631968. Epub 2006/04/25. eng.
33. Gupta AK, Gover MD, Nouri K, Taylor S. The treatment of melasma: a review of clinical trials. J Am Acad Dermatol. 2006;55(6):1048–65. PubMed PMID: 17097400. Epub 2006/11/14. eng.

34. Kircik LH. Efficacy and safety of azelaic acid (AzA) gel 15% in the treatment of post-inflammatory hyperpigmentation and acne: a 16-week, baseline-controlled study. J Drugs Dermatol. 2011;10(6):586–90. PubMed PMID: 21637899. Epub 2011/06/04. eng.
35. Woolery-Lloyd H, Friedman A. Optimizing patient care with "natural" products: treatment of hyperpigmentation. J Drugs Dermatol. 2009;8(6 Suppl):s10–3. PubMed PMID: 19562884. Epub 2009/07/01. eng.
36. Hantash BM, Jimenez F. A split-face, double-blind, randomized and placebo-controlled pilot evaluation of a novel oligopeptide for the treatment of recalcitrant melasma. J Drugs Dermatol. 2009;8(8):732–5. PubMed PMID: 19663110. Epub 2009/08/12. eng.
37. Khemis A, Kaiafa A, Queille-Roussel C, Duteil L, Ortonne JP. Evaluation of efficacy and safety of rucinol serum in patients with melasma: a randomized controlled trial. Br J Dermatol. 2007;156(5):997–1004. PubMed PMID: 17388924. Epub 2007/03/29. eng.
38. Maeda K, Naganuma M. Topical trans-4-aminomethylcyclohexanecarboxylic acid prevents ultraviolet radiation-induced pigmentation. J Photochem Photobiol B. 1998;47(2–3):136–41. PubMed PMID: 10093913. Epub 1999/03/27. eng.
39. Briganti S, Camera E, Picardo M. Chemical and instrumental approaches to treat hyperpigmentation. Pigment Cell Res. 2003;16(2):101–10. PubMed PMID: 12622786. Epub 2003/03/08. eng.
40. Paine C, Sharlow E, Liebel F, Eisinger M, Shapiro S, Seiberg M. An alternative approach to depigmentation by soybean extracts via inhibition of the PAR-2 pathway. J Invest Dermatol. 2001;116(4):587–95. PubMed PMID: 11286627. Epub 2001/04/05. eng.
41. Hakozaki T, Minwalla L, Zhuang J, Chhoa M, Matsubara A, Miyamoto K, et al. The effect of niacinamide on reducing cutaneous pigmentation and suppression of melanosome transfer. Br J Dermatol. 2002;147(1):20–31. PubMed PMID: 12100180. Epub 2002/07/09. eng.
42. Yamakoshi J, Sano A, Tokutake S, Saito M, Kikuchi M, Kubota Y, et al. Oral intake of proanthocyanidin-rich extract from grape seeds improves chloasma. Phytother Res. 2004;18(11):895–9. PubMed PMID: 15597304. Epub 2004/12/15. eng.
43. Rigopoulos D, Gregoriou S, Katsambas A. Hyperpigmentation and melasma. J Cosmet Dermatol. 2007;6(3):195–202. PubMed PMID: 17760699. Epub 2007/09/01. eng.
44. Sarkar R, Kaur C, Bhalla M, Kanwar AJ. The combination of glycolic acid peels with a topical regimen in the treatment of melasma in dark-skinned patients: a comparative study. Dermatol Surg. 2002;28(9):828–32. PubMed PMID: 12269877. discussion 32. Epub 2002/09/25. eng.
45. Erbil H, Sezer E, Tastan B, Arca E, Kurumlu Z. Efficacy and safety of serial glycolic acid peels and a topical regimen in the treatment of recalcitrant melasma. J Dermatol. 2007;34(1):25–30. PubMed PMID: 17204097. Epub 2007/01/06. eng.
46. Javaheri SM, Handa S, Kaur I, Kumar B. Safety and efficacy of glycolic acid facial peel in Indian women with melasma. Int J Dermatol. 2001;40(5):354–7. PubMed PMID: 11555002. Epub 2001/09/14. eng.
47. Burns RL, Prevost-Blank PL, Lawry MA, Lawry TB, Faria DT, Fivenson DP. Glycolic acid peels for postinflammatory hyperpigmentation in black patients. A comparative study. Dermatol Surg. 1997;23(3):171–4. PubMed PMID: 9145958. discussion 5. Epub 1997/03/01. eng.
48. Lee HS, Kim IH. Salicylic acid peels for the treatment of acne vulgaris in Asian patients. Dermatol Surg. 2003;29(12):1196–9. PubMed PMID: 14725662. discussion 9. Epub 2004/01/17. eng.
49. Grimes PE. The safety and efficacy of salicylic acid chemical peels in darker racial-ethnic groups. Dermatol Surg. 1999;25(1):18–22. PubMed PMID: 9935087. Epub 1999/02/06. eng.
50. Ahn HH, Kim IH. Whitening effect of salicylic acid peels in Asian patients. Dermatol Surg. 2006;32(3):372–5. PubMed PMID: 16640681. discussion 5. Epub 2006/04/28. eng.
51. Joshi SS, Boone SL, Alam M, Yoo S, White L, Rademaker A, et al. Effectiveness, safety, and effect on quality of life of topical salicylic acid peels for treatment of postinflammatory hyperpigmentation in dark skin. Dermatol Surg. 2009;35(4):638–44. PubMed PMID: 19400885. discussion 44. Epub 2009/04/30. eng.

52. Terrell S, Aires D, Schweiger ES. Treatment of acne vulgaris using blue light photodynamic therapy in an African-American patient. J Drugs Dermatol. 2009;8(7):669–71. PubMed PMID: 19588644. Epub 2009/07/11. eng.
53. Sherling M, Friedman PM, Adrian R, Burns AJ, Conn H, Fitzpatrick R, et al. Consensus recommendations on the use of an erbium-doped 1,550-nm fractionated laser and its applications in dermatologic laser surgery. Dermatol Surg. 2010;36(4):461–9. PubMed PMID: 20187898. Epub 2010/03/02. eng.
54. Rahman Z, Alam M, Dover JS. Fractional Laser treatment for pigmentation and texture improvement. Skin Therapy Lett. 2006;11(9):7–11. PubMed PMID: 17075654. Epub 2006/11/01. eng.
55. Robins P, Battle Jr EF, Alexis AF, Cook-Bolden F, Alqubaisy Y, McLeod MP, et al. Unique laser techniques in patients with skin of color. J Drugs Dermatol. 2011;10(12):4–26. PubMed PMID: 22134557. Epub 2011/12/03. eng.
56. Callender VD. Acne in ethnic skin: special considerations for therapy. Dermatol Ther. 2004;17(2):184–95. PubMed PMID: 15113286. Epub 2004/04/29. eng.

Chapter 41
Pseudofolliculitis Barbae

Angela Lamb and Gregory N. Yañez

41.1 Introduction

Pseudofolliculitis barbae (PFB), also known as razor bumps or barber's itch, is a common inflammatory condition of shaved areas that predominately affects darkly pigmented men with curly hair [1, 2]. The classic presentation is an African American man presenting with painful and/or pruritic inflammatory papules and pustules in distribution of the shaven beard. The mustache area is usually spared [3]. One survey of patients at a New York City clinic found that among women with PFB, the most common hair removal methods were tweezing followed by shaving, electrolysis, waxing, depilatory use, and laser treatments [4]. The only definitive treatment is to stop all attempts at hair removal to allow the epidermis time to recover from the inflammatory state. In chronic cases or cases where patients continue to shave the affected areas, firm papules and even keloid scars may be appreciated on exam.

41.2 Background

In darkly pigmented men of African ancestry, PFB has an estimated prevalence of 45–85 % [2, 5]. The prevalence and severity of symptoms is diminished in lighter patients. Women also develop this disorder in groomed areas where the hair is

A. Lamb, M.D. (✉)
Department of Dermatology, Mount Sinai Hospital, 638 Columbus Avenue,
New York, NY 10024, USA
e-mail: angela.lamb@mountsinai.org

G.N. Yañez, B.A.
Icahn School of Medicine at Mount Sinai Class of 2015, New York, NY, USA
e-mail: gregory.yanez@mssm.edu

J.A. Zeichner (ed.), *Acneiform Eruptions in Dermatology: A Differential Diagnosis*,
DOI 10.1007/978-1-4614-8344-1_41, © Springer Science+Business Media New York 2014

tightly curled such as the axilla and groin regions [4, 6]. Some authors have also noted perimenopausal women can suffer from PFB as higher androgen levels simulate hair growth in the beard area [4]. A survey of patients at the Skin of Color Center in New York found that 83 % of their patients with PFB were between ages 11 and 30 with the average age of 22, and among female patients 98 % were of African ancestry and 2 % were Hispanic [4].

There are two types of lesions in pseudofolliculitis barbae: intrafollicular and transfollicular lesions. The initiating event in the pathogenesis of pseudofolliculitis barbae is generally thought to be shaving; however it should be noted that female PFB patients report grooming via tweezing, electrolysis, waxing, and use of depilatory agents [4]. A better working understanding may be to consider any grooming technique that causes trauma as a potential inciting event in PFB pathogenesis.

Since most patients develop PSB secondary to shaving, an understanding of how shaving in particular leads to PFB is helpful. Shaving leaves an oblique cut at the distal end of the hair strand [7]. The curved morphology of the hair and hair follicle in patients with curly hair contributes to formation of lesions as the hair grows. Instead of growing straight out, it curves back into the epidermis or dermis. Helical and spiral hair types are the most likely to cause these lesions [4]. Intrafollicular lesions occur when the growing hair penetrates the dermis while still growing within its follicle of origin. Transfollicular lesions occur when the distal end of the hair penetrates the skin outside the follicle. Transfollicular lesions typically penetrate the skin 1.5–2 mm from the originating hair follicle [7].

German researchers have also discovered a genetic risk factor that partially contributes to the PFB phenotype. They found that a single-nucleotide polymorphism resulting in an abnormal Ala12Thr substitution in the 1A α(alpha)-helical segment of the accompanying layer-specific keratin K6hf was responsible for a 6.12 odds ratio increased risk of PFB compared to wild type [8]. In contrast, a curved hair follicle was associated with a 51.27 odds ratio for expression of the PFB phenotype in the German study population [8]. These researchers note that most other disruptive keratin mutations are phenotypically silent, and the mutations are only unmasked phenotypically secondary to mechanical trauma to the tissue [9]. The German researchers postulate that the stretching of the skin involved with shaving results in trauma that unmasks PFB, which explain why in many cases, allowing the beard to grow normally resolves symptoms.

In pseudofolliculitis, inflammation occurs as a result of the body's inflammatory response to the ingrown hair. Suppurative parafollicular foci form at the sites where infiltration occurs [10]. As lesions progress, small, foreign body granulomas and a mixed inflammatory cell infiltrate become evident [10]. The lesions are sometimes cleared by a process of transepithelial elimination in which the surface epithelium grows around the lesion to encase the inflammatory response along with the inciting ingrown hair [10].

41.3 Clinical Presentation

The prototypical patient population is darkly pigmented men often of African or Hispanic ancestry who shave. On presentation, inflamed papules are apparent on the beard and anterolateral neck (Fig. 41.1). Pustules and abscesses may also be seen. The mustache area, even when it is shaved daily, is typically spared [3]. The lesions of acne vulgaris can be distinguished from those of pseudofolliculitis barbae by the presence of comedones. Firm papules can develop hyperpigmentation, hypertrophic scars, and, in chronic disease, keloids [3].

41.4 Work-Up

PFB is primarily a clinical diagnosis. In the setting of hirsutism in women with associated PFB, a hormonal work-up could be considered to rule out an endocrine disorder. DHEAS and LH/FSH ratio are among the tests to be ordered. If the lesions have become infected, bacterial culture for selection of appropriate topical or systemic antibiotic therapy may be appropriate. Biopsies are also rarely performed.

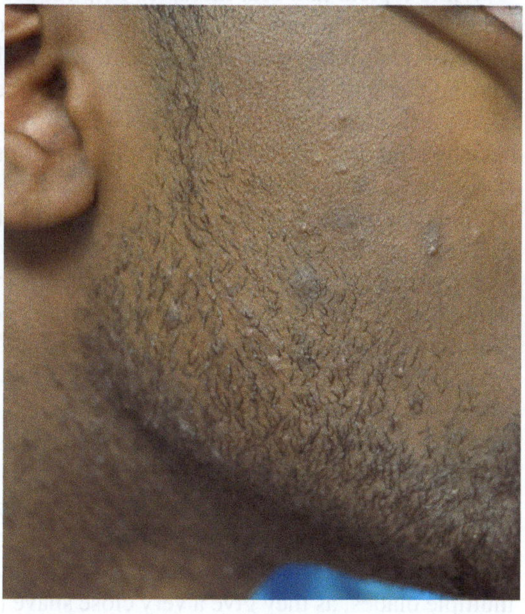

Fig. 41.1 Flesh colored papules and pustules in the beard of an African American man (Photo credit: Joshua A. Zeichner, M.D.)

41.5 Treatment

It is important to understand that in the acute stage of PFB, medical intervention is warranted as patients can experience significant morbidity from pain and pruritus. Additionally, patients may struggle to comply with workplace policies that require employees to be clean shaven. Indeed, military physicians have studied this condition to resolve conflicts between servicemen with PFB and their commanders over adherence to military policy that servicemen should be clean shaven [2].

If a patient has a folliculitis along with PFB, a course of systemic antibiotics, such as minocycline or doxycycline, is warranted. Topical antibiotic therapy with clindamycin or mupirocin may also be considered. Bacterial cultures of pustules should be taken prior to commencing antibiotic therapy.

Initial treatment of pustular and papular PFB should be directed towards minimizing inflammation and preventing bacterial superinfection. To that end a course of topical combined clindamycin benzoyl peroxide is helpful. Additionally, low potency topical corticosteroids, such as hydrocortisone valerate or desonide, can be used. Potent topical corticosteroids or intralesional triamcinolone injections should be reserved for more advanced lesions and should be used cautiously on the face. Topical retinoids are useful as therapy as well. Kligman and Mills found that tretinoin 0.05 % solution applied twice a day for 8 weeks improved symptom of papules in 78.95 % of study patients. The treatment worked best in those with more mild cases of PFB. They speculated that tretinoin's efficacy was due to a reduction of hyperkeratosis caused by repeated trauma to the epidermis [11].

While topical and oral therapies help reduce inflammation, they do not address the underlying pathophysiology of PFB. The root causes are attempts to groom the beard whether it be by shaving, plucking, etc. The patient should be counseled that shaving contributes to the lesions. Some sources contend that most inflammatory papules resolve after 1 month of not shaving [7]. It can take 2–6 weeks of shaving cessation for complete resolution of symptoms [4]. The author's approach is to advise the patient to discontinue shaving until he sees resolution of papules and pustules in concert with therapies recommended above.

In patients who need to maintain a clean-shaven appearance for work or personal preference, education must be provided on proper grooming practices. Patients should take a shower then apply a warm water compress to the face before shaving. This hydrates the skin and the hairs so that they can be more easily shaved. Additionally patients should shave with the grain, avoid pulling the skin taut to reduce tension and minimize trauma, and clean the blade frequently to avoid traction from hair buildup [4]. Some authors also recommend applying a cool compress after shaving [4].

Patients should select grooming tools that minimize trauma to the skin. A manual razor, clipper, or electric razor that does not give an extremely close shave is best. While somewhat controversial, some authors suggest avoiding razors with multiple blades, as they give a very close shave [4]. Manual razors with a guard that prevents a close shave and electric razors have been shown to be good choices for

PFB patients. In one study, use of one such manual razor specially made for PFB patients conferred a 25 % or greater reduction in the number of lesions for 72.7 % of study participants with 86.4 % of patients reporting some improvement [12]. A study of electric rotary razors found that 90 % of the 300 participants switched to use the razors after the trial period [13].

For women with PFB, topical eflornithine is an option that can help decrease the rate of hair growth and thickness of individual hairs. This often decreases the frequency of hair removal techniques. Unfortunately, hair growth rate resumes to its normal rate after cessation. Laser hair removal is another frequently recommended option. This addresses both the desire to be clean shaven along with addressing the root cause of PFB.

41.6 Conclusion

Pseudofolliculitis barbae is a chronic condition resulting from an interplay of both the hair and the skin. Chronic inflammation from ingrown hairs is the primary cause. Treatment is directed at reducing this inflammation as well as minimizing the underlying trauma caused by hair removal processes. This condition has a large psychosocial and emotional impact, so proper education of patients is extremely important.

References

1. Garcia Rl Jr WJW. PSeudofolliculitis barbae in a woman. Arch Dermatol. 1978;114(12):1856.
2. Alexander WID AM. Pseudofolliculitis barbae in the military. A medical, administrative and social problem. J Natl Med Assoc. 1974;66(6):459–64, 79. Pubmed Central PMCID: PMC2609333.
3. Edlich RF, Haines PC, Nichter LS, Silloway KA, Morgan RF. Pseudofolliculitis barbae with keloids. J Emerg Med. 1986;4(4):283–6.
4. Perry PK, Cook-Bolden FE, Rahman Z, Jones E, Taylor SC. Defining pseudofolliculitis barbae in 2001: a review of the literature and current trends. J Am Acad Dermatol. 2002;46(2 Suppl 2):S113–9.
5. Brauner GI, Flandermeyer KL. Pseudofolliculitis barbae 2. Treatment. Int J Dermatol. 1977;16(6):520–5.
6. Alexander A. PSeudofolliculitis diathesis. Arch Dermatol. 1974;109(5):729–30.
7. Strauss JSKA. Pseudofolliculitis of the beard. AMA Arch Dermatol. 1956;74:533–42.
8. Winter H, Schissel D, Parry DAD, Smith TA, Liovic M, Birgitte Lane E, et al. An unusual Ala12Thr polymorphism in the 1A [alpha]-helical segment of the companion layer-specific keratin K6hf: evidence for a risk factor in the etiology of the common hair disorder pseudofolliculitis barbae. J Investig Dermatol. 2004;122(3):652–7.
9. Irvine AD, McLean WHI. Human keratin diseases: the increasing spectrum of disease and subtlety of the phenotype–genotype correlation. Br J Dermatol. 1999;140(5):815–28.
10. Pinkus H. Chronic scarring pseudofolliculitis of the negro beard. Arch Derm Syphilol. 1943;47(6):782–92.

11. Kligman Am Jr MOH. Pseudofolliculitis of the beard and topically applied tretinoin. Arch Dermatol. 1973;107(4):551–2.
12. Alexander AM. Evaluation of a foil-guarded shaver in the management of pseudofolliculitis barbae. Cutis. 1981;27(5):534–7, 40–2. PubMed PMID: 7238107. Epub 1981/05/01. eng.
13. Garcia R, Henderson R. The adjustable rotary electric razor in the control of pseudofolliculitis barbae. J Assoc Milit Dermatol. 1978;4:28.

Chapter 42
Pustular Psoriasis

Sebastian Bernardo and Mark Lebwohl

42.1 Introduction

Psoriasis is a polygenic, chronic inflammatory skin disease linked to dysregulation of the immune system that classically presents as sharply demarcated erythematous plaques with silvery scale [1, 2]. In some patients, the condition can manifest as a generalized pustular variant that can follow a severe, potentially life-threatening course that demands urgent dermatological evaluation and treatment [1]. While pustules may be a part of the clinical picture in both pustular psoriasis and acne vulgaris, comedones are classically absent in the former. Further, pustular psoriasis commonly spares the face, even in its generalized form. Unlike severe acne, patients presenting with pustular psoriasis may be toxic appearing on physical exam and be found to have hematological abnormalities and electrolyte imbalances that represent a true dermatologic emergency.

42.2 Background

Psoriasis is the most prevalent autoimmune disease in the United States. Affecting approximately 2.2 % of the American population, psoriasis is associated with significant patient morbidity and is estimated to cost $11.25 billion in direct and indirect health care costs annually [3, 4].

S. Bernardo, M.D.
Department of Dermatology, Mt. Sinai School of Medicine,
161 West 86th Street, Apt 1a, New York, NY 10024, USA

M. Lebwohl, M.D. (✉)
Department of Dermatology, Mt. Sinai School of Medicine,
5 East 98th Street, 5th Floor, New York, NY 10029, USA
e-mail: Lebwohl@aol.com

J.A. Zeichner (ed.), *Acneiform Eruptions in Dermatology: A Differential Diagnosis*,
DOI 10.1007/978-1-4614-8344-1_42, © Springer Science+Business Media New York 2014

Although pustular psoriasis is reported to occur in less than 5 % of individuals with psoriasis, its potential for severe complications and mortality warrants immediate workup and appropriate management [1, 2]. Pustular psoriasis can present in childhood but is more commonly seen in middle-aged adults [5, 6]. While adult men and women are affected equally, pustular psoriasis is more common in boys than girls by a ratio of 3:2 among pediatric patients [1, 6, 7]. When all psoriatic variants are included, Caucasians are more commonly affected than African Americans (2.5 % vs. 1.3 %) [8]. As an individual subtype, however, pustular psoriasis has no racial predilection [9, 10].

The pathophysiology underlying pustular psoriasis has not been clearly delineated. Cutaneous cytokine and immune dysregulation coupled with environmental triggers are most likely responsible. HLA-B27, HLA-Aw19, and HLA-Bw35 have all been described as haplotypes that increase the likelihood of a pustular psoriatic phenotype [2]. Genetic predispositions that contribute to alterations in the cytokine milieu of the skin may help to explain the complex tissue alterations associated with pustular psoriasis. Upregulation of proinflammmatory cytokines such as TNF-α, Il-8, VEGF, and growth-related oncogene (Gro)-alpha in conjunction with reduced activity of anti-inflammatory molecules such as Il-36Ra increase microvascular permeability and allow leukocytes to interact with keratinocytes and endothelial cells [11–15].

In addition to what is occurring under the skin's surface, several environmental triggers have been associated with pustular psoriasis. Withdrawal of systemic corticosteroids is the most common precipitating cause and has been consistently documented in the literature as inducing or aggravating this condition [1, 16–20]. Specific medications such as lithium, antimalarials, beta-blockers, and irritating topical therapies have been implicated as well [20]. TNF-α inhibitors, which have emerged as effective therapeutic options for pustular psoriasis, have also been documented as inducing this condition for unknown reasons [21–25]. Other precipitating factors include infections (especially group B strep), pregnancy, hypocalcemia, seasonal variation, stress, exposure to sunlight, and menstruation [2, 5, 6, 17, 26].

42.3 Clinical Presentation

Psoriasis is a disease with a broad spectrum of clinical presentations that include pustular psoriasis, a variant characterized by sterile pustules forming on erythematous, inflamed skin that desquamates as the pustules dry (Fig. 42.1) [12, 27]. Pustules in psoriasis may occur in many settings and may be generalized or localized.

Generalized subtypes of pustular psoriasis include the von Zumbusch, annular, and exanthematic variants. In von Zumbusch, or acute GPP, disease onset is abrupt, explosive, and characterized by burning erythema that quickly spreads to affect large areas of skin [28, 29]. Clusters of pinpoint, sterile pustules develop and coalesce to form circinate lakes of pus. As these pustules rupture, crusting and scaling soon follow with new crops of pustules appearing after these crusts have been

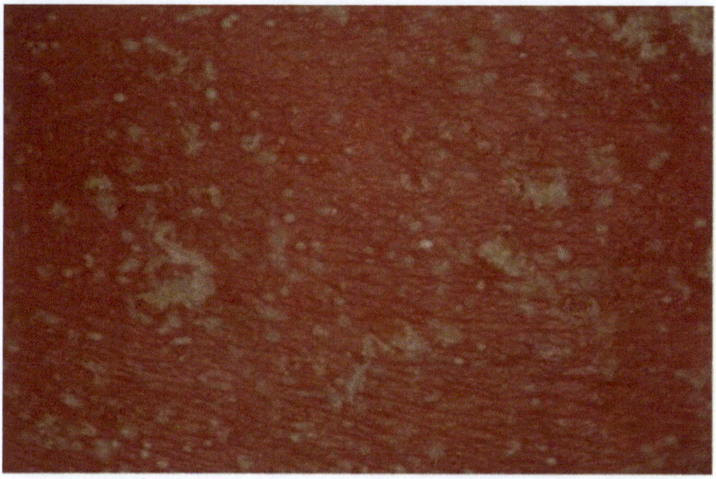

Fig. 42.1 Pustular psoriasis—sterile pustules on erythematous skin. *Borrowed from the Mount Sinai Dermatology collection*

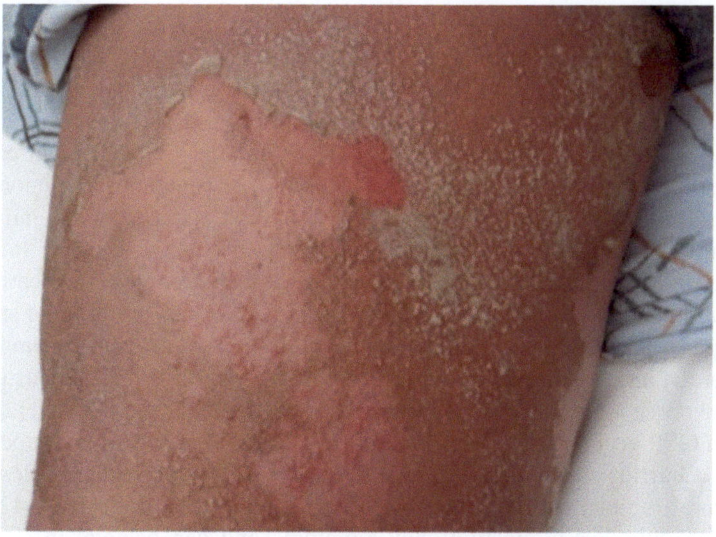

Fig. 42.2 Pustular psoriasis—von Zumbusch variant. *Borrowed from the Mount Sinai Dermatology collection*

shed (Fig. 42.2) [27]. The acute phase is associated with fever, fatigue, headache, chills, malaise, onycholysis, and burning [29]. With large areas of skin involved, patients are susceptible to infection, fluid loss, hypothermia, and electrolyte abnormalities, a combination that represents a medical emergency that demands immediate workup and appropriate treatment.

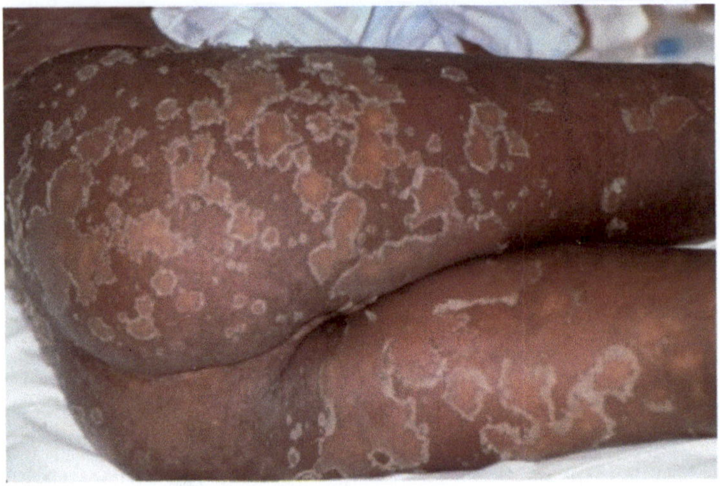

Fig. 42.3 Pustular psoriasis—annular variant. *Borrowed from the Mount Sinai Dermatology collection*

The annular subtype of pustular psoriasis is characterized by scattered gyrate or annular lesions consisting of erythema and scaling with pustulation at advancing edges. Over a period of hours to days, lesions enlarge by centrifugal expansion while healing occurs centrally (Fig. 42.3) [2, 9, 27]. It is the most common form of GPP in children and is associated with fever, malaise, and systemic manifestations that are milder than cases of von Zumbusch [6, 9].

The exanthematic variant is typically triggered by infection or medications such as lithium in patients without a history of psoriasis. An acute eruption of small pustules appears and recedes within a couple of days without systemic symptoms [2, 27]. There is an overlap with this form of pustular psoriasis and the pustular drug eruption known as acute generalized exanthematous pustulosis (AGEP) [2].

When GPP occurs during pregnancy, it is referred to as impetigo herpetiformis. Usually occurring in the third trimester, lesions usually begin in the flexural and genitocrural regions and tend to cluster, enlarging centrifugally (Fig. 42.4). It is associated with severe constitutional symptoms and can be fatal in some cases [30–32].

Pustules in psoriasis may be localized to the palms and soles, paronychial tissues, or occur at the periphery of plaque-like lesions [31]. In palmoplantar pustulosis, lesions can reach 0.5 cm in diameter and are localized to the hands and feet (Figs. 42.5 and 42.6). Pustular content can turn brown while involuting beneath caloused skin of the palms and soles (Fig. 42.7) [27]. Desquamation follows soon thereafter [2]. The disease is chronic and in one series, only 28 % of patients were disease free upon reexamination 10 years later [2]. Stress and focal infections have been described as triggering factors [2].

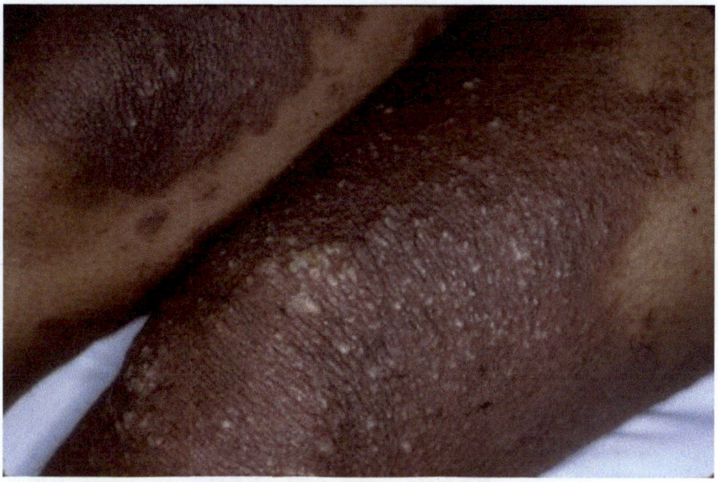

Fig. 42.4 Impetigo herpetiformis. *Borrowed from "The Skin and Systemic Disease: A Color Atlas and Text"* [66]

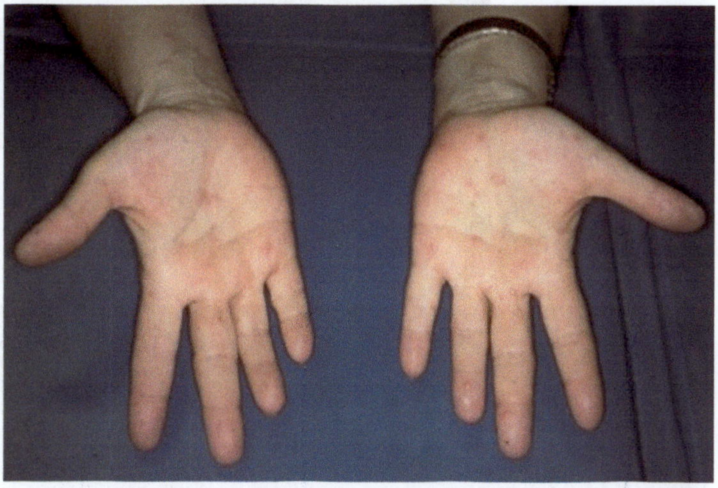

Fig. 42.5 Palmar pustular psoriasis. *Borrowed from the Mount Sinai Dermatology collection*

In acrodermatitis of hallopeau, pustulation of the distal portions of the fingers and toes is followed by scaling and crust formation [2]. Paronychia, skin atrophy, onychodystrophy, onycholysis, and osteolysis of the distal phalanges may be seen [33] (Fig. 42.8). Following a chronic-relapsing course, this variant of pustular psoriasis is frequently difficult to treat and patients may transition into developing other subtypes of psoriasis [2].

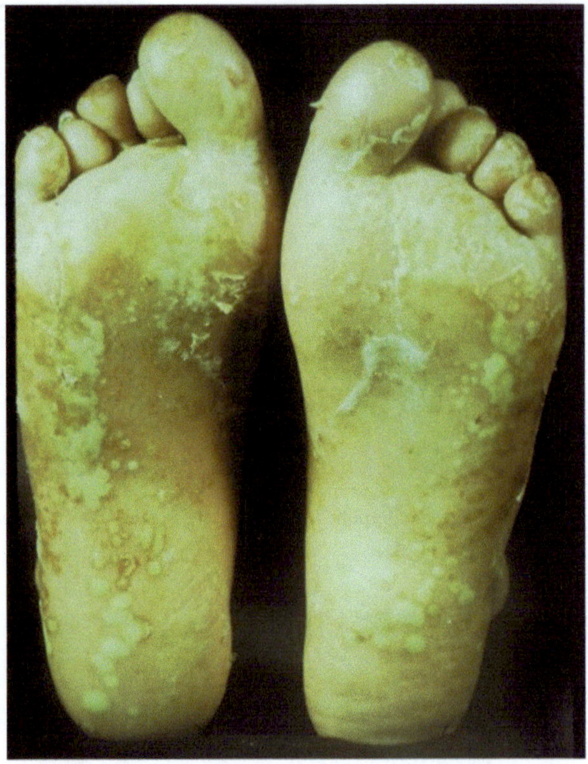

Fig. 42.6 Plantar pustular psoriasis. *Borrowed from "The Skin and Systemic Disease: A Color Atlas and Text"* [66]

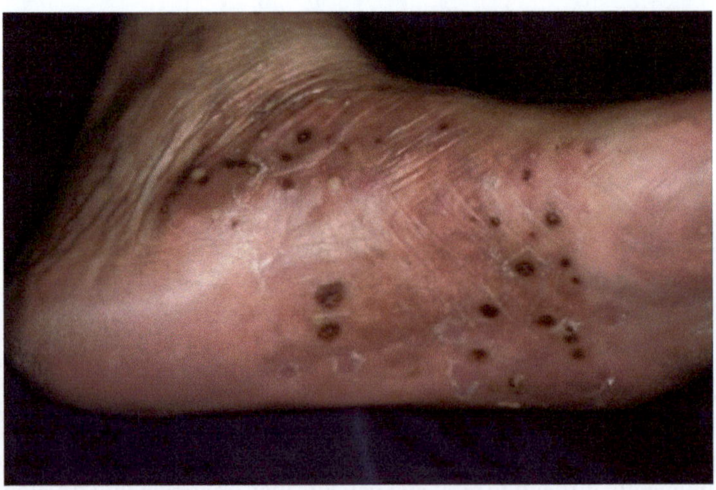

Fig. 42.7 Plantar pustular psoriasis with involuting lesions. *Borrowed from the Mount Sinai Dermatology collection*

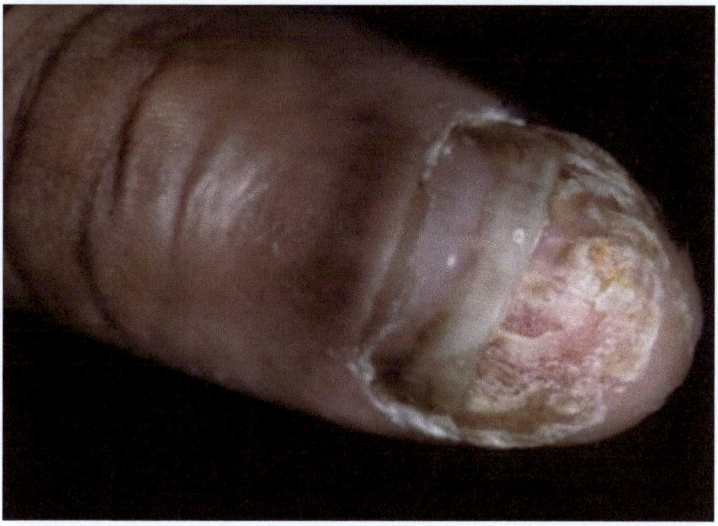

Fig. 42.8 Acrodermatitis of hallopeau. *Borrowed from the Mount Sinai Dermatology collection*

42.4 Workup

The diagnosis of pustular psoriasis can usually be made on the basis of its clinical features. However, when the diagnosis is in question, pustular psoriasis has unique pathological and laboratory findings that allow it to be distinguished from other psoriatic variants. A punch biopsy allows for optimal visualization of disease histology, which is predominantly characterized by neutrophil accumulation [2]. Migrating from sinuous, dilated capillaries within the dermis, neutrophils collect between residual keratinocyte plasma membranes accompanied by intercellular edema [31]. This forms a macropustule in the epidermis that begins as a spongiform pustule of Kogoj and develops into a large munro macroabscess [27]. Histological features of psoriasis vulgaris may also be present and include parakeratosis, elongation of epidermal rete ridges, and a perivascular lymphocytic or mixed inflammatory infiltrate within the papillary dermis [27, 34]. Laboratory findings associated with pustular psoriasis include neutrophilia with WBC counts as high as 30,000, absolute lymphopenia, hypoalbuminemia, hypocalcemia, anemia, decreased creatinine clearance, and elevations in ESR, transaminases, alkaline phosphatase, and bilirubin [9, 29, 35, 36]. Cultures of pustules are sterile. However, since the protective functions of the skin are lost in GPP, patients have succumbed to staphylococcal sepsis and blood cultures may be warranted.

42.5 Treatment

Although many systemic and topical treatments have been described as effective management options for patients with pustular psoriasis, no evidence-based consensus has been reached regarding the correct therapeutic hierarchy

Table 42.1 Systemic therapies

Medication class	Medication	Dosing
Retinoids	Acitretin	25–50 mg PO daily [9, 60]
	Isotretinoin	1 mg/kg PO daily [9]
Antimetabolites	Methotrexate	Single weekly PO dose: 7.5–25 mg (37.5 mg maximum in severe cases) [2]
		Divided weekly PO dose: 2–5 mg three times every 12 h for 3 doses for cumulative total dose of 6–15 mg weekly (30 mg maximum in severe cases) [2]
		Parenteral dosing: 40–50 mg maximum dose IM or IV weekly [2]
Alkylating agents	Cyclosporine	3 mg/kg/day PO in two divided doses (5 mg/kg/day maximum in severe cases) [2]
Biologics	Infliximab	One 5 mg/kg IV dose at weeks 0, 2, and 6. Then every 8 weeks up to week 46 [53]
	Adalimumab	40 mg SC every one or two weeks [50, 64]
	Etanercept	25–50 mg sq once or twice weekly [49]
Psoralens	8-MOP	0.4–0.6 mg/kg PO given 1–3 h before phototherapy [65]

Table 42.2 Topical therapies

Medication class	Medication	Dosing	
Corticosteroids	Fluocinonide	Apply cream or ointment twice daily [9]	15, 30, 60, 120 g [9]
	Desoximetasone		15, 60, 120 g [9]
	Halcinonide		15, 60, 240 g [9]
	Clobetasol		15, 30, 45, 60 g [9]
Vitamin D3 analogues	Calcipotriol	Available as ointment, cream, or lotion formulation. Apply twice daily (50 μg/g concentration). Maximum weekly dose 100 g [2]	
	Calcitriol	Apply ointment twice daily (3 μg/g concentration). Maximum weekly dose 210 g [2]	
Bath PUVA	8-MOP (solution)	15–20 min immersion in 0.5–5 mg/L 8-MOP bathwater immediately followed by phototherapy [2]	

to follow. In all cases, effective treatment begins by removing precipitating factors that may induce or aggravate the condition, many of which had been discussed previously [37]. Recommendations for generalized and localized disease will be discussed. For specific medication dosing, refer to Tables 42.1 and 42.2.

42.5.1 Generalized Disease

In the acute setting, topical therapies are frequently ineffective in patients with generalized disease, and management with systemic agents in an experienced burn unit is often necessary to prevent patient morbidity and mortality (Table 42.1). In conjunction with starting therapy for GPP, supportive measures such as bedrest, compresses, fluid replacement, correction of electrolyte abnormalities, as well as antibiotics and serial blood cultures are essential in urgent cases [9, 29]. First-line therapy includes oral retinoids such as acitretin and isotretinoin [1, 38]. Retinoid therapy was effective in 84 % of patients in one large retrospective study [39]. Side effects include hypertriglyceridemia, xerosis, hair loss, hepatotoxicity, and cheilitis [6, 40, 41].

Methotrexate or cyclosporine are also first-line therapies for GPP [1]. Both have been consistently documented as valuable treatment options for GPP and were effective in 76.2 % and 71.2 % of patients, respectively, in a large, multicenter study of 385 patients with GPP in Japan [1, 9, 16, 32, 39, 42–47]. Before initiating therapy with either agent, it is necessary to obtain a detailed medical history and frequent blood tests to prevent potentially severe side effects such as methotrexate-induced bone marrow toxicity [1]. Advantages of methotrexate are its efficacy, affordability, and convenient weekly oral dose [40]. It is limited by its teratogenicity and side effects, which include myelosuppression, hepatotoxicity, and pulmonary toxicity [48]. Cyclosporine has been used safely during pregnancy and its rapid onset makes it effective in managing acute GPP [1, 32]. However, the side effects of nephrotoxicity, hypertension, and immunosuppression limit its use [48].

The advent of biological agents has added another medication class to the dermatologist's armamentarium in the treatment of GPP. The efficacy of infliximab, adalimumab, and etanercept has been documented in several reports in the literature, including cases that were refractory to methotrexate, acitretin, and other systemic therapies [6, 49–53]. With a faster onset of action than adalimumab or etanercept, infliximab may be particularly useful in life-threatening cases of GPP with systemic involvement [1]. As a class, the biologics are generally well tolerated. They potentially increase the risk of infections and carcinogenesis so baseline testing with a complete metabolic panel, CBC, LFTs, and tuberculosis screening should be performed with appropriate follow-up [1, 50].

42.5.2 Localized Disease

Localized cases may be managed with superpotent topical steroids or light therapies but may require systemic treatment with retinoids, methotrexate, cyclosporine, or biologics in refractory cases [46, 54–58] (Table 42.2). Topical corticosteroids can be given as monotherapy, used under occlusion for increased penetration, or combined with newer vitamin D analogues such as calcitriol or calcipotriene [1]. Unfortunately, many patients fail to respond to topical therapy and other treatment modalities are required. Both oral and bath "soak" PUVA therapies have been consistently shown to be effective management options for patients with palmoplantar pustulosis [1, 29, 59–61]. In the first 4 weeks of treatment, oral PUVA has been found to be slightly more effective than bath PUVA but the former has more systemic side effects such as nausea [59]. Combination therapy with PUVA and retinoids has been found to be more effective than PUVA alone and is associated with a reduction in the number of PUVA sessions and UVA dose required for clearing [60, 62, 63].

42.6 Conclusion

Several effective therapies for pustular psoriasis have emerged since von Zumbusch described his case over 100 years ago. Going forward, much remains to be learned and the development of evidence-based guidelines for treatment is imperative. Continued research will yield a better understanding of the complex interactions underlying disease pathogenesis and identify new targets for improved therapy.

References

1. Roosevelt L, Emer J. Pustular psoriasis: a practical review of the literature. Psoriasis Forum. 2011;17(1):33–41.
2. Van de Kerkhof PCM. Psoriasis. In: Bolognia JL, Jorizzo JL, Rapini RP, editors. Dermatology. New York, NY: Mosby [Elsevier]; 2003. p. 125–46.
3. National Psoriasis Foundation—Psoriasis statistics, prevalence, severity, age of onset and psoriasis research. The National Psoriasis Foundation Website. http://www.psoriasis.org/learn_statistics. Accessed 29 Sept 2011.
4. Stern RS, Nijsten T, Feldman SR, Margolis DJ, Rolstad T. Psoriasis is common, carries a substantial burden even when not extensive, and is associated with widespread treatment dissatisfaction. J Investig Dermatol Symp Proc. 2004 Mar;9(2):136–9.
5. Zelickson BD, Muller SA. Generalized pustular psoriasis: a review of 63 cases. Arch Dermatol. 1991;127:1339–45.
6. de Oliveira ST, Maragno L, Arnone M, Fonseca Takahashi MD, Romiti R. Generalized pustular psoriasis in childhood. Pediatr Dermatol. 2010;27:349–54.
7. Liao PB, Rubinson R, Howard R, Sanchez G, Frieden IJ. Annular pustular psoriasis—most common form of pustular psoriasis in children: report of three cases and review of the literature. Pediatr Dermatol. 2002;19:19–25.
8. Gelfand JM, Stern RS, Nijsten T, et al. The prevalence of psoriasis in african americans: results from a population-based study. J Am Acad Dermatol. 2005;52:23–6.
9. Visual Dx—adult rash: psoriasis, pustular. Visual Dx website. http://www.visualdx.com/visualdx/visualdx6/getDiagnosisText.do?moduleId=7&diagnosisId=52229. Accessed 12 Sept 2011.
10. Gudjonsson JE, Elder JT. Psoriasis. In: Fitzpatrick TB, Wolff K, editors. Fitzpatrick's dermatology in general medicine. 7th ed. New York, NY: McGraw-Hill; 2008. p. 169–93.
11. Schon MP, Boehncke WH. Psoriasis. N Engl J Med. 2005;352:1899–912.
12. Benoit S, Toksoy A, Bröcker EB, Gillitzer R, Goebeler M. Treatment of recalcitrant pustular psoriasis with infliximab: effective reduction of chemokine expression. Br J Dermatol. 2004;150(5):1009–12.

13. Yamamoto M, Tada Y, Asahina A, et al. Severe generalized pustular psoriasis accompanied by bullae formation with increased serum vascular endothelial growth factor level. J Dermatol. 2012;39(2):183–5. 2011 July 18. [Epub ahead of print].
14. Marrkchi S, Guigue P, Renshaw BR, et al. Interleukin-36-receptor antagonist deficiency and generalized pustular psoriasis. N Engl J Med. 2011;365(7):620–8.
15. Onoufriadis A, Simpson MA, Pink AE, et al. Mutations in Il36RN/Il1F5 are associated with the severe episodic inflammatory skin disease known as generalized pustular psoriasis. Am J Hum Genet. 2011;89(3):432–7.
16. Umezawa Y, Ozawa A, Kawasima T, et al. Therapeutic guidelines for the treatment of generalized pustular psoriasis (GPP) based on a proposed classification of disease severity. Arch Dermatol Res. 2003;295(1):S43–54.
17. Freedberg IM, Eisen AZ, Wolff K, Austen KF, Goldsmith LA, Katz SI, editors. Dermatology in general medicine. 6th ed. New York, NY: McGraw Hill; 2003.
18. Brenner M, Molin S, Ruebsam K, Weisenseel P, Ruzicka T, Prinz JC. Generalized pustular psoriasis induced by systemic glucocorticosteroids: four cases and recommendations for treatment. Br J Dermatol. 2009;161(4):964–6.
19. Ryan T, Baker H. Systemic corticosteroids and folic acid antagonists in the treatment of generalized pustular psoriasis evaluation and prognosis based on the study of 104 cases. Br J Dermatol. 1969;81:134–45.
20. Rongioletti F, Fiorucci C, Parodi A. Psoriasis induced or aggravated by drugs. J Rhematol Suppl. 2009;83:59–61.
21. Park JJ, Lee SC. A case of tumor necrosis factor-α inhibitors-induced pustular psoriasis. Ann Dermatol. 2010;22:212–5.
22. Wenk KS, Claros JM, Ehrlich A. Flare of pustular psoriasis after initiating ustekinumab therapy. J Dermatolog Treat. 2012;23(3):212–4. 2011 Jan 22 [Epub ahead of print].
23. Pourciau C, Shwayder T. Occurrence of pustular psoriasis after treatment of Crohn disease with infliximab. Pediatr Dermatol. 2010;27(5):539–40.
24. Collamer AN, Guerrero KT, Henning JS, Battafarano DF. Psoriatic skin lesions induced by tumor necrosis factor antagonist therapy: a literature review and potential mechanisms of action. Arthritis Rheum. 2008;59(7):996–1001.
25. Shmidt E, Wetter DA, Ferguson SB, Pittelkow MR. Psoriasis and palmoplantar pustulosis associated with tumor necrosis factor-α inhibitors: The Mayo Clinic experience, 1998 to 2010. J Am Acad Dermatol. 2012;67(5):e179–85. 2011 Jul 11 [Epub ahead of print].
26. Gudjonsson JE, Thorarinsson AM, Sigurgeirsson B, Kristinsson KG, Valdimarsson H. Streptococcal throat infections and exacerbation of chronic plaque psoriasis: a prospective study. Br J Dermatol. 2003;149:530–4.
27. Prystowsky JH, Cohen PR. Pustular and erytherodermic psoriasis. Psoriasis. 1995;13:757–70.
28. Katz M, Seidenbaum M, Weinrauch L. Penicillin-induced generalized pustular psoriasis. J Am Acad Dermatol. 1987;17:918–20.
29. Fitzpatrick TB, Johnson RA, Wolff K, Suurmond D, editors. Color atlas and synopsis of clinical dermatology common and serious diseases. New York, NY: McGraw-Hill; 2001.
30. Maize JC, Burgdorf WHC, Hurt MA, et al. Cutaneous pathology. 1st ed. Philadelphia, PA: Churchill Livingstone; 1998.
31. Barnhill RL, Crowson AN, Magro CM, Piepkorn MW. Dermatopathology. 3rd ed. China: McGraw-Hill; 2010. p. 66–7.
32. Hazarika D. Generalized pustular psoriasis of pregnancy successfully treated with cyclosporine. Indian J Dermatol Venereol Leprol. 2009;75(6):638–41.
33. Puig L, Barco D, Vilarrasa E, Alomar A. Treatment of acrodermatitis continua of hallopeau with TNF-blocking agents: case report and review. Dermatology. 2010;220(2):154–8.
34. Zelickson BD, Muller SA. Generalized pustular psoriasis in childhood: report of thirteen cases. J Am Acad Dermatol. 1991;24:186–94.
35. Viguier M, Allez M, Zagdanski AM, et al. High frequency of cholestasis in generalized pustular psoriasis: evidence for neutrophilic involvement of the biliary tract. Hepatology. 2004;40:452–8.

36. Borges-Costa J, Silva R, Goncalves L, et al. Clinical and laboratory features in acute generalized pustular psoriasis. Am J Clin Dermatol. 2011;12(4):271–6.
37. Lebwohl MG, Heymann WR, Berth-Jones J, Coulson I. Treatment of skin disease. 2nd ed. China: Mosby-Elsevier; 2006.
38. Sofen HL, Moy RL, Lowe NJ. Treatment of generalised pustular psoriasis with isotretinoin. Lancet. 1984;7:40.
39. Ozawa A, Ohkido M, Haruki Y, et al. Treatments of generalized pustular psoriasis: a multicenter study in Japan. J Dermatol. 1999;26:141–9.
40. Gollnick HPM. Oral retinoids—efficacy and toxicity in psoriasis. Br J Dermatol. 1996;135(49):6–17.
41. Dogra S, Kaur I. Childhood psoriasis. Indian J Dermatol Venereol Leprol. 2010;76(4): 357–65.
42. Kalb RE, Strober B, Weinstein G, Lebwohl M. Methotrexate and psoriasis: 2009 national psoriasis foundation consensus conference. J Am Acad Dermatol. 2009;60(5):824–37.
43. Meinardi MM, Westerhof W, Bos JD. Generalized pustular psoriasis (von zumbusch) responding to cyclosporine A. Br J Dermatol. 1987;116(2):269–70.
44. Rosmarin DM, Lebwohl M, Elewski BE, Gottlieb AB. Cyclosporine and psoriasis: 2008 national psoriasis foundation consensus conference. J Am Acad Dermatol. 2010;62(5): 838–53.
45. Dogra S, Kumaran MS, Handa S, Kanwar AJ. Methotrexate for generalized pustular psoriasis in a 2-year-old child. Pediatr Dermatol. 2005;22(1):85–6.
46. Maza A, Montaudie H, Sbidian E, et al. Oral cyclosporine in psoriasis: a systematic review on treatment modalities, risk of kidney toxicity and evidence for use in non-plaque psoriasis. J Eur Acad Dermatol Venereol. 2011;25(2):19–27.
47. Paul C, Gallini A, Maza A, et al. Evidence-based recommendations on conventional systemic treatments in psoriasis: systemic review and expert opinion of a panel of dermatologists. J Eur Acad Dermatol Venereol. 2011;25(2):2–11.
48. Gottlieb A, Korman NJ, Gordon KB, et al. Guidelines of care for the management of psoriasis and psoriatic arthritis: section 4: guidelines of care for the management and treatment of psoriasis with traditional systemic agents. J Am Acad Dermatol. 2008;58:851–64.
49. Esposito M, Mazzotta A, Casciello C, Chimenti S. Etanercept at different dosages in the treatment of generalized pustular psoriasis: a case series. Dermatology. 2008;216(4):355–60.
50. Zangrilli A, Papoutsaki M, Talamonti M, Chimenti S. Long-term efficacy of adalimumab in generalized pustular psoriasis. J Dermatolog Treat. 2008;19(3):185–7.
51. Alvarez AC, Rodriguez-Nevado I, de Argila D. Recalcitrant pustular psoriasis successfully treated with adalimumab. Pediatr Dermatol. 2011;28(2):195–7.
52. Chandran NS, Chong WS. A dramatic response to a single dose of infliximab as rescue therapy in acute generalized pustular psoriasis of von Zumbusch associated with a neutrophilic cholangitis. Australas J Dermatol. 2010;51(1):29–31.
53. Torii H, Nakagawa H. Long-term study of infliximab in Japanese patients with plaque psoriasis, psoriatic arthritis, pustular psoriasis and psoriatic erythroderma. J Dermatol. 2011;38(4): 321–34.
54. Visual Dx—pustulosis, palmoplantar. Visual Dx website. http://www.visualdx.com/visualdx/visualdx6/getDiagnosisText.do?moduleId=7&diagnosisId=52240. Accessed 29 Sept 2011.
55. Thielen AM, Barde C, Marazza G, Saurat JH. Long-term control with etanercept (Enbrel) of a severe acrodermatitis continua of hallopeau refractory to infliximab (Remicade). Dermatology. 2008;217(2):137–9.
56. Lee CS, Koo J. A review of acitretin, a systemic retinoid for the treatment of psoriasis. Expert Opin Pharmacother. 2005;6(10):1725–34.
57. Di Lernia V, Guareschi E. Successful treatment of hand and foot psoriasis with infliximab. Dermatol Online J. 2010;16(7):8.
58. Adişen E, Tekin O, Gülekon A, Gürer MA. A retrospective analysis of treatment responses of palmoplantar psoriasis in 114 patients. J Eur Acad Dermatol. 2009;23(7):814–9.

59. Hofer A, Fink-Puches R, Kerl H, Quehenberger F, Wolf P. Paired comparison of bathwater versus oral delivery of 8-methoxypsoralen in psoralen plus ultraviolet: a therapy for chronic palmoplantar psoriasis. Photodermatol Photoimmunol Photomed. 2006;22(1):1–5.
60. Sbidian E, Maza A, Montaudie H, et al. Efficacy and safety of oral retinoids in different psoriasis subtypes: a systematic literature review. J Eur Acad Dermatol Venereol. 2011;25(2): 28–33.
61. Behrens S, von Kobyletzki G, Gruss C, Reuther T, Altmeyer P, Kerscher M. Puva-bath photochemotherapy (PUVA-soak therapy) of recalcitrant dermatoses of the palms and soles. Photodermatol Photoimmunol Photomed. 1999;15(2):47–51.
62. Ettler K, Richards B. Acitretin therapy for palmoplantar pustulosis combined with UVA and topical 8-MOP. Int J Dermatol. 2001;40:541–2.
63. Lauharanta J, Geiger JM. A double-blind comparison of acitretin and etretinate in combination with bath PUVA in the treatment of extensive psoriasis. Br J Dermatol. 1989;121:107–12.
64. Yawalkar N, Hunger RE. Succesful treatment of recalcitrant palmoplantar pustular psoriasis with sequential use of infliximab and adalimumab. Dermatology. 2009;218(1):79–83.
65. Honigsmann H, Schwartz T. In: Bolognia JL, Jorizzo JL, Rapini RP, editors. Dermatology. New York, NY: Mosby [Elsevier]; 2003. p. 2109–25.
66. Lebwohl MG. The skin and systemic disease: a color atlas and text. 2nd ed. New York, NY: Churchill Livingstone; 2004.

Chapter 43
Rosacea

Joseph Bikowski

43.1 Introduction

Rosacea, a chronic, inflammatory skin condition, is estimated to affect ten million Americans [1]. Characterized by a centrofacial distribution of acneiform papules and pustules, diffuse erythema, and frequently but not always telangiectases [2], rosacea is a highly visible disease that has been associated with negative influences on affected individuals' quality of life [3, 4]. Although the disease is generally thought to be of primarily cosmetic consequence, patients have reported stinging and pain associated with rosacea [5], and functional impairments may result from severe rhinophyma [6]. A number of treatment options are available—both topical and systemic—for the management of rosacea in its various presentations. With a proper diagnosis, a rational therapeutic strategy, and supportive skin care and patient education, control of rosacea is possible.

43.2 Background

Rosacea is generally considered a disease that affects individuals in middle age; the incidence is shown to increase with age and peak in those over age 65 [7]. While the majority of individuals with rosacea are women (69 %), men may be prone to more severe presentations [8]. The vast majority of rosacea patients (96 %) are Caucasian [8].

J. Bikowski, M.D. (✉)
Director, Bikowski Skin Care Center, 500 Chadwick Street, Sewickley, PA, USA
e-mail: drb@bikowskimd.com

J.A. Zeichner (ed.), *Acneiform Eruptions in Dermatology: A Differential Diagnosis*,
DOI 10.1007/978-1-4614-8344-1_43,

The pathophysiology of rosacea is not well elucidated, although the clinical features of the disease are well documented. Based on recent molecular studies, current understanding holds that vascular and inflammatory manifestations of the disease are mediated by an altered innate immune response [1, 9]. Recently, the antimicrobial peptide cathelicidin and its activator kallikrein-5 have been found to contribute to the exacerbated immune response in rosacea [10]. Neutrophils have also been shown to induce inflammation associated with rosacea and are thought to promote the release of reactive oxygen species [11]. Other inflammatory mediators implicated in the development of rosacea include histamine, serotonin, bradykinin, or prostaglandins [1].

Chronic UV exposure has been suggested to play a role in the pathophysiology of rosacea, causing damage to dermal connective tissues, which facilitates and exacerbates the effects of vasodilation and vascular pooling [12]. A recent study involving 1,000 patients, however, failed to demonstrate an association between UV exposure and papulopustular rosacea [13].

Environmental trigger factors may be associated with exacerbation of rosacea and may initiate the flushing and blushing response in susceptible individuals. The degree to which any individual is affected, if at all, by a given trigger is variable. Commonly cited triggers include thermally hot beverages or foods, alcoholic drinks, and/or spicy foods [14].

43.3 Clinical Presentation

The classic presentation of rosacea includes a primarily centrofacial distribution of acneiform papules and pustules on a background of erythema and telangiectases [2]. However, rosacea presents across a continuum from mild signs and symptoms, such as transient flushing and dryness, to severe manifestations of persistent erythema, edema, and phymatous formations. Ocular involvement is common but potentially under-recognized [15, 16].

A National Rosacea Society Expert Committee has identified four primary rosacea subtypes [5]. Subtype 1, erythematotelangiectatic rosacea (ETR) is a common presentation, characterized by flushing and persistent facial erythema. Telangiectases are common but not always present (Fig. 43.1). Subtype 2, papulopustular rosacea (PPR) often coexists with ETR. It is characterized by persistent central facial erythema with transient papules, pustules, or both in a central facial distribution (Fig. 43.2). Phymatous rosacea constitutes Subtype 3 and may include thickened skin, nodules, and anatomical enlargement (Fig. 43.3). Although rhinophyma (enlargement of the nose) is most common, other manifestations include phymas of the chin, forehead, and ears. Only a minority of patients will progress to phymatous rosacea. Most, if not all, of these will be men.

Ocular rosacea, symptoms of which include interpalpebral conjunctival hyperemia, foreign-body sensation, burning or stinging, dryness, itching, light sensitivity, blurred vision, telangiectasia of the conjunctiva and lid margin, is Subtype 4 (Fig. 43.4).

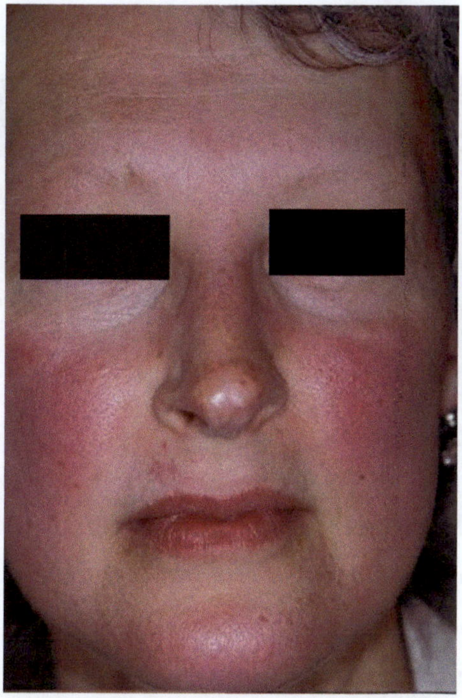

Fig. 43.1 Erythematotelangiectatic rosacea (ETR, Subtype 1) is characterized by flushing and persistent central facial erythema. Telangiectases are common but not always present

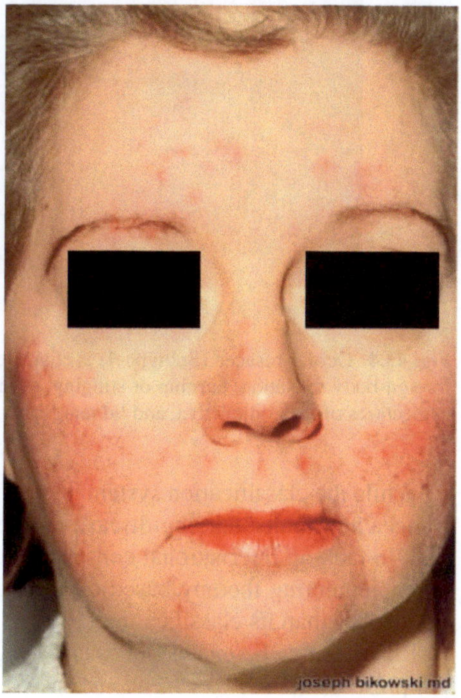

Fig. 43.2 Papulopustular rosacea (PPR, Subtype 2) is characterized by persistent central facial erythema with transient papules and/or pustules

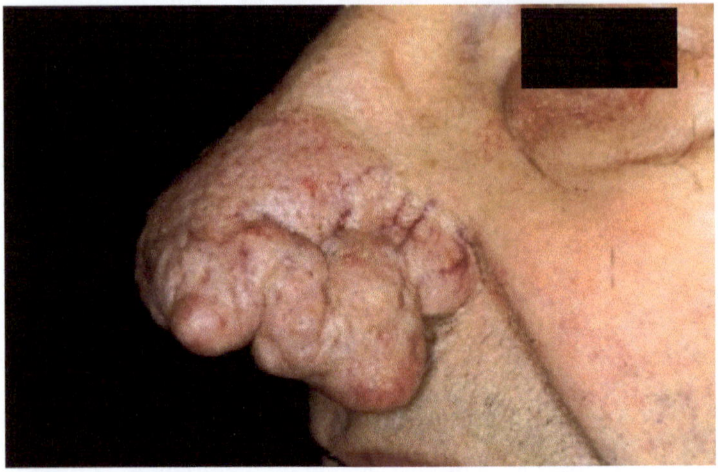

Fig. 43.3 Phymatous rosacea (Subtype 3) is characterized by thickened skin, nodules, and anatomical enlargement

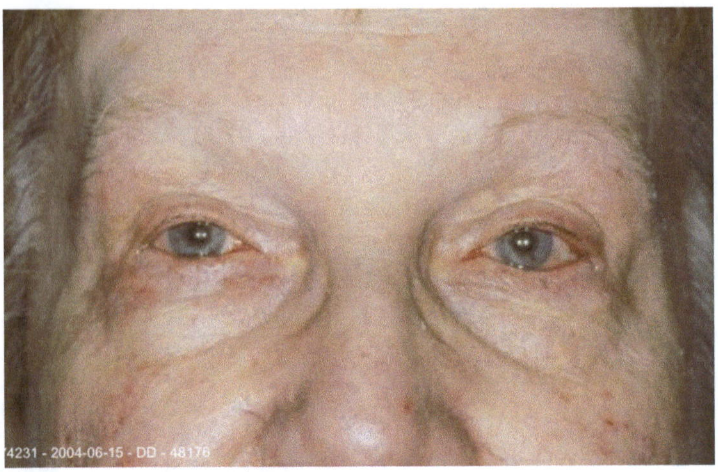

Fig. 43.4 Ocular rosacea (Subtype 4) is characterized by interpalpebral conjunctival hyperemia, foreign-body sensation, burning or stinging, dryness, itching, light sensitivity, blurred vision, telangiectases of the conjunctiva, and lid margin

While the classification system is helpful for recognizing signs and symptoms of rosacea and understanding disease progression, its clinical relevance may be limited. In fact, an international consensus committee has emphasized the importance of implementing therapy based on signs and symptoms of the specific presenting case rather than its classification [10].

Rosacea may be mistaken for acne vulgaris, though the two are distinguished by the presence (acne) or absence (rosacea) of comedones. Furthermore, while rosacea's centrofacial distribution includes the forehead, lesions are not typically

Table 43.1 Differential diagnosis of rosacea

Condition	Distinguishing feature
Acne vulgaris	Presence of comedones
Perioral dermatitis	Involvement about the mouth (sparing the vermillion border), nasolabial folds, and chin
Steroid-induced dermatitis	History of topical application of corticosteroids to the face Involvement of skin adjacent to the vermillion border
Demodex dermatitis	+/– Papules/pustules Responds to treatment with topical crotamiton or permethrin

present at the hairline. By contrast, lesions may be concentrated at the hairline in some acne presentations.

Perioral dermatitis and steroid induced dermatitis, sometimes erroneously termed steroid rosacea, should also be ruled out. As its name indicates, perioral dermatitis is focused about the mouth, nasolabial folds, and chin, sparing a clear area between the eruption and the vermillion border [17]. Steroid-induced dermatitis, which frequently mimics this distribution of lesions, is most easily recognized via patient questioning, admitted history of topical application of corticosteroids to the face, and involvement of the skin adjacent to the vermillion border [18] (Table 43.1).

43.4 Work-Up

There are no diagnostic tests for rosacea. When ocular rosacea is suspected, patients may be referred for ophthalmic evaluation and treatment. Patients with rosacea should be educated about ocular involvement and be encouraged to attend to their ocular health.

Despite historic associations of rosacea with acne vulgaris, the two are of distinctly different etiologies, and there is no microorganism widely accepted as causative in rosacea. An association between rosacea and the *Demodex folliculorum* mite has been identified, although no evidence has elevated this correlation to causation [19]. In fact, there is some evidence that a distinct condition termed *Demodex* dermatitis may exist that is frequently inaccurately diagnosed as rosacea [20]. This condition, which is characterized by facial erythema, dryness, scaling, and roughness with or without papules/pustules, responds to treatment with topical crotamiton or permethrin; such therapeutic response may confirm the diagnosis of *Demodex* dermatitis rather than rosacea.

43.5 Treatment

Among the treatment options for rosacea are both topical and systemic formulations (Table 43.2). Increasingly, laser and light-based interventions are emerging for the management of vascular and phymatous irregularities, which are generally not

Table 43.2 Rosacea therapies

Treatment	Known or suspected activities in rosacea
Topical antimicrobial formulations: sodium sulfacetamide/sulfur, metronidazole	Antibacterial, anti-inflammatory
Azelaic acid	Antibacterial, keratolytic, anti-inflammatory
Systemic antibiotics (conventional)	Anti-inflammatory
Anti-inflammatory dose doxycycline (40 mg, controlled release)	Anti-inflammatory
Oral isotretinoin	Anti-inflammatory, immunomodulatory
Laser and Light devices (pulsed dye laser and IPL)	Destroy vessels/vascular structures, reduce erythema
Surgical correction and ablative laser surgery	Mechanical debulking of phymas

amenable to pharmacologic intervention. Topical agents for rosacea include various formulations of sodium sulfacetamide and sulfur, metronidazole, azelaic acid, and benzoyl peroxide/clindamycin. Oral agents include antibiotics in conventional and subantimicrobial doses as well as isotretinoin.

Given the potential influence of triggers in exacerbating rosacea, treatment should be aimed at identifying and avoiding these as much as possible. Additionally, because rosacea is associated with dysfunction of the epidermal barrier [21], skincare intended to cleanse and moisturize without causing irritation or dryness is considered essential to successful management. Soap-free moisturizing cleansers and scientifically formulated moisturizers containing ceramides may help restore epidermal barrier function [22]. Cosmetics, specifically a green-tinted foundation, may be used to camouflage the redness of rosacea.

Topical antimicrobial formulations, including sodium sulfacetamide and sulfur, metronidazole, and clindamycin, are thought to provide benefit primarily via anti-inflammatory effects. More than 60 years ago, topical sodium sulfacetamide 10 % and sulfur 5 % were the first agents approved for the treatment of acne vulgaris, seborrheic dermatitis, and rosacea. Sodium sulfacetamide is a sulfonamide with antibacterial activity, while sulfur is keratolytic.

Topical metronidazole is available in both 0.75 % and 1 % topical formulations that have been shown to be safe and effective for the treatment of PPR either used alone or in combination with oral antibiotics [23]. Metronidazole's mechanism of action in rosacea is hypothesized to involve anti-inflammatory and antimicrobial properties [23].

Azelaic acid is a naturally occurring dicarboxylic acid originally used as a 20 % cream to treat acne vulgaris. Azelaic acid 15 % aqueous gel was approved in 2002 for the treatment of mild to moderate papulopustular rosacea. The efficacy of azelaic acid 15 % gel in rosacea may be linked to the inhibition of neutrophil-mediated reactive oxygen species [24]. Azelaic acid also has antibacterial, keratolytic, and anti-inflammatory properties. Its efficacy in the management of PPR has been demonstrated in various studies [25].

A meta-analysis of available data on topical rosacea therapies suggests that either topical metronidazole or azelaic acid is appropriate for the management of rosacea subtype 2 [26]. These agents do not offer significant efficacy for diffuse erythema, telangiectases, or phymatous formations.

A first-in-class topical alpha-agonist received FDA approval for the treatment of the erythema of rosacea in August 2013. Brimonidine gel 0.33 % is a once-daily topical agent that was shown in clinical trials to provide a significantly greater improvement in the facial redness of rosacea than vehicle gel. The drug has vasoconstrictive properties that are believed to confer the redness reducing effects. Additional topical vasoconstrictors are in development for use in rosacea. Conventional antibiotics are still used in the management of rosacea, with their efficacy presumed to be associated with their anti-inflammatory effects. The availability of anti-inflammatory dose doxycycline (40 mg, controlled release) has modified the approach to systemic rosacea therapy [27]. Anti-inflammatory dose doxycycline is shown to be at least as effective as conventional doxycycline doses for the treatment of PPR but with a reduction in side effects [26] and no risk of contributing to the development of bacterial resistance [27]. Like topical interventions, oral antibiotics confer greatest efficacy in managing the signs and symptoms of PPR rather than the other subtypes.

Use of topical and systemic agents in combination is expected to enhance therapeutic responses and maintain results [27, 28]. Topical and systemic agents may also be used in combination with devices, which are increasingly used for the reduction of erythema and telangiectases associated with rosacea. Specifically, pulsed dye laser and intense-pulsed light (IPL) devices that target hemoglobin as the target chromophore are used to treat erythema and telangiectases [29].

Oral isotretinoin, which has both anti-inflammatory and immunomodulatory properties, has been used as a treatment for severe rosacea, particularly phymatous presentations [30, 31]. Surgical correction and ablative laser surgery may also be used to manage phymas.

43.6 Conclusion

Rosacea is a chronic, inflammatory facial dermatosis frequently confused with acne vulgaris. While the papulopustular subtype of rosacea presents with pustules, other clinical features (such as centrofacial erythema and a lack of comedones) distinguish rosacea from acne. Both topical and oral therapies can help reduce inflammation in rosacea, but light-based treatments are required to address underlying erythema.

References

1. Yamasaki K, Gallo RL. The molecular pathology of rosacea. J Dermatol Sci. 2009;55:77–81.
2. Diamantis S, Waldorf HA. Rosacea: clinical presentation and pathophysiology. J Drugs Dermatol. 2006;5:8–12.
3. Balkrishnan R, McMichael AJ, Hu JY, Camacho FT, Shew KR, Bouloc A, et al. Correlates of health-related quality of life in women with severe facial blemishes. Int J Dermatol. 2006;45:111–5.

4. Aksoy B, Altaykan-Hapa A, Egemen D, Karagöz F, Atakan N. The impact of rosacea on quality of life: effects of demographic and clinical characteristics and various treatment modalities. Br J Dermatol. 2010;163:719–25.
5. Wilkin J, Dahl M, Detmar M, et al. Standard grading system for rosacea: report of the National Rosacea Society Expert Committee on the classification and staging of rosacea. J Am Acad Dermatol. 2004;50:907–12.
6. Hoasjoe DK, Stucker FJ. Rhinophyma: review of pathophysiology and treatment. J Otolaryngol. 1995;24:51–6.
7. Wollina U. Rosacea and rhinophyma in the elderly. Clin Dermatol. 2011;29:61–8.
8. Feldman SR, Hollar CB, Gupta AK, Fleischer Jr AB. Women commonly seek care for rosacea: dermatologists frequently provide the care. Cutis. 2001;68:156–60.
9. Elsaie ML, Choudhary S. Updates on the pathophysiology and management of acne rosacea. Postgrad Med. 2009;121:178–86.
10. Elewski BE, Draelos Z, Dréno B, Jansen T, Layton A, Picardo M. Rosacea-global diversity and optimized outcome: proposed international consensus from the Rosacea International Expert Group. J Eur Acad Dermatol Venereol. 2011;25:188–200.
11. Jones DA. Rosacea, reactive oxygen species, and azelaic acid. J Clin Aesthet Dermatol. 2009;2:26–30.
12. Marks R. The enigma of rosacea. J Dermatolog Treat. 2007;18(6):326–8.
13. McAleer MA, Fitzpatrick P, Powell FC. Papulopustular rosacea: prevalence and relationship to photodamage. J Am Acad Dermatol. 2010;63:33–9.
14. National Rosacea Society website. http://www.rosacea.org/patients/materials/tripwires.php. Accessed 21 Sept 2011.
15. Oltz M, Check J. Rosacea and its ocular manifestations. Optometry. 2011;82:92–103.
16. Ghanem VC, Mehra N, Wong S, Mannis MJ. The prevalence of ocular signs in acne rosacea: comparing patients from ophthalmology and dermatology clinics. Cornea. 2003;22:230–3.
17. Lipozencic J, Ljubojevic S. Perioral dermatitis. Clin Dermatol. 2011;29:157–61.
18. Ljubojeviae S, Basta-Juzbasiae A, Lipozenèiae J. Steroid dermatitis resembling rosacea: aetiopathogenesis and treatment. J Eur Acad Dermatol Venereol. 2002;16:121–6.
19. Zhao YE, Wu LP, Peng Y, Cheng H. Retrospective analysis of the association between Demodex infestation and rosacea. Arch Dermatol. 2010;146:896–902.
20. Bikowski JB, Del Rosso JQ. Demodex dermatitis: a retrospective analysis of clinical diagnosis and successful treatment with topical crotamiton. J Clin Aesthet Dermatol. 2009;2:20–5.
21. Draelos ZD. Treating beyond the histology of rosacea. Cutis. 2004;74(3 Suppl):28–31. 32–34.
22. Bikowski J. The use of therapeutic moisturizers in various dermatologic disorders. Cutis. 2001;68(5 Suppl):3–11.
23. Conde JF, Yelverton CB, Balkrishnan R, Fleischer Jr AB, Feldman SR. Managing rosacea: a review of the use of metronidazole alone and in combination with oral antibiotics. J Drugs Dermatol. 2007;6:495–8.
24. Del Rosso JQ, Baum EW, Draelos ZD, et al. Azelaic acid gel 15%: clinical versatility in the treatment of rosacea. Cutis. 2006;78(5 Suppl):6–19.
25. Del Rosso JQ, Bhatia N. Azelaic acid gel 15% in the management of papulopustular rosacea: a status report on available efficacy data and clinical application. Cutis. 2011;88:67–72.
26. van Zuuren EJ, Kramer S, Carter B, Graber MA, Fedorowicz Z. Interventions for rosacea. Cochrane Database Syst Rev. 2011;16:CD003262.
27. Bikowski JB. The pharmacologic therapy of rosacea: a paradigm shift in progress. Cutis. 2005;75(3):27–32.
28. Wolf Jr JE. Present and future rosacea therapy. Cutis. 2005;75(3 Suppl):4–7.
29. Kennedy Carney C, Cantrell W, Elewski BE. Rosacea: a review of current topical, systemic and light-based therapies. G Ital Dermatol Venereol. 2009;144:673–88.
30. Jansen T, Plewig G. Clinical and histological variants of rhinophyma, including nonsurgical treatment modalities. Facial Plast Surg. 1998;14:241–53.
31. Park H, Del Rosso JQ. Use of oral isotretinoin in the management of rosacea. J Clin Aesthet Dermatol. 2011;4:54–61.

Chapter 44
Rosacea Fulminans

Cristina Caridi and Joshua A. Zeichner

44.1 Introduction

Rosacea fulminans is a rare dermatosis characterized by the sudden onset of coalescing nodules and draining sinuses on the face, typically affecting young women. First reported in 1940 by the name pyoderma faciale, it was thought to be an infiltrative pyoderma, possibly caused by tuberculosis, despite being unable to identify a cause [1]. It was not until 1992 that it was suggested that the condition was a form of rosacea, as all patients also experienced flushing and blushing along with the rapid and volatile onset. The term rosacea fulminans was then proposed [2]. Despite research, a bacterial infection has not been shown to play a pathogenic role, further evidence that the condition is not a pyoderma, but rather a severe variant of rosacea [3]. Rosacea fulminans has also been referred to as granulomatous rosacea.

44.2 Background

The pathophysiology of rosacea fulminans is unknown. Hyperactivity of the innate immune system, severe emotional stress, hormonal changes (including those during pregnancy), and an association with inflammatory bowel disease have all been suggested [2, 4–7]. *Helicobacter pylori* bacteria have been identified in the gastric mucosa of patients with both rosacea and rosacea fulminans and is thought to stimulate production of vasoactive molecules, including prostaglandins, histamine, and various cytokines [8, 9]. A more in-depth review of the pathophysiology may be found in the rosacea chapter of this book.

C. Caridi, B.A. (✉) • J.A. Zeichner, M.D.
Department of Dermatology, Mt. Sinai School of Medicine, New York, NY, USA

J.A. Zeichner (ed.), *Acneiform Eruptions in Dermatology: A Differential Diagnosis*,
DOI 10.1007/978-1-4614-8344-1_44,

While extremely rare, rosacea fulminans is also assumed to be highly underreported. Approximately 80 cases have been published since the 1940s. It occurs almost exclusively in healthy females in the second to third decades, but ages range from the teens into the 50s [1, 2]. There is no associated history with acne vulgaris [3], but many patients may have an underlying diagnosis of rosacea [10, 11].

44.3 Clinical Presentation

Rosacea fulminans is characterized by a sudden and explosive onset of large indurated erythematous plaques, nodules, papules, pustules, and draining sinuses restricted to the face (Fig. 44.1). Patients generally has previously unblemished skin [1, 2, 11]. The most severely affected areas of the face include the forehead, nasal bridge, cheeks, and chin [3]. Comedones are characteristically absent and the trunk is spared. Large abscesses may be interconnected through sinus tracts that discharge copious amounts of pus [2].

No true prodrome exists prior to the onset of the disease. However, there are reports of patients who develop a sudden onset of excessive skin oiliness prior to the eruption [1, 2]. Patients are otherwise healthy, though some experience fatigue, discomfort, or general malaise. One patient has been reported to develop rosacea fulminans in association with erythema nodosum [12]. Another report documented a case of severe ocular involvement presenting with blurry vision. Ophthalmologic exam revealed severe blepharitis with advanced keratitis and ocular perforation. While ocular involvement is common in traditional rosacea, it is not usually present in rosacea fulminans [11].

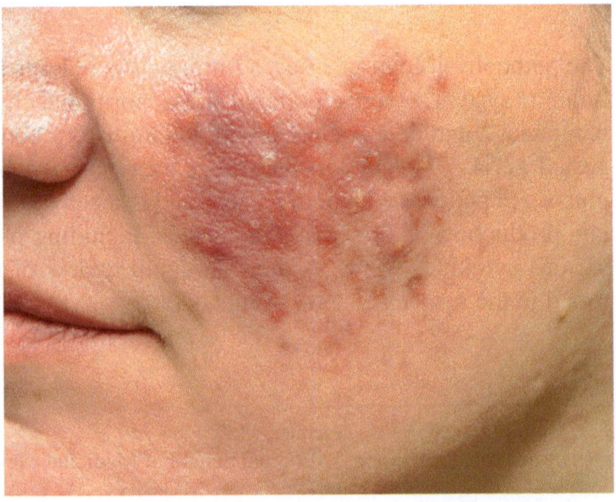

Fig. 44.1 An indurated, erythematous plaque on the left cheek of a woman in her 30s. Pustules and papules are evident within the plaque, and the patient complains of tenderness in the area (Photo credit: Joshua A. Zeichner, M.D.

Because of the particularly ferocious nature of the disease, patients may become depressed, anxious, and isolated because of the appearance [2, 13]. Scarring is common and expected and can range from minimal damage to keloids [2, 14].

44.4 Work-up

The diagnosis of rosacea fulminans is largely clinical, although supportive labs and a skin biopsy can be performed. Some patients have been documented to have a mild anemia, leukocytosis, increased erythrocyte sedimentation rate (ESR), elevated C-reactive protein (CRP), and positive rheumatoid factor and antinuclear antibodies [1, 2, 4, 14, 15]. Skin biopsy reveals evidence of inflammation, with massive neutrophil infiltration in early stages and epithelioid cell granulomas in older lesions [4, 12, 16]. Bacterial pathogens have not been consistently recovered, and most bacteria identified are commensal skin flora [2, 3]. Isolated cases report identification of *Staphylococcus aureus* and gram-negative bacteria [3, 5].

44.5 Treatment

If untreated, rosacea fulminans generally resolves after approximately 1 year, although aggressive therapy is usually given to avoid the development of permanent scars. The most commonly effective treatment for rosacea fulminans is oral isotretinoin, usually in combination with oral corticosteroids to reduce the risk of an initial flare. Isotretinoin is typically dosed at 0.5 mg/kg/day for the first month then increased to 1 mg/kg/day at month 2, depending on the clinical appearance. Just as in acne vulgaris, the target cumulative dose is 120–150 mg/kg [2, 4, 11, 17–19]. Oral dapsone, oral and topical antibiotics, benzoyl peroxide, and topical and systemic corticosteroids, among others, have all been reported as well [2, 5, 6, 18, 20]. Oral azithromycin has also been shown to be effective in a pregnant woman [15].

Surgical interventions have been associated with poor outcomes. Incision and drainage of abscesses and sinus should not be performed as it can lead to excessive scarring [2]. Early biopsy, however, can help correctly diagnose a patient early in the course of the disease and ultimately results in a more rapid treatment [16].

44.6 Conclusion

Rosacea fulminans is a rapidly occurring, severe facial dermatosis thought to be an extreme variant of rosacea. It results in significant scarring, both physically and emotionally. Early diagnosis with prompt treatment (usually with oral isotretinoin) is important to minimize long-term sequelae.

References

1. O'Leary PA, Kierland RR. Pyoderma faciale. Arch Dermatol. 1940;41:451–62.
2. Plewig G, Jansen T, Kligman AM. Pyoderma faciale a review and report of 20 additional cases: is it rosacea? Arch Dermatol. 1992;128:1611–7.
3. Sudy E, Urbina F. Pyoderma faciale: gram-negative recovery by means of needle aspiration. Cont Med Educ. 2002;69:261–4.
4. Ferahbas A, Utas S, Mistik S, Uksal U, Peker D. Rosacea fulminans in pregnancy case report and review of the literature. Am J Clin Dermatol. 2006;7(2):141–4.
5. Massa MC, Su WP. Pyoderma faciale: a clinical study of twenty-nine patients. J Am Acad Dermatol. 1982;6:84–91.
6. Dessoukey MW. Pyoderma faciale: manifestation of inflammatory bowel disease. Int J Dermatol. 1996;35:724–6.
7. Manna V, Marks R, Holt P. Involvement of immune mechanisms in the pathogenesis of rosacea. Br J Dermatol. 1982;107:203–8.
8. Rebora A, Drago F, Parodi A. May helicobacter pylori be important for dermatologists? Dermatology. 1995;191:6–8.
9. Szlachcic A, Sliwowski Z, Karczewska E, Bielana W, Pytko-Poloncyzk J, Konturek SJ. *Helicobacter pylori* and its eradication in rosacea. J Physiol Pharmacol. 1999;50:777–86.
10. Ormond P, Rogers S. Case 3: pyoderma faciale (PF) (rosacea fulminans). Clin Exp Dermatol. 2003;28:107–8.
11. de Morais e Silva FA, Bonassi M, Steiner D, Ribeiro da Cunha TV. Rosacea fulminans in pregnancy with ocular perforation. J Ger Soc Dermatol. 2011;9:542–3.
12. Akhyani M, Daneshpazhooh M, Ghandi N. The association of pyoderma faciale and erythema nodosum. Clin Exp Dermatol. 2007;32:275–7.
13. Fender AB, Ignatovitch Y, Mercurio MG. Pyoderma faciale. Cutis. 2008;81:488–90.
14. Firooz A, Firoozabadi MR, Dowlati Y. Rosacea fulminans (pyoderma faciale): successful treatment of a 3-year-old girl with oral isotretinoin. Int J Dermatol. 2001;40:203–5.
15. Fuentalsaz V, Ara M, Corredera C, et al. Rosacea fulminans in pregnancy: successful treatment with azithromycin. Clin Exp Dermatol. 2011;36(6):674–6.
16. Helm TA, Schechter J. Biopsy may help identify early pyoderma faciale (rosacea fulminans). Cutis. 2006;77:225–7.
17. Lewis VJ, Holme SA, Wright A, Antsey AV. Rosacea fulminans in pregnancy. Br J Dermatol. 2004;151:917–9.
18. Marks VJ, Briggaman RA. Pyoderma faciale: successful treatment with isotretinoin. J Am Acad Dermatol. 1987;17:1062–3.
19. Ortonne JP. Oral isotretinoin treatment policy: do we all agree? Dermatology. 1997;195 Suppl 1:34–7.
20. Bormann G, Gaber G, Fischer M, Marsch WC. Dapsone in rosacea fulminans. J Eur Acad Dermatol Venereol. 2001;15(5):465–7.

Chapter 45
Sarcoidosis

Laura Thornsberry and Joseph English III

45.1 Introduction

Sarcoidosis is a multiorgan noninfectious granulomatous disease which can manifest in the integumentary system in a variety of ways, one of the most common being a maculopapular, acneiform facial eruption. Although sarcoidosis is generally categorized as a pulmonary disease, it involves the skin in approximately 25–30 % of cases. The etiology of sarcoidosis remains unknown. The polymorphic cutaneous lesions are grouped into specific and nonspecific lesions. The characteristic histological finding in sarcoidosis, the noncaseating granuloma, is present in the specific lesions of cutaneous sarcoidosis, including macules, papules, plaques, subcutaneous nodules, infiltrative scars, and lupus pernio. The nonspecific lesions of cutaneous sarcoidosis, such as erythema nodosum (EN), calcifications, erythema multiforme, and clubbing, lack this feature. Sarcoidosis is a diagnosis of exclusion based on a combination of clinical, histological, and radiographic evidence. Since cutaneous sarcoidosis is frequently present at the onset of systemic disease, the dermatologist is often the first health-care provider to evaluate the patient. Biopsy-proven cutaneous sarcoidosis warrants a further workup for systemic disease. Corticosteroids are the mainstay of treatment for symptomatic sarcoidosis, followed by antimalarial and immunosuppressive medications.

L. Thornsberry, M.D. (✉)
Department of Internal Medicine, PGY-1, UPMC Montefiore Hospital, University of Pittsburgh, N-713, 200 Lothrop Street, Pittsburgh, PA 15213, USA
e-mail: thornsberryla@upmc.edu

J. English III, M.D.
Department of Dermatology, University of Pittsburgh, Pittsburgh, PA USA
e-mail: englishjc@upmc.edu

J.A. Zeichner (ed.), *Acneiform Eruptions in Dermatology: A Differential Diagnosis*,
DOI 10.1007/978-1-4614-8344-1_45,

45.2 Background

There are many theories surrounding the etiology of sarcoidosis, but the cause(s) of the disease is still unknown. A multicenter trial of over 700 patients, entitled "A Case Control Etiologic Study of Sarcoidosis (ACCESS)," was unable to identify a specific antigen in sarcoidosis but did establish an increased risk of the disease with exposure to mold and musty odors, agricultural chemicals and aerosols, and insecticides [1]. In sarcoidosis, normal tissue function is disrupted by noncaseating granulomas. The formation of the noncaseating granuloma begins with macrophages and dendritic cells (antigen-presenting cells) using class II major histocompatibility (MHC) complexes to present an unknown antigen(s) to CD4+ T cells [2]. Through interactions with the MHC and costimulatory molecules, the T cell becomes activated and ignites a T_H1 inflammatory response. The T cells release IL-2 and IFN-γ to recruit additional T cells, as well as stimulate macrophages to produce TNF-α, leading to the differentiation of macrophages into epithelioid cells and formation of multinucleated giant cells [2].

In the United States, there are two peaks for sarcoidosis, in people between 25 and 35 years and in women between 45 and 65 years [3]. Sarcoidosis is more common in African Americans (although all races can be affected), and this group is more likely to present with advanced disease and have a poorer prognosis [4]. The highest incidence of disease in the United States in African American women in their fourth decade of life [3]. Sarcoidosis persists as a progressive disease in 30 % but has a mortality of less than 5 % [5]. The most common causes of death are progressive pulmonary fibrosis or other pulmonary or cardiac complications [4]. The first-degree relatives of people with sarcoidosis are at a 5-time increased risk for developing the disease [6]. Recent research has proposed certain genetic susceptibilities associated with the disease. An increased risk of sarcoidosis is associated with HLA-DRB1 and a splice site mutation in the gene butyrophilin-like 2 (BTNL2) [7].

45.3 Clinical Presentation

Cutaneous sarcoidosis is a clinically polymorphic disease. Many atypical presentations of cutaneous sarcoidosis have been reported, including but not limited to ichthyosiform, ulcerative, erythrodermic, hypopigmented, photo-distributed, verrucous, morpheaform, and lichenoid sarcoidosis [8]. Maculopapular eruptions are the most common specific lesion and tend to occur on the head, neck, perioral region, eyelids, and nasolabial folds. The papules are usually small (3–5 mm), monomorphic, and flesh-colored without epidermal change. The papules may also be red, violaceous, or hyperpigmented, and groups of papules may coalesce into annular lesions or plaques. This presentation of sarcoidosis may present similar to other acneiform eruptions of the face (Figs. 45.1 and 45.2). The differential diagnosis includes acne,

Fig. 45.1 Papular sarcoidosis in the T zone

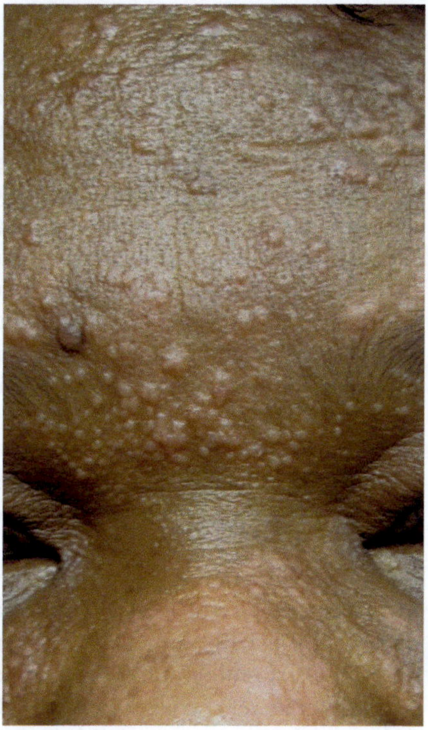

Fig. 45.2 Papular sarcoidosis of the malar checks

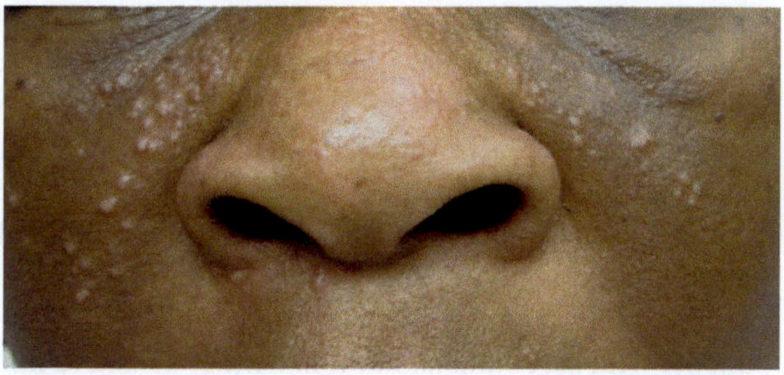

rosacea, granulomatous periorificial dermatitis, and granulomatous rosacea. Sarcoidosis differs from acne vulgaris in that there is no comedonal component and lesions are not pustular in nature. The majority of the time the difference can be determined clinically but biopsy can easily distinguish these entities. Although maculopapular sarcoidosis may not seem significant, Mana [9] reported a series in which four out of 14 patients with maculopapular lesions developed chronic cutaneous, pulmonary, or ocular sarcoidosis [9].

45.4 Workup

The diagnosis of sarcoidosis requires careful integration of clinical, radiographic, and histological information, as well as the exclusion of other granulomatous diseases. Evaluation begins with a thorough history and physical examination focusing on the skin, lungs, heart, eyes, lymph nodes, and nervous system. When sarcoidosis is suspected, the skin is often the most accessible and least invasive option available for obtaining a biopsy. If the biopsy reveals noncaseating granulomas, the stains and tissue cultures must be negative for infectious agents, such as Mycobacteria, fungi, leishmaniasis, and syphilis, and foreign body granulomas must also be excluded [9]. When a diagnosis of cutaneous sarcoidosis is suspected, the patient needs to be evaluated for systemic sarcoidosis. This will require consultation with several specialty physicians.

Evaluation for pulmonary sarcoidosis begins with a chest radiograph and pulmonary function tests. Pulmonary manifestations are present in approximately 90 % of patients with sarcoidosis. The radiograph most commonly reveals bilateral hilar lymphadenopathy, but may also show infiltrates or fibrosis, while the pulmonary function tests may demonstrate a restrictive pattern with decreased diffusing capacity [10, 11]. High-resolution computed tomography (CT) of the chest is not usually indicated, but can be used to further evaluate patients with atypical chest radiographs [10]. Cardiac sarcoidosis is initially evaluated by electrocardiogram and echocardiogram [10]. Heart failure or symptoms such as palpitations and syncope are only present in 5 % of patients and usually indicate advanced disease [12]. Cardiac magnetic resonance imaging (MRI) is a specific but not sensitive test for detecting structural cardiac disease [12]. Ocular sarcoidosis most commonly presents as uveitis, but can ultimately result in blindness, thus a complete ophthalmologic evaluation is recommended [10]. Neurosarcoidosis is present in up to 15 % of patients with systemic disease [8]. Evaluation may include radiographs of the skull, electroencephalography, CT scan, and/or MRI of the central nervous system [8].

In addition laboratory testing includes complete blood counts, liver and kidney function tests, serum calcium level, creatinine kinase and aldolase, and urinalysis. The serum angiotensin-converting enzyme (SACE) level is increased in 60 % of patients with sarcoidosis, but it is neither sensitive nor specific, and can be elevated in common diseases, such as diabetes and osteoarthritis [4, 9].

45.5 Treatment

There is no FDA-approved treatment for sarcoidosis, and there is limited evidence-based medicine regarding the treatment of cutaneous sarcoidosis [13]. In terms of cutaneous sarcoidosis, corticosteroids (oral and intralesional) are the mainstay of treatment [14, 15]. Corticosteroids provide anti-inflammatory and immunosuppressive effects, theoretically decreasing granuloma formation [16]. The dosing ranges and schedules of corticosteroids are highly variable, and there is not adequate evidence supporting their use for cutaneous sarcoidosis [11]. Historically, oral prednisone has been reported as effective for cutaneous sarcoidosis, but randomized controlled trials are needed [14, 17, 18]. Given the extensive side effects of systemic corticosteroids, they are generally only used for expansive disfiguring cutaneous lesions after local steroids have failed [3]. Corticosteroids must be tapered slowly over weeks to months to avoid disease flares.

Hydroxychloroquine is an antimalarial agent which is thought to work by decreasing antigen presentation by APCs, resulting in decreased T-cell activation and decreased granuloma formation [19]. The efficacy of antimalarials in cutaneous sarcoidosis has been reported since the 1960s, but there have not been any randomized controlled trials for this indication [20, 21]. More recent studies have reported regression of cutaneous sarcoidosis with hydroxychloroquine (2–3 mg/kg/day for up to 12 weeks) [22] or chloroquine (500 mg daily for 14 days, then 250 mg for long-term maintenance) [23]. Antimalarial medications require frequent eye exams (at least yearly) for ototoxicity. Methotrexate, a dihydrofolate reductase inhibitor, has emerged as a second-line treatment for cutaneous sarcoidosis, typically prescribed at doses of 10–30 mg/week [16]. Webster [24] reported clearing of refractory cutaneous sarcoidosis in three patients with 15 mg/week for up to 11 months [24]. Baughman [25] reported improvement in 16 out of 17 patients treated with methotrexate over a period of 2 years and with average doses of 28 mg/week [25]. Minocycline (200 mg/day) has been reported in one open prospective study of 12 patients with refractory cutaneous sarcoidosis, with 8 patients experiencing complete regression and 2 with partial regression after 12 months, but with 3 suffering relapse of disease after stopping this therapy [26].

Other medications that have been reported for the treatment of sarcoidosis include pentoxifylline [27], thalidomide [28–32], allopurinol [33, 34], isotretinoin [35, 36], infliximab [37, 38], adalimumab [39], azathioprine [40], cyclophosphamide [40], cyclosporine [41], chlorambucil [42, 43], leflunomide [44, 45], and melatonin [46], but randomized controlled trials are needed to evaluate these treatments. Non-pharmaceutical options include lasers, dermabrasion, excision, and phototherapy (PUVA, UVB, and photodynamic therapy).

45.6 Conclusion

Sarcoidosis is a systemic disease affecting multiple organ systems. Cutaneous lesions may be mistaken for acne but can be distinguished based on the lack of comedones and the distinct histological appearance. Prompt diagnosis is important, as the skin may be a presenting sign of widespread disease. Multiple therapies are effective, and patients often require oral medications for internal disease as well as topicals for cutaneous lesions.

References

1. Newman L, ACCESS Research Group. A case control etiologic study of sarcoidosis: environmental and occupational risk factors. Am J Respir Crit Care Med. 2004;170(12):1324–30.
2. Noor A. Immunopathogenesis of sarcoidosis. Clin Dermatol. 2007;25:250–8.
3. English J. Sarcoidosis. J Am Acad Dermatol. 2001;44(5):725–43.
4. Heath C. Sarcoidosis: are there differences in your skin of color patients? J Am Acad Dermatol. 2012;66(1):121.e1–14.
5. Morgenthau A. Recent advances in sarcoidosis. Chest. 2011;139:174–82.
6. Judson M. The diagnosis of sarcoidosis. Clin Chest Med. 2008;29:415–27.
7. Valentonyte R. Sarcoidosis is associated with a truncating splice site mutation in BTNL2. Nat Genet. 2005;37:357–64.
8. English J. Sarcoidosis. In: Callen J, editor. Dermatologic signs of internal disease. China: Saunders Elsevier; 2009.
9. Mana J. Cutaneous involvement in sarcoidosis. Arch Dermatol. 2007;133:882–8.
10. Costabel U. Systemic evaluation of a potential cutaneous sarcoidosis patient. Clin Dermatol. 2007;25:303–11.
11. Izikson A, English JC. Cutaneous sarcoidosis. In: Williams H, editor. Evidence-based dermatology. 2nd ed. London: Wiley-Blackwell; 2008.
12. Skold C. Determination of cardiac involvement in sarcoidosis by magnetic resonance imaging and Doppler echocardiography. J Intern Med. 2002;252(5):465–71.
13. Iannuzzi M. Sarcoidosis. JAMA. 2011;305(4):391–9.
14. Russo G. Cutaneous sarcoidosis: diagnosis and treatment. Complement Ther. 1994;20:418–21.
15. Wilson N. Cutaneous sarcoidosis. Postgrad Med J. 1998;74:649–52.
16. Badgwell C. Cutaneous sarcoidosis therapy updated. J Am Acad Dermatol. 2007;56:69–83.
17. Albertini J. Ulcerative sarcoidosis: case report and review of the literature. Arch Dermatol. 1997;133:215–9.
18. Veien N. Cutaneous sarcoidosis: prognosis and treatment. Clin Dermatol. 1986;4:75–87.
19. Fox R. Mechanism of action of antimalarial drugs: inhibition of antigen processing and presentation. Lupus. 1993;2 Suppl 1:S9–12.
20. Morse S. The treatment of sarcoidosis with chloroquine. Am J Med. 1961;1961:779–84.
21. Siltzbach L. Chloroquine therapy in 43 patients with intrathoracic and cutaneous lesions. Acta Med Scand. 1964;176 Suppl 425:302–6.
22. Jones E. Hydroxychloroquine is effective therapy for control of cutaneous sarcoidal granulomas. J Am Acad Dermatol. 1990;23:487–9.
23. Zic J. Treatment of cutaneous sarcoidosis with chloroquine. Arch Dermatol. 1991; 127:1034–40.
24. Webster G. Weekly low-dose methotrexate for cutaneous sarcoidosis. J Am Acad Dermatol. 1991;24:451–4.
25. Lower E. Prolonged use of methotrexate for sarcoidosis. Arch Intern Med. 1995;155:846–51.
26. Bachelez H. The use of tetracyclines for the treatment of sarcoidosis. Arch Dermatol. 2001;137:69–73.
27. Zabel P. Pentoxifylline in treatment of sarcoidosis. Am J Respir Crit Care Med. 1997;155: 1665–9.
28. Carlesimo M. Treatment of cutaneous and pulmonary sarcoidosis with thalidomide. J Am Acad Dermatol. 1995;32:866–9.
29. Rousseau L. Cutaneous sarcoidosis successfully treated with low doses of thalidomide. Arch Dermatol. 1998;134:1045–6.
30. Lee J. Disfiguring cutaneous manifestation of sarcoidosis treated with thalidomide: a case report. J Am Acad Dermatol. 1998;39:835–8.
31. Baughman R. Thalidomide for chronic sarcoidosis. Chest. 2002;122:227–32.
32. Nguyen Y. Treatment of cutaneous sarcoidosis with thalidomide. J Am Acad Dermatol. 2004;50:235–41.

33. Samuel M. Sarcoidosis: initial results on six patients treated with allopurinol. Br J Dermatol. 1984;111 Suppl 26:20.
34. Voelter-Mahlknecht S. Treatment of subcutaneous sarcoidosis with allopurinol. Arch Dermatol. 1999;135:1560–1.
35. Waldinger T. Treatment of cutaneous sarcoidosis with isotretinoin. Arch Dermatol. 1983;119:1003–5.
36. Georgiou S. Cutaneous sarcoidosis: complete remission after oral isotretinoin therapy. Acta Derm Venereol. 1998;78:457–9.
37. Baughman R. Infliximab in cutaneous sarcoidosis. Sarcoidosis Vasc Diffuse Lung Dis. 2001;18:70–4.
38. Meyerle J. The use of infliximab in cutaneous sarcoidosis. J Drugs Dermatol. 2003;2:413–4.
39. Heffernan M. Adalimumab for treatment of cutaneous sarcoidosis. Arch Dermatol. 2006;142:17–9.
40. Baughman R. Alternatives to corticosteroids in the treatment of sarcoidosis. Sarcoidosis Vasc Diffuse Lung Dis. 1997;14:121–30.
41. Rebuck A. Cyclosporin in pulmonary sarcoidosis. Lancet. 1987;1:1486.
42. Kataria Y. Chlorambucil in sarcoidosis. Chest. 1980;78:36–43.
43. Isreal H. Chlorambucil treatment of sarcoidosis. Sarcoidosis. 1991;8:35–41.
44. Baughman R. Leflunomide for chronic sarcoidosis. Sarcoidosis Vasc Diffuse Lung Dis. 2004;21:43–8.
45. Majithia V. Successful treatment of sarcoidosis with leflunomide. Rheumatology. 2003;42:700–2.
46. Cagnoni M. Melatonin for treatment of chronic refractory sarcoidosis. Lancet. 1995;346: 1229–30.

Chapter 46
Seborrheic Dermatitis

Elizabeth Farhat and Linda Stein Gold

46.1 Introduction

Seborrheic dermatitis is a chronic inflammatory papulosquamous skin condition that commonly involves the sebum-rich areas of the scalp, ears, face, chest, and skinfolds. It typically has a chronic, relapsing course that can range in severity from asymptomatic dandruff of the scalp to extensive skin involvement resulting in exfoliative erythroderma. Patients are otherwise healthy, but it has been noted to be a marker for human immunodeficiency virus (HIV) infection as well as some neurologic diseases. It is thought to be linked to a reaction to *Malassezia furfur* (*Pityrosporum ovale*), but the relationship is complex.

46.2 Background

46.2.1 Epidemiology

Seborrheic dermatitis peaks during time periods of increased sebum production initially during infancy and later during adolescence and adulthood. It is generally divided into infantile seborrheic dermatitis and adult seborrheic dermatitis which generally occurs in those aged 30–60 years [1]. Up to 70 % of infants may develop seborrheic dermatitis within the first 3 months of life which usually resolves by 1 year of age [2]. The prevalence in healthy adults is between 1 % and 3 %, more commonly seen in males than females, and typically worsens during the winter

E. Farhat, M.D. • L.S. Gold, M.D. (✉)
Department of Dermatology, Henry Ford Health System, 6530 Farmington Road, West Bloomfield, MI 48322, USA
e-mail: lstein1@hfhs.org

J.A. Zeichner (ed.), *Acneiform Eruptions in Dermatology: A Differential Diagnosis*, DOI 10.1007/978-1-4614-8344-1_46, © Springer Science+Business Media New York 2014

months [3]. Many consider dandruff, pityriasis simplex, to be the mildest form of seborrheic dermatitis which may affect up to 50 % of the population [4].

Seborrheic dermatitis has been noted to be a marker for HIV infection and may be the presenting sign [5, 6]. The prevalence of seborrheic dermatitis in early HIV infection is 36 % and 50–83 % in patients with acquired immunodeficiency syndrome (AIDS) [7–9]. Patients with Parkinson's disease have increased sebum production as well as an increased prevalence of seborrheic dermatitis. Treatment with L-dopa results in with both quantitative sebum reduction and clinical improvement of seborrhea [10]. This increased prevalence also occurs in patients with neuroleptic-induced Parkinsonism after the use of neuroleptic drugs such as chlorpromazine hydrochloride and haloperidol and in those with mood disorders such as schizophrenia, depression, and anxiety [11, 12]. Seborrheic dermatitis is seen in other genetic disorders including familial amyloidosis with polyneuropathy and Down's syndrome [13–15].

The role of ultraviolet (UV) light on seborrheic dermatitis is unclear. Patients frequently report improvement after exposure to sunlight [16]. Also, seborrheic dermatitis is noted to flare during the winter months [17]. However, mountain guides who have increased UV exposure were noted to have increased prevalence of seborrheic dermatitis thought to be secondary to UV-induced immunosuppression [18]. Additionally psoralen plus UVA (PUVA) light treatment can induce seborrheic dermatitis, whereas narrowband UVB (NBUVB) has been used to successfully treat severe disease [19, 20].

46.2.2 Pathophysiology

The etiology of seborrheic dermatitis is controversial with no genetic disposition noted. It appears to be related to active sebaceous glands given the predilection for body sites with increased sebaceous distribution. There also may be a hormonal influence as the disease emerges at puberty and is more common in men, which may be secondary to androgenic stimulation of the pilosebaceous unit increasing sebum production [3]. However, the amount of sebum excretion in patients with seborrheic dermatitis is not increased compared to unaffected individuals, and sebaceous glands themselves are not actively involved in its pathogenesis [21]. It is thought that sebaceous glands may instead have a more permissive role that allows for growth of lipophilic *Malassezia* fungi (formerly *Pityrosporum ovale*) [22].

The relationship between *Malassezia* yeast and seborrheic dermatitis has been debated for years. *Malassezia* yeasts are lipid-dependent components of normal skin flora. Initially it was thought that these yeasts were the underlying cause of seborrheic dermatitis because scalp cultures from patients with dandruff revealed increased amounts of *Pityrosporum*. Later investigations, however, revealed no correlation between the amount of *P. ovale* present and disease severity [23, 24]. Others believed that an initial impairment of desquamation led to increased nutrient availability allowing yeast to flourish. The yeasts, themselves, are not pathogenic [25].

Nevertheless, antifungal medications have been shown to improve scaling and itching of the scalp associated with seborrheic dermatitis [26].

The current thought is that seborrheic dermatitis occurs in susceptible individuals caused by an inflammatory process mediated by oleic acid which is released from sebaceous triglycerides in the presence of *Malassezia* yeast [27]. Analysis of genomes from *M. globosa* and *M. restricta* revealed a functional lipase gene (LIP1) and several phospholipase genes with expression detected on the human scalp [28, 29]. The lipase and phospholipase activity of the yeast cleaves sebaceous gland triglycerides into free fatty acids which induces flaking and inflammation in patients with an altered stratum corneum. Other proposed mechanisms include direct release of proinflammatory cytokines (IL-6, IL-8, IL-1alpha) and a decrease in anti-inflammatory cytokines (IL-10) from keratinocytes in response to *Malassezia* species [30]. This is possibly due to an irritant non-immunogenic stimulation induced by the yeast [31].

46.3 Clinical Presentation

Seborrheic dermatitis presents as well-demarcated erythematous patches or plaques with a greasy, white or yellow scale located on the sebum-rich areas of the body including the scalp, external auditory meatus, postauricular area, face, central chest, and intertriginous areas including axillae and groin folds (Figs. 46.1 and 46.2). Rarely, it can present as a solitary lesion in the male external genital area [23]. It may be associated with blepharoconjunctivitis with scaling and erythema of the eyelid margin and inflammation of the conjunctiva. Itching is usually minimal and may be confined to the scalp. In infants it can present as cradle cap of the scalp or as diaper dermatitis. In patients with HIV the clinical presentation can be more explosive and dramatic and may be presenting sign in some patients. The differential diagnosis is extensive (Table 46.1). Scalp psoriasis can be differentiated from seborrheic dermatitis using dermoscopy which demonstrates red dots and globules,

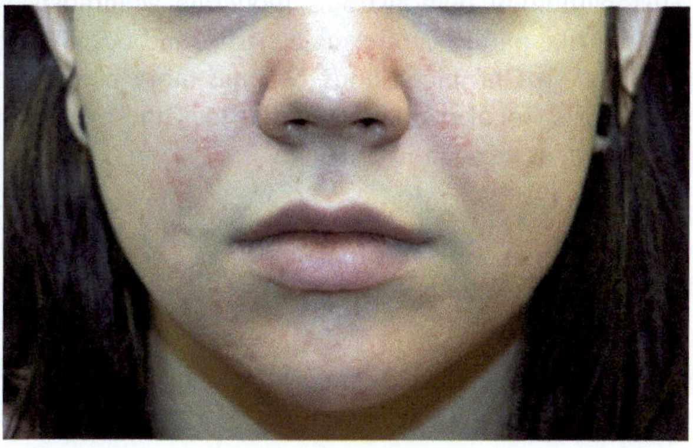

Fig. 46.1 Erythematous, scaly patches primarily affected the medial cheeks and nasolabial folds. While the patient complained of acne, she did not present with any comedonal lesions. She also had scale in the eyebrows and scalp. Her rash improved with use of topical ketoconazole cream

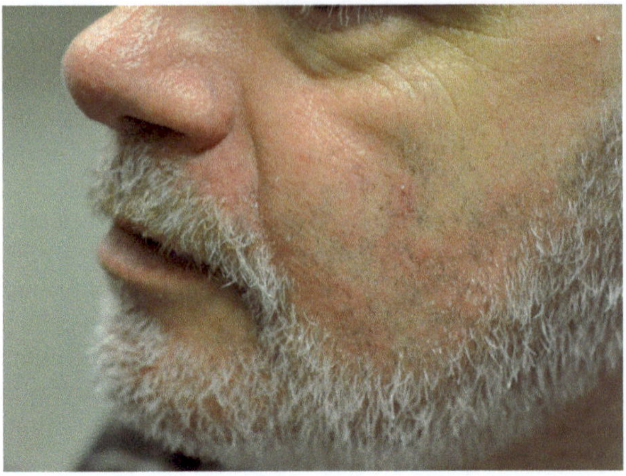

Fig. 46.2 Typical erythematous scaly patches in the beard and nasolabial folds

twisted red loops, and glomerular vessels in psoriasis in contrast to arborizing vessels and atypical or absent vascular patterns in seborrheic dermatitis [32].

46.4 Work-Up

46.4.1 Laboratory

Seborrheic dermatitis is a clinical diagnosis based on history and physical examination. For definitive diagnosis biopsy can be performed for histopathologic examination.

46.4.2 Biopsies

Histopathology demonstrates moderate acanthosis with accentuated rete ridges, mound-like parakeratotic scale crusts, and occasional foci of suprapapillary spongiosis [33]. Chronic lesions become more psoriasiform appearing with irregular acanthosis, focal parakeratosis but lack the exocytosis of neutrophils or Munro's microabscesses seen in psoriasis.

46.4.3 Cultures

Fungal culture or potassium hydroxide preparation can be performed to rule out tinea capitis or tinea versicolor.

Table 46.1 Clinical presentation and differential diagnosis of seborrheic dermatitis

Diagnosis	Clinical findings	Differentiation
Infantile seborrheic dermatitis	Erythematous patches and plaques on scalp with greasy scaling and crusting (cradle cap) and patches in axillae; inguinal folds may have oozing, crusting, satellite lesions	
Atopic dermatitis	Erythematous eczematous patches located on the face, scalp, and extensor surfaces of the body with crusting	Later onset after 3rd month, more inflammation, more pruritus; patients are much more uncomfortable, irritable
Irritant diaper dermatitis	Erythematous patches confined to diaper area	Spares skinfolds, less scaling
Candidiasis of diaper area	Beefy red patches with satellite pustules	Potassium hydroxide preparation or fungal culture
Infantile psoriasis	Sharply demarcated erythematous patches in diaper area	Difficult to distinguish, may be more well demarcated
Langerhans' cell histiocytosis	Letterer-Siwe in infants <1 year: skin-colored papules, scaling and crusting of scalp, flexural neck, axilla, perineum	Multisystem disease with osteolytic bone lesions, diabetes insipidus, tender lesions, petechiae, purpura, nail changes
Wiskott-Aldrich syndrome	Dermatitis involving face, scalp, flexural areas	X-linked recessive disorder, low platelets, infections
Leiner's disease	Poorly defined seborrheic dermatitis-like erythroderma	Fever, anemia, diarrhea, infection, C3 and C5 deficiency
Pityriasis simplex (dandruff)	Fine scaling of the scalp and hair-bearing areas of the face with minimal underlying erythema	
Tinea capitis	Diffuse scaling of the scalp especially *Trichophyton tonsurans* can occur without hair loss and can be patchy	Direct microscopic exam or fungal culture is diagnostic
Pityriasis amiantacea	Thick, asbestos-like scales adherent to tufts of scalp hairs	May be associated with psoriasis in 1/3, atopic dermatitis, seborrheic dermatitis, or tinea capitis
Adult seborrheic dermatitis	Erythematous symmetric patches with greasy scales on the eyebrows, nasolabial creases, postauricular, scalp, chest	
Psoriasis	Well-demarcated erythematous patches with thick silvery-white micaceous adherent scale on scalp, extensor surfaces	Look for involvement of elbows and knees in psoriasis, nail involvement, arthritis; dermoscopic findings (see above)
Dermatomyositis	May present with erythema and scaling of posterior scalp	Poikiloderma, hair loss, muscle weakness; skin biopsy

(continued)

Table 46.1 (continued)

Diagnosis	Clinical findings	Differentiation
Rosacea	May have erythematous patches or papules on the nose and cheeks with subsequent development of telangiectasias	May occur with seborrheic dermatitis or blepharitis; less scaling; associated with flushing and specific triggers
Drug-related seborrheic dermatitis-like eruption	Scaly erythema or papulopustules on glabella, eyebrows, nasolabial creases, posterior-auricular area, and scalp with or without swelling, erythema, and pain of palms and soles	Reported in patients with hand-foot syndrome associated with erlotinib [84] or sorafenib [84], also seen with recombinant IL-2 [84], PUVA, [20] isotretinoin [84], and cimetidine [84]
Systemic lupus erythematosus	Malar rash on face can mimic seborrheic dermatitis	Systemic symptoms, photosensitivity, positive ANA, biopsy
Tinea versicolor	Scaly hyper- or hypopigmented macules on trunk	Direct microscopic examination reveals spores and hyphae
Pityriasis rosea	Erythematous scaly macules in "Christmas tree" distribution	Inverse variant may mimic, look for larger herald patch

46.5 Treatment

Seborrheic dermatitis is a chronic intermittent condition often requiring long-term therapeutic options for maintenance treatment. Topical treatments including antifungals, corticosteroids, keratolytics, and topical immunomodulator medications are typically used (Table 46.2). Rarely, systemic antifungals or phototherapy can be employed for severe or refractory cases.

46.5.1 Antifungals

Topical antifungals are the mainstay of seborrheic dermatitis treatment. The mechanism of azole antifungals involves inhibition of ergosterol (a fungal cell wall component) via the cytochrome P450 system in addition to anti-inflammatory properties through blockage of 5-lipoxygenase production [10]. Ketoconazole 2 % has been shown to be effective in randomized controlled studies with improvement in erythema, scaling, and pruritus using the cream, gel, foam, and shampoo formulations [34–37]. A recent meta-analysis also showed strong evidence for the effectiveness of ketoconazole when compared to vehicle [38]. Bifonazole has also demonstrated efficacy in randomized controlled trials using both the 1 % shampoo and 1 % cream preparations [39, 40]. This may be augmented if used in conjunction with urea 40 % ointment which acts as a keratolytic and enhances penetration [41].

Table 46.2 Topical treatments for seborrheic dermatitis

Medication	Formulation	Use	Other info/adverse reactions
Ketoconazole	Cream 2 %	Twice daily	Pregnancy Category C
	Gel 2 %	Once daily	Burning and irritation (<3 %)
	Foam 2 %	Twice daily	
	Shampoo 1 %/2 %	1–2× weekly	
Bifonazole	Cream 1 %	Once daily	Not available in the United States
	Shampoo 1 %	3× per week	
Ciclopirox	Gel 0.77 %	Twice daily	Pregnancy Category B
	Shampoo 1 %	Twice weekly	Burning and pruritus
Hydrocortisone	Cream 1 %/2.5 %	Twice daily	Pregnancy Category C
Fluocinolone	Solution 0.01 %	1–2× daily	Pregnancy Category C
	Scalp oil 0.01 %	Nightly	Oil is in peanut oil vehicle but thought to be safe in peanut allergy
	Shampoo 0.01 %	Daily	
Metronidazole	Gel 0.75 %/1 %	1–2× daily	Pregnancy Category B
			Burning, stinging, pruritus
Tacrolimus	Ointment 0.1 %	Twice daily	Pregnancy Category C
Pimecrolimus	Cream 1 %	Twice daily	Black-box warning: lymphoma and skin cancer
Lithium	Ointment 8 %	Twice daily	Not available in the United States

Ciclopirox is a hydroxypyridone derivative with antifungal, antibacterial, and anti-inflammatory properties. Its mechanism of action involves inhibition of uptake of essential compounds which alters cellular permeability [42]. Ciclopirox 1 % shampoo and 1 % cream have demonstrated improvement for scalp and facial seborrheic dermatitis in randomized, double-blind trials [43, 44]. The frequency of treatment using ciclopirox 1 % shampoo is one to two times weekly with maintenance every 1–2 weeks [45]. Ciclopirox 1 % cream had similar efficacy as ketoconazole 2 % foaming gel, and ciclopirox 1.5 % shampoo was as effective as ketoconazole 2 % shampoo in randomized trials [46, 47].

There are also multiple over-the-counter antifungal preparations. A randomized, placebo-controlled, double-blinded trial comparing ketoconazole and selenium sulfide demonstrated similar efficacy of selenium sulfide 2.5 % shampoo for irritation and itching associated with moderate to severe seborrheic dermatitis, but ketoconazole 2 % shampoo was better tolerated [48]. Adverse effects include xanthotrichia or yellow hair discoloration [49]. Zinc pyrithione 1 % shampoo did demonstrate benefit but was inferior to ketoconazole 2 % shampoo in an open-label comparison trial [50]. A combination ciclopirox 1.5 %/zinc pyrithione 1 % shampoo was more effective than ketoconazole 2 % foaming gel in a clinical trial investigating erythema, pruritus, global efficacy, and quality of life [51]. Tea tree oil 5 % shampoo showed benefit when compared to placebo for mild to moderate dandruff [52].

46.5.2 Antibiotics

Topical metronidazole 1 % gel was shown to be superior to placebo, but metronidazole 0.75 % gel was no different than placebo in several double-blind randomized trials [53–56]. In contrast, an additional study found metronidazole 0.75 % gel to be as effective as ketoconazole 2 % cream [57].

46.5.3 Corticosteroids

Short-term topical corticosteroid treatment can be employed for severe inflammation or pruritus. Side effects including atrophy, telangiectasias, dyspigmentation, and steroid-induced rosacea limit their use. Twice-daily application of hydrocortisone 1 % cream showed similar improvement to ketoconazole 2 % cream in double-blind comparative studies [58, 59]. A single-blind study of ketoconazole 2 % foaming gel or betamethasone dipropionate 0.05 % lotion demonstrated superiority of ketoconazole for symptoms, tolerability, and global evaluation by both patient and physician for areas on the scalp, eyelashes, nasolabial folds, and chest with significant reduction in *P. ovale* [60]. The combination of ketoconazole 2 % shampoo twice weekly with clobetasol proprionate 0.05 % shampoo twice weekly provided greater efficacy than ketoconazole alone for severe scalp disease [61]. Fluocinolone acetonide 0.01 % solution, shampoo, and oil have been helpful for patients with scalp involvement [62, 63].

46.5.4 Immunomodulators

Tacrolimus and pimecrolimus are nonsteroidal anti-inflammatory agents that inhibit calcineurin and decrease subsequent cytokine production and can be used off label as steroid-sparing agents. Tacrolimus 0.1 % ointment showed improvement in seborrheic dermatitis in open-label pilot studies with side effects of burning and irritation [64, 65]. Tacrolimus was also as effective as topical betamethasone 17-valerate lotion [66]. Pimecrolimus cream 1 % was superior to vehicle and as effective as betamethasone 17-valerate 0.1 % cream in randomized clinical trials [67, 68]. The black-box warning for rare cases of lymphoma seen in animal models has limited use of these agents.

46.5.5 Lithium Salts

The activity of lithium salts on seborrheic dermatitis is thought to be anti-inflammatory, possibly secondary to reduction of expression of Toll-like receptor 2 by keratinocytes [69]. Randomized, placebo-controlled, multicenter trials using lithium succinate 8 % or lithium gluconate 8 % ointment twice daily showed improvement in all symptoms of seborrheic dermatitis [70, 71]. Furthermore, a trial of lithium gluconate 8 % ointment was more effective than ketoconazole 2 % emulsion twice weekly [72]. Lithium succinate 8 % ointment was also effective in treating HIV-positive patients [73].

46.5.6 Other Topical Treatments

Coal tar 4 % shampoo was shown to be superior to placebo in a small randomized controlled trial [74]. Other shampoos include lipohydroxy acid (LHA) 0.1 % and 1.3 % salicylic acid which showed improvement in global efficacy and cosmetic acceptability [75].

Topical emollients have also been employed for treatment of seborrheic dermatitis including Promiseb™ topical cream which maintains moisture in the affected areas. Similarly, MAS064D (Sebclair) includes a compound of emollients, anti-inflammatory and antimycotic agents with improvement in erythema, scaling, and pruritus when compared to vehicle in a small randomized, double-blind trial [76].

A novel agent contains Regul™, a topical modulator of toll-like receptor 2, which is involved in IL-8 expression after contact with Malassezia yeast, may prevent relapses of seborrheic dermatitis [77]. Cecropin A(1–8)-magainin2(1–12) hybrid peptide analog P5, an antimicrobial peptide, was also shown to inhibit the expression of IL-8 and toll-like receptor 2 in *M. furfur*-infected keratinocytes and furthermore downregulated NF-kB activation [78]. This may be a potential therapeutic agent in the future.

46.5.7 Oral Antifungals

Itraconazole showed efficacy in open non-comparative trials at 200 mg daily for 1 week followed by 200 mg every 2 weeks or 200 mg for 2 consecutive days monthly [79–81]. A randomized trial using weekly fluconazole 300 mg did not show improvement compared to placebo [82]. Terbinafine 250 mg daily showed significant improvement when compared to placebo in a subpopulation of patients with unexposed areas including scalp, sternum, and interscapular areas but no benefit in those with exposed areas such as face involved [83]. The use of systemic antifungals is limited by the adverse side effect profile.

46.5.8 Phototherapy

In a small open prospective trial, narrowband ultraviolet B phototherapy given three times weekly starting at 70 % of the minimal erythema dose, increasing by 20 % per treatment for 8 weeks, led to marked improvement or complete clearance in patients with severe seborrheic dermatitis [84].

References

1. Elish D, Silverberg N. Infantile seborrheic dermatitis. Cutis. 2006;77:297–300.
2. Foley P, Zuo Y, Plunkett A, Merlin K, Marks R. The frequency of common skin conditions in preschool-aged children in Australia. Arch Dermatol. 2003;139:318–22.
3. Gupta AK, Bluhm R. Seborrheic dermatitis. J Eur Acad Dermatol Venereol. 2004;28:13–26.
4. Bikowski J. Facial seborrheic dermatitis: a report on current status and therapeutic horizons. J Drugs Dermatol. 2009;8:125–33.
5. Mahe A, Simon F, Coulibaly S, Tounkara A, Bobin P. Predictive value of seborrheic dermatitis and other common dermatoses for HIV infection in Bamako Mali. J Am Acad Dermatol. 1996;34:1084–6.
6. Coopman SA, Johnson RA, Platt R, Stern RS. Cutaneous disease and drug reactions in HIV infection. N Engl J Med. 1993;328:1670–4.
7. Berger RS, Stoner MF, Hobbs ER, Hayes TJ, Boswell RN. Cutaneous manifestations of early human immunodeficiency virus exposure. J Am Acad Dermatol. 1988;19:298–303.
8. Coldiron BM, Bergstresser PR. Prevalence and clinical spectrum of skin disease in patients infected with human immunodeficiency virus. Arch Dermatol. 1989;125:357–61.
9. Mathes BM, Douglass MC. Seborrheic dermatitis in patients with acquired immunodeficiency syndrome. J Am Acad Dermatol. 1985;13:947–51.
10. Kohn SR, Pochi PE, Strauss JS, Sax DS, Feldman RG, Timberlake WH. Sebaceous gland secretion in Parkinson's disease during L-DOPA treatment. J Invest Dermatol. 1973; 60:134–6.
11. Binder RL, Jonelis FJ. Seborrheic dermatitis in neuroleptic-induced parkinsonism. Arch Dermatol. 1983;119:473–5.
12. Maietta G, Fornaro P, Rongioletti F, Reobra A. Patients with mood depression have a high prevalence of seborrheic dermatitis. Acta Derm Venereol. 1990;70:432–4.
13. Rocha N, Velho G, Horta M, Martins A, Massa A. Cutaneous manifestations of familial amyloidotic polyneuropathy. J Eur Acad Dermatol Venereol. 2005;19:605–7.
14. Barankin B, Guenther L. Dermatological manifestations of Down's syndrome. J Cutan Med Surg. 2001;5:289–93.
15. Ercis M, Balci S, Atakan N. Dermatological manifestations of 71 Down syndrome children admitted to a clinical genetics unit. Clin Genet. 1996;50:317–20.
16. Berg M. Epidemiological studies of the influence of sunlight on the skin. Photodermatol. 1989;6:80–4.
17. Banerjee S, Gangopadhyay DN, Jana S, Chanda M. Seasonal variation in pediatric dermatoses. Indian J Dermatol. 2010;55:44–6.
18. Moehrle M, Dennenmoser B, Schalagenhauff B, Thomma S, Garbe C. High prevalence of seborrheic dermatitis on the face and scalp in mountain guides. Dermatology. 2000; 201:146–7.
19. Tegner E. Seborrheic dermatitis of the face induced by PUVA treatment. Acta Derm Venereol. 1983;63:335–9.
20. Pirkhammer D, Seeber A, Honigsmann H, Tanew A. Narrow-band ultraviolet B (TL-01) phototherapy is an effective and safe treatment option for patients with severe seborrheic dermatitis. Br J Dermatol. 2000;143:964–8.
21. Burton JL, Pye RJ. Seborrhoea is not a feature of seborrheic dermatitis. Br Med J. 1983;286:1169–70.
22. Naldi L, Rebora A. Seborrheic dermatitis. N Eng J Med. 2009;360:387–96.
23. McGinely KJ, Leyden JJ, Marples RR, Kligman AM. Quantitative microbiology of the scalp in non-dandruff, dandruff, and seborrheic dermatitis. J Invest Dermatol. 1975;64:401–5.
24. Whitlock FA. Pityrosporum ovale and some scaly conditions of the scalp. Br Med J. 1953;1:484–7.
25. Leyden JJ, McGinely KJ, Kligman AM. Role of microorganisms in dandruff. Arch Dermatol. 1976;112:333–8.

26. Carr MM, Pryce DM, Ive FA. Treatment of seborrhoeic dermatitis with ketoconazole: I. Response of seborrhoeic dermatitis of the scalp to topical ketoconazole. Br J Dermatol. 1987;116:213–6.
27. DeAngelis YM, Gemmer CM, Kaczvinsky JR, Kenneally DC, Schwartz JR, Dawson Jr TL. Three etiologic facets of dandruff and seborrheic dermatitis: Malassezia fungi, sebaceous lipids, and individual sensitivity. J Investig Dermatol Symp Proc. 2005;10:295–7.
28. DeAngelis YM, Saudners CW, Johnstone KR, Reeder NL, Coleman CG, Kaczvinsky JR, et al. Isolation and expression of a Malassezia globosa lipase gene, LIP1. J Invest Dermatol. 2007;127:2138–46.
29. Xu J, Saunders CW, Hu P, Grant RA, Boekhout T, Kuramae EE, et al. Dandruff-associated Malassezia genomes reveal convergent and divergent virulence traits shared with plant and human fungal pathogens. Proc Natl Acad Sci USA. 2007;104:18730–5.
30. Thomas DS, Ingham E, Bojar RA, Holland KT. In vitro modulation of human keratinocyte pro-and anti-inflammatory cytokine production by the capsule of Malassezia species. FEMS Immunol Med Microbiol. 2008;54:203–14.
31. Faergemann J, Bergbrant IM, Dohse M, Scott A, Westgate G. Seborrhoeic dermatitis and Pityrosporum (Malassezia) folliculitis: characterization of inflammatory cells and mediators in the skin by immunohistochemistry. Br J Dermatol. 2001;144:549–56.
32. Kim GW, Jung HJ, Ko HC, Kim MB, Lee WJ, Lee SJ, et al. Dermoscopy can be useful in differentiating scalp psoriasis from seborrheic dermatitis. Br J Dermatol. 2011;164:652–6.
33. Pinkus H, Mehregan AH. The primary histologic lesion of seborrheic dermatitis and psoriasis. J Invest Dermatol. 1965;46:109–16.
34. Skinner Jr RB, Noah PW, Taylor RM, Zanolli MD, West S, Guin JD, et al. Double-blind treatment of Seborrheic dermatitis with 2% ketoconazole cream. J Am Acad Dermatol. 1985;12:852–6.
35. Elewski B, Ling MR, Phillips TJ. Efficacy and safety of a new once-daily topical ketoconazole 2% gel in the treatment of seborrheic dermatitis: a phase III trial. J Drugs Dermatol. 2006;5:646–50.
36. Elewski BE, Abramovits W, Kempers S, Schlessinger J, Rosen T, Gupta AK, et al. A novel foam formulation of ketoconazole 2% for the treatment of seborrheic dermatitis on multiple body regions. J Drugs Dermatol. 2007;6:1001–8.
37. Faergemann J. Treatment of seborrhoeic dermatitis of the scalp with ketoconazole shampoo. A double-blind study. Acta Derm Venereol. 1990;70:171–2.
38. Apasrawirote W, Udompataikul M, Rattanamongkolgul S. Topical antifungal agents for seborrheic dermatitis: systematic review and meta-analysis. J Med Assoc Thai. 2011;94:756–60.
39. Segal R, David M, Ingber A, Lurie R, Sandbank M. Treatment with bifonazole shampoo for seborrhea and seborrheic dermatitis: a randomized, double-blind study. Acta Derm Venereol. 1992;72:454–5.
40. Zienicke H, Korting HC, Braun-Falco O, Effendy I, Hagedorn M, Küchmeister B, et al. Comparative efficacy and safety of bifonazole 1% cream and the corresponding base preparation in the treatment of seborrhoeic dermatitis. Mycoses. 1993;36:325–31.
41. Shemer A, Nathansohn N, Kaplan B, Weiss G, Newman N, Trau H. Treatment of scalp seborrheic dermatitis and psoriasis with an ointment of 40% urea and 1% bifonazole. Int J Dermatol. 2000;39:532–4.
42. Abrams BB, Hänel H, Hoehler T. Ciclopirox olamine: a hydroxypyridone antifungal agent. Clin Dermatol. 1991;9:471–7.
43. Lebwohl M, Plott T. Safety and efficacy of ciclopirox 1% shampoo for the treatment of seborrheic dermatitis of the scalp in the US population: results of a double-blind, vehicle-controlled trial. Int J Dermatol. 2004;43:17–20.
44. Dupuy P, Maurette C, Amoric JC, Chosidow O, Study Investigator Group. Randomized, placebo-controlled, double-blind study on clinical efficacy of ciclopiroxolamine 1% cream in facial seborrhoeic dermatitis. Br J Dermatol. 2001;144:1033–7.
45. Shuster S, Meynadier J, Kerl H, Nolting S. Treatment and prophylaxis of seborrheic dermatitis of the scalp with antipityrosporal 1% ciclopirox shampoo. Arch Dermatol. 2005;141:47–52.

46. Chosidow O, Maurette C, Dupuy P. Randomized, open-labeled, non-inferiority study between ciclopiroxolamine 1% cream and ketoconazole 2% foaming gel in mild to moderate facial seborrheic dermatitis. Dermatology. 2003;203:233–40.
47. Ratnavel RC, Squire RA, Boorman GC. Clinical efficacies of shampoos containing ciclopirox olamine (1.5%) and ketoconazole (2.0%) in the treatment of seborrhoeic dermatitis. J Dermatolog Treat. 2007;18:88–96.
48. Danby FW, Maddin WS, Margesson LJ, Rosenthal D. A randomized, double-blind, placebo-controlled trial of ketoconazole 2% shampoo versus selenium sulfide 2.5% shampoo in the treatment of moderate to severe dandruff. J Am Acad Dermatol. 1993;29:1008–12.
49. Prevost N, English 3rd JC. Xanthotrichia (yellow hair) due to selenium sulfide and dihydroxyacetone. J Drugs Dermatol. 2008;7:689–91.
50. Piérard-Franchimont C, Goffin V, Decroix J, Piérard GE. A multicenter randomized trial of ketoconazole 2% and zinc pyrithione 1% shampoos in severe dandruff and seborrheic dermatitis. Skin Pharmacol Appl Skin Physiol. 2002;15:434–41.
51. Lorette G, Ermosilla V. Clinical efficacy of a new ciclopiroxolamine/zinc pyrithione shampoo in scalp seborrheic dermatitis treatment. Eur J Dermatol. 2006;16:558–64.
52. Satchell AC, Saurajen A, Bell C, Barnetson RS. Treatment of dandruff with 5% tea tree oil shampoo. J Am Acad Dermatol. 2002;47:852–5.
53. Parsad D, Pandhi R, Negi KS, Kumar B. Topical metronidazole in seborrheic dermatitis—a double-blind study. Dermatology. 2001;202:35–7.
54. Siadat AH, Iraji F, Shahmoradi Z, Enshaieh S, Taheri A. The efficacy of 1% metronidazole gel in facial seborrheic dermatitis: a double blind study. Indian J Dermatol Venereol Leprol. 2006;72:266–9.
55. Koca R, Altinyazar HC, Eştürk E. Is topical metronidazole effective in seborrheic dermatitis? A double-blind study. Int J Dermatol. 2003;42:632–5.
56. Ozcan H, Seyhan M, Yologlu S. Is metronidazole 0.75% gel effective in the treatment of seborrhoeic dermatitis? A double-blind, placebo controlled study. Eur J Dermatol. 2007;17:313–6.
57. Seckin D, Gurbuz O, Akin O. Metronidazole 0.75% gel vs. ketoconazole 2% cream in the treatment of facial seborrheic dermatitis: a randomized, double-blind study. J Eur Acad Dermatol Venereol. 2007;21:345–50.
58. Stratigos JD, Antoniou C, Katsambas A, Böhler K, Fritsch P, Schmölz A, et al. Ketoconazole 2% cream versus hydrocortisone 1% cream in the treatment of seborrheic dermatitis. A double-blind comparative study. J Am Acad Dermatol. 1988;19:850–3.
59. Katsambas A, Antoniou C, Frangouli E, Avgerinou G, Michailidis D, Stratigos J. A double-blind trial of treatment of seborrhoeic dermatitis with 2% ketoconazole cream compared with 1% hydrocortisone cream. Br J Dermatol. 1989;121:353–7.
60. Ortonne JP, Lacour JP, Vitetta A, Le Fichoux Y. Comparative study of ketoconazole 2% foaming gel and betamethasone dipropionate 0.05% lotion in the treatment of seborrhoeic dermatitis in adults. Dermatology. 1992;184:275–80.
61. Ortonne JP, Nikkels AF, Reich K, Ponce Olivera RM, Lee JH, Kerrouche N, et al. Efficacious and safe management of moderate to severe scalp seborrhoeic dermatitis using clobetasol propionate shampoo 0·05% combined with ketoconazole shampoo 2%: a randomized, controlled study. Br J Dermatol. 2011;165:171–6.
62. Falk MS. Fluocinolone acetonide in propylene glycol. Arch Dermatol. 1963;88:928–9.
63. Kircik L. The evolving role of therapeutic shampoos for targeting symptoms of inflammatory scalp disorders. J Drugs Dermatol. 2010;9:41–8.
64. Meshkinpour A, Sun J, Weinstein G. An open pilot study using tacrolimus ointment in the treatment of seborrheic dermatitis. J Am Acad Dermatol. 2003;49:145–7.
65. Braza TJ, DiCarlo JB, Soon SL, McCall CO. Tacrolimus 0.1% ointment for seborrhoeic dermatitis: an open-label pilot study. Br J Dermatol. 2003;148:1242–4.
66. Shin H, Kwon OS, Won CH, Kim BJ, Lee YW, Choe YB, et al. Clinical efficacies of topical agents for the treatment of seborrheic dermatitis of the scalp: a comparative study. J Dermatol. 2009;36:131–7.

67. Warshaw EM, Wohlhuter RJ, Liu A, Zeller SA, Wenner RA, Bowers S, et al. Results of a randomized, double-blind, vehicle-controlled efficacy trial of pimecrolimus cream 1% for the treatment of moderate to severe facial seborrheic dermatitis. J Am Acad Dermatol. 2007;57:257–64.
68. Rigopoulos D, Ioannides D, Kalogeromitros D, Gregoriou S, Katsambas A. Pimecrolimus cream 1% vs. betamethasone 17-valerate 0.1% cream in the treatment of seborrhoeic dermatitis. A randomized open-label clinical trial. Br J Dermatol. 2004;151:1071–5.
69. Ballanger F, Tenaud I, Volteau C, Khammari A, Dréno B. Anti-inflammatory effects of lithium gluconate on keratinocytes: a possible explanation for efficiency in seborrhoeic dermatitis. Arch Dermatol Res. 2008;300:215–23.
70. Efalith Multicenter Trial Group. A double-blind, placebo-controlled, multicenter trial of lithium succinate ointment in the treatment of seborrheic dermatitis. J Am Acad Dermatol. 1992;26:452–7.
71. Dreno B, Moyse D. Lithium gluconate in the treatment of seborrhoeic dermatitis: a multicenter, randomised, double-blind study versus placebo. Eur J Dermatol. 2002;12:549–52.
72. Dreno B, Chosidow O, Revuz J, Moyse D, Study Investigator Group. Lithium gluconate 8% vs ketoconazole 2% in the treatment of seborrhoeic dermatitis: a multicentre, randomized study. Br J Dermatol. 2003;148:1230–6.
73. Langtry JA, Rowland Payne CM, Staughton RC, Stewart JC, Horrobin DF. Topical lithium succinate ointment (Efalith) in the treatment of AIDS-related seborrhoeic dermatitis. Clin Exp Dermatol. 1997;22:216–9.
74. Davies DB, Boorman GC, Shuttleworth D. Comparative efficacy of shampoos containing coal tar (4.0% w/w; Tarmed), coal tar (4.0% w/w) plus ciclopirox olamine (1.0% w/w/; Tarmed) and ketoconazole 92.0% w/w/; Nizoral) for the treatment of dandruff/seborrheic dermatitis. J Deramtol Treat. 1999;10:177–83.
75. Seite S, Rougier A, Talarico S. Randomized study comparing the efficacy and tolerance of a lipohydroxy acid shampoo to a ciclopiroxolamine shampoo in the treatment of scalp seborrheic dermatitis. J Cosmet Dermatol. 2009;8:249–53.
76. Veraldi S, Menter A, Innocenti M. Treatment of mild to moderate seborrhoeic dermatitis with MAS064D (Sebclair), a novel topical medical device: results of a pilot, randomized, double-blind, controlled trial. J Eur Acad Dermatol Venereol. 2008;22:290–6.
77. Ionescu MA, Baroni A, Brambilla L, Cannavò SP, Cristaudo A, Vedove CD, et al. Double blind clinical trial in a series of 115 patients with seborrheic dermatitis: prevention of relapses using a topical modulator of Toll like receptor 2. G Ital Dermatol Venereol. 2011;146:185–9.
78. Ryu S, Choi SY, Acharya S, Chun YJ, Gurley C, Park Y, et al. Antimicrobial and anti-inflammatory effects of cecropin A(1–8)-magainin2(1–12) hybrid peptide analog P5 against Malassezia furfur infection in human keratinocytes. J Invest Dermatol. 2011;131:1677–83.
79. Shemer A, Kaplan B, Nathansohn N, Grunwald MH, Amichai B, Trau H. Treatment of moderate to severe facial seborrheic dermatitis with itraconazole: an open non-comparative study. Isr Med Assoc J. 2008;10:417–8.
80. Kose O, Erbil H, Gur AR. Oral itraconazole for the treatment of seborrhoeic dermatitis: an open, noncomparative trial. J Eur Acad Dermatol Venereol. 2005;19:172–5.
81. Baysal V, Yildirim M, Ozcanli C, Ceyhan AM. Itraconazole in the treatment of seborrheic dermatitis: a new treatment modality. Int J Dermatol. 2004;43:63–6.
82. Cömert A, Bekiroglu N, Gürbüz O, Ergun T. Efficacy of oral fluconazole in the treatment of seborrheic dermatitis: a placebo-controlled study. Am J Clin Dermatol. 2007;8:235–8.
83. Vena GA, Micali G, Santoianni P, Cassano N, Peruzzi E. Oral terbinafine in the treatment of multi-site seborrhoic dermatitis: a multicenter, double-blind placebo-controlled study. Int J Immunopathol Pharmacol. 2005;18:745–53.
84. Pirkhammer D, Seeber A, Hönigsmann H, Tanew A. Narrow-band ultraviolet B (ATL-01) phototherapy is an effective and safe treatment option for patients with severe seborrhoeic dermatitis. Br J Dermatol. 2000;143:964–8.

Chapter 47
Steatocystoma Multiplex

Alejandra Vivas and Jonette Keri

47.1 Introduction

Steatocystoma multiplex (SM) is one of the infrequent forms of keratin disorders characterized by multiple benign sebaceous gland papules and/or nodules, usually located in hair-covered areas where pilosebaceous glands are well developed; however this condition may occur anywhere on the body. Though it is mostly thought to be a hereditary autosomal dominant disease associated to missense mutations of the keratin 17 (K17) gene, many sporadic cases have been reported. This suggests the disease may have a multifactorial etiology. Steatocystoma simplex is the sporadic solitary tumor counterpart to SM and has no hereditary tendency. Diagnosis is mainly clinical, but histopathology is characteristic and aids to confirmation of diagnosis when uncertain. Some of the frequent locations of SM include neck, chest, upper back, proximal extremities, and face, which are also common areas for acne to present. Due to the many similarities of these two conditions, SM should be included in the differential diagnosis when evaluating an acneiform eruption.

A. Vivas, M.D. (✉)
Department of Dermatology, University of Miami, 1321 NW 14th Street, Room 505, Miami, FL 33136, USA
e-mail: avivas@med.miami.edu

J. Keri, M.D., Ph.D.
Department of Dermatology and Cutaneous Surgery, Veterans Hospital, University of Miami, Miami, FL, USA

J.A. Zeichner (ed.), *Acneiform Eruptions in Dermatology: A Differential Diagnosis*, DOI 10.1007/978-1-4614-8344-1_47,

47.2 Background

The exact etiopathogenesis has not been completely elucidated, but keratin 17 (K17) has been proposed as a central element in the formation of hereditary steatocystomas. This protein of keratin-containing intermediate filaments is found in several epithelial structures such as the ungual bed, hair follicles, and sebaceous glands. The area where the mutations of the gene K17 occur in SM is identical to mutations found in patients with pachyonychia congenita type 2 (PC-2) [1]. A variety of mutations have been described in patients with either steatocystoma multiplex or PC-2, and all of them are localized to the helix initiation 1A domain of the K17 gene [2]. Therefore these two conditions are thought to be connected and can present simultaneously with the additional typical features of PC-2, i.e., hypertrophic nail dystrophy and focal hyperkeratosis of the palms, soles, knees, and elbows [3]. Hybrid lesions with histological features of both conditions have been described [4]. SM has also been reported to be related to acrokeratosis verruciformis, hypertrophic lichen planus [5], and eruptive vellus hair cysts (EVHCs) [6]. Some authors suggest that SM and EVHCs belong to one spectrum of the same disease that should be referred as to "multiple pilosebaceous cysts" which would be a more appropriate diagnosis than the terms of EVHCs and steatocystoma multiplex [7]. On the other hand, some state that they are two separate entities based on the expression of different keratins. Lesions of SM express keratins 10 and 17, in contrast to EVHCs which express only keratin 17 [8].

Recently two missense mutations (R94H and N92S) of the K17 gene were identified in two Chinese pedigrees. N92S is a novel mutation for SM, whereas R94H is a recurrent mutation. Interestingly R94H was also previously found in a sporadic case of PC-2 [2].

Other hypotheses have been formulated to explain this rare condition including hamartomatous malformation of the pilosebaceous duct junction [9, 10] sebaceous retention cysts, a variant of a dermoid cyst or a nevoid formation of abortive hair follicles where sebaceous glands attach [11]. Also the occurrence of trauma, infection, or immunological conditions might be implicated [12].

SM usually begins in adolescence or early adult life and seems to be equally distributed among both genders although it has been proposed that it is more frequently found in males [13]. Although rarely, this condition has been described in newborns [14] as well as in elderly [15]. The association of SM to the development of sebaceous glands and common presentation during puberty suggest a hormonal trigger for lesion growth.

47.3 Clinical Presentation

SM present in a monomorphous fashion as numerous asymptomatic round-to-oval, skin-colored to yellowish papules or nodules with smooth surface. The sites of predilection are the trunk (especially the presternal area), neck, axilla, inguinal region,

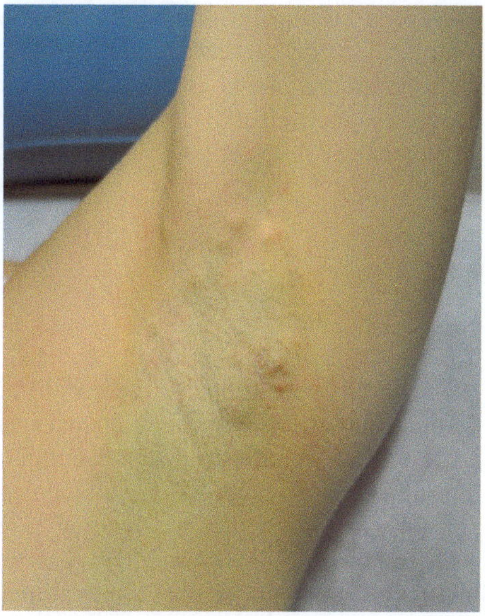

Fig. 47.1 Non-tender, flesh-colored, subcutaneous nodules in the axilla (Photo credit: Joshua A. Zeichner, M.D.)

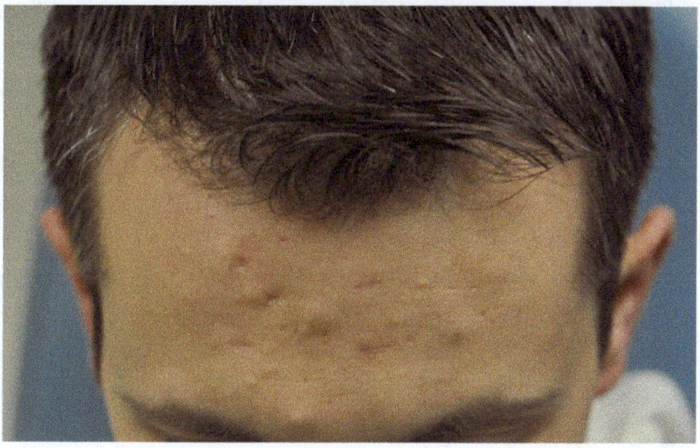

Fig. 47.2 Non-tender, flesh-colored, subcutaneous nodules on the forehead (Photo credit: Joshua A. Zeichner, M.D.)

scalp, and proximal extremities (Fig. 47.1). Less common locations include face, scrotum [16], acral distribution in which involvement of distal extremities is more prominent [17], and breasts [18] among others (Fig. 47.2). In more severe cases the lesions can be generalized, polymorphous, and present with joint symptoms and deteriorated general status, as described in one of the variants referred as to SM generalisata [19].

Lesions are variable in size, tend to grow slowly, and have a sebum content that can appear as a clear oily liquid or as a yellowish creamy material [11]. Although usually asymptomatic, complication with secondary inflammatory changes can occur. One of the distinctive characteristics that may differentiate this condition from others, specifically from acne, is the absence of surface punctum.

Several localized forms of SM have been described such as eruptive SM of the scalp [20], facial papular variant [21, 22], and sebocystomatosis, which comprises multiple lesions of SM confined to the forehead and frontal scalp accompanied by congenital alopecia [23]. Steatocystoma suppurativa is a scarring inflammatory version of this disorder [24].

47.4 Workup

The diagnosis of SM is primarily clinical. However for some cases a biopsy may be needed. The typical histopathological finding of these lesions is seen in the mid-dermis with the presence of an encapsulated dermal cyst with infolded walls composed of stratified, squamous epithelium without a granular layer. In addition there are flattened sebaceous gland lobules arising from the wall and cellular hyaline eosinophilic cuticles on the luminal side of the cyst wall similar to that of the sebaceous duct [25]. Occasionally keratin, vellus hairs, hair follicles, and smooth muscle components are noted in the lumen [23, 26] adding further evidence to the hypothesis that SM is a hamartomatous condition [27].

Electron microscopy shows cyst wall cells undergoing trichilemmal keratinization similar to that of the isthmus portion of the outer hair sheath [24]. Immunohistochemical analysis has demonstrated that the inner epithelial layer of the cysts is positive for the specific marker calretinin which could be useful in identifying these lesions when equivocal [28].

The combined mammographic and sonographic findings can aid in confirming the diagnosis of the subtype of SM involving the breast [18].

The clinical differential diagnosis of SM includes different forms of acne, eruptive vellus hair cysts, epidermoid or dermoid cysts, hidradenitis suppurativa, milia, pseudofolliculitis barbae, neurofibromatosis, and lipomas [11].

47.5 Treatment

Treatment options are limited and only few present satisfactory results; therefore this condition carries therapeutic challenge. As the lesions are characteristically asymptomatic, treatment is usually not necessary. However as previously mentioned some lesions can grow larger, present with inflammation, and develop symptoms such as discomfort or pain and even can rupture with concomitant drainage [29]. In addition this condition can be cosmetically undesirable representing a psychological burden for the patient, especially when lesions are located in visible areas. In these cases surgical excision or incision and drainage are the standard treatments. However conventional excision techniques have shown to be impractical when treating multiple lesions; therefore new surgical procedures with the use of different instruments have emerged [30, 31] to increase effectiveness of treatment and patient satisfaction and minimize scarring and recurrence. Alternatives to surgery include needle aspiration which decreases the size of the lesions, but the result may last only for a relatively short period of time [32]. Oral retinoids have been used for their anti-inflammatory properties which may be effective in suppurative lesions and also can reduce the frequency of new lesions, but the outcomes have been variable and not particularly encouraging [11]. Limited success and poor cosmetic outcome has been reported with the use of liquid nitrogen cryotherapy [33]. Other option treatments include intralesional steroids and lasers [23]. Successful use of carbon dioxide laser (CO_2 laser) [34] and Er:Yag laser has been recently reported with excellent cosmetic results. The laser wave creates a punctum for subsequent drainage of the content of the cyst using appropriate devices [35]. Combination treatments are encouraged as long as satisfactory results are achieved.

References

1. Oh SW, Kim MY, Lee JS, Kim SC. Keratin 17 mutation in pachyonychia congenita type 2 patient with early onset steatocystoma multiplex and Hutchinson-like tooth deformity. J Dermatol. 2006;33:161–4.
2. Wang JF, Lu WS, Sun LD, et al. Novel missense mutation of keratin in Chinese family with steatocystoma multiplex. Eur Acad Dermatol Venereol. 2009;23:723–4.
3. Kanda M, Natsuga K, Nishie W, et al. Morphological and genetic analysis of steatocystoma multiplex in an Asian family with pachyonychia congenita type 2 harbouring a KRT17 missense mutation. Br J Dermatol. 2009;160:465–8.
4. Hurlimann AF, Panizzon RG, Burg G. Eruptive vellus hair cyst and steatocystoma multiplex: hybrid cysts. Dermatology. 1996;192:64–6.
5. Moritz DL, Silverman RA. Steatocystoma multiplex treated with isotretinoin: a delayed response. Cutis. 1988;42:437–9.
6. Ahn SK, Chung J, Lee WS, Lee SH, Choi EH. Hybrid cysts showing alternate combination of eruptive vellus hair cyst, steatocystoma multiplex, and epidermoid cyst, and an association among the three conditions. Am J Dermatopathol. 1996;18:645–9.
7. Yoshida M, Oiso N, Kurokawa I, Tsubura A, Kimura M, Kawada A. A case of multiple pilosebaceous cysts. Case Rep Dermatol. 2010;2:116–9.
8. Tomkova H, Fujimoto W, Arata J. Expression of keratins (K 10 and K 17) in steatocystoma multiplex, eruptive vellus hair cysts, and epidermoid and trichilemmal cysts. Am J Dermatopathol. 1997;19:250–3.
9. Sabater-Marco V, Perez-Ferriols A. Steatocystoma multiplex with smooth muscle. A hamartoma of the pilosebaceous apparatus. Am J Dermatopathol. 1996;18:548–50.
10. Plewig G, Wolff HH, Braun-Falco O. Steatocystoma multiplex: anatomic reevaluation, electron microscopy, and autoradiography. Arch Dermatol Res. 1982;272:363–80.
11. Lima AM, Rocha SP, Batista CM, Reis CM, Leal II, Azevedo LE. Case for diagnosis. Steatocystoma multiplex. An Bras Dermatol. 2011;86:165–6.
12. Setoyama M, Mizoguchi S, Usuki K, Kanzaki T. Steatocystoma multiplex: a case with unusual clinical and histological manifestation. Am J Dermatopathol. 1997;19:89–92.
13. Magid ML, Wentzell JM, Roenick Jr HH. Multiple cystic lesions: steatocystoma multiplex. Arch Dermatol. 1990;126:101. 104.
14. Park YM, Cho SH, Kang H. Congenital linear steatocystoma multiplex of the nose. Pediatr Dermatol. 2000;17:136–8.
15. Rongioletti F, Cattarini G, Romanelli P. Late onset vulvar steatocystoma multiplex. Clin Exp Dermatol. 2002;27:445–7.

16. Stollery N. Photo quiz. Case 2. Steatocystoma multiplex. Practitioner. 2007;251(1701):31. 34.
17. Rollins T, Levin RM, Heymann WR. Acral steatocystoma multiplex. J Am AcadDermatol. 2000;43:396–9.
18. Mester J, Darwish M, Deshmukh SM. Steatocystoma multiplex of the breast: mammographic and sonographic findings. AJR Am J Roentgenol. 1998;170:115–6.
19. Fekete GL, Fekete JE. Steatocystoma multiplex generalisata partially suppurativa-case report. Acta Dermatovenerol Croat. 2010;18:114–9.
20. Kumakiri M, Yajima C. Eruptive steatocystoma multiplex on the scalp. J Dermatol. 1991;18:537–9.
21. Nishimura M, Kohda H, Urabe A. Steatocystoma multiplex. A facial papular variant. Arch Dermatol. 1986;122:205–7.
22. Requena L, Martin L, Renedo G, et al. A facial variant of steatocystoma multiplex. Cutis. 1993;51:449–52.
23. Kim SJ, Park HJ, Oh ST, Lee JY, Cho BK. A case of steatocystoma multiplex limited to the scalp. Ann Dermatol. 2009;21:106–9.
24. Davey MA. Steatocystoma multiplex treatment & management. In: Elston DM; editor. Medscape reference. http://emedicine.medscape.com/article/1059725-treatment. Accessed 11 Dec 2011.
25. Yamada A, Saga K, Jimbow K. Acquired multiple pilosebaceous cysts on the face having the histopathological features of steatocystoma multiplex and eruptive vellus hair cysts. Int J Dermatol. 2005;44:861–3.
26. Thomas VD, Swanson NA, Lee KK. Benign epithelial tumors, hamartomas, and hyperplasias. In: Wolff K, Goldsmith LA, Katz SI, Gilchrest BA, Paller AS, Leffell DJ, editors. Fitzpatrick's dermatology in general medicine. 7th ed. New York, NY: McGraw-Hill; 2008. p. 1065–6.
27. Cho S, Chang SE, Choi JH, Sung KJ, Moon KC, Koh JK. Clinical and histologic features of 64 cases of steatocystoma multiplex. J Dermatol. 2002;29:152–6.
28. Riedel C, Brinkmeier T, Kutzne H, Plewig G, Frosch PJ. Late onset of a facial variant of steatocystoma multiplex—calretinin as a specific marker of the follicular companion cell layer. J Dtsch Dermatol Ges. 2008;6:480–2.
29. Cuperus E, Leguit RJ, Sigurdsson V. Steatocystoma multiplex, a rare distribution of a rare disease. Eur J Dermatol. 2010;20:402–3.
30. Choudhary S, Koley S, Salodkar A. A modified surgical technique for steatocystoma multiplex. J Cutan Aesthet Surg. 2010;3:25–8.
31. Lee SJ, Choe YS, Park BC, Lee WJ, Kim do W. The vein hook successfully used for eradication of steatocystoma multiplex. Dermatol Surg. 2007;33:82–4.
32. Düzova AN, Sentürk GB. Suggestion for the treatment of steatocystoma multiplex located exclusively on the face. Int J Dermatol. 2004;43:60–2.
33. Apaydin R, Bilen N, Bayramgürler D, Başdaş F, Harova G, Dökmeci S. Steatocystoma multiplex suppurativum: oral isotretinoin treatment combined with cryotherapy. Australas J Dermatol. 2000;41:98–100.
34. Madan V, August PJ. Perforation and extirpation of steatocystoma multiplex. Int J Dermatol. 2009;48:329–30.
35. Mumcuoğlu CT, Gurel MS, Kiremitci U, Erdemir AV, Karakoca Y, Huten O. Er: yag laser therapy for steatocystoma multiplex. Indian J Dermatol. 2010;55:300–1.

Chapter 48
Xanthomas

Libby Rhee and Mark Kaufmann

48.1 Introduction

Cutaneous xanthomas result from the localized accumulation of lipid within the dermis or connective tissue. They can present anywhere on the body with a variety of morphologies ranging from discrete macules and papules to nodules and diffuse plaques, typically with a yellow-to-orange color due to the lipid deposition. In darker skin types, however, the lesions may appear more red-to-brown in color.

Xanthomas are most commonly associated with hyperlipemic states, which may be due to primary genetic causes or secondary to other metabolic derangements. Less frequently, normolipemic xanthomas have been reported in association with monoclonal gammopathies or without any associated underlying disease.

The major subtypes of xanthomas associated with disorders of lipid metabolism include tuberous, tendinous, eruptive, planar, and palmar. Xanthelasmas, a type of planar xanthoma, may or may not be associated with a hyperlipidemia. Prompt recognition and early diagnosis of the lesions can significantly aid in the management and prognosis of any potential underlying disease as cutaneous lesions may sometimes precede any systemic signs of symptoms. Moreover, the morphology and distribution of the xanthomas can suggest a particular lipoproteinemia or another systemic disease.

L. Rhee, D.O. (✉)
Department of Dermatology, St. Barnabas Hospital, 4422 Third Avenue,
Bronx, NY 10457, USA
e-mail: libbyrhee@gmail.com

M. Kaufmann, M.D.
Department of Dermatology, Icahn School of Medicine at Mt. Sinai,
New York, NY, USA

J.A. Zeichner (ed.), *Acneiform Eruptions in Dermatology: A Differential Diagnosis*,
DOI 10.1007/978-1-4614-8344-1_48,

48.2 Background

Xanthomatosis is a pan-ethnic phenomenon that affects men and women equally. They are more common in persons over the age of 50 but have been reported in all age groups from infancy to the elderly. Despite the high prevalence of hyperlipidemia in the general population, which is reported to affect slightly more than half of all Americans, cutaneous xanthomas only affect a relative minority of individuals [1]. The precise incidence of xanthomatous skin lesions remains unknown, and it is difficult to predict who will develop them. It is presumable that patients may not seek dermatologic care for their skin lesions, which may resolve spontaneously or with treatment of the underlying lipid abnormality or another associated disease. The lesions, while pathognomonic or suggestive of specific dyslipidemias, largely remain a cosmetic concern and can be quite disfiguring depending on their size and location. Morbidity and mortality are related to elevated serum lipids and the ensuing atherosclerotic disease or pancreatitis.

The precise mechanism of xanthoma formation is yet to be fully elucidated. A basic understanding of normal lipid metabolism helps to understand the possible pathogenesis of xanthomas and underlying disorders of lipid metabolism. In general, it is believed that circulating plasma lipoproteins are able to cross dermal capillary blood vessels where they are subsequently phagocytosed by macrophages, forming lipid-laden foam cells. The steps regulating this chain of events still remain unclear [2, 3].

Since lipids are naturally hydrophobic, they are transported in complex structures known as lipoproteins, which contain a hydrophilic shell composed of phospholipids, free cholesterol, and specific proteins called apolipoproteins or apoproteins. The triglycerides and cholesterol esters remain within the core for storage or usage of lipids.

Lipoproteins vary in their inner lipid content and are classified by their density. Triglycerides comprise the major lipid core of chylomicrons and very low-density lipoproteins (VLDLs). Cholesterol esters are the main component of low-density lipoproteins (LDLs) and high-density lipoproteins (HDLs) and remnants of chylomicrons and VLDLs. Apoproteins present on the surface confer specificity and allow for binding of the respective apoproteins to a particular receptor or target tissue.

There are two major pathways of lipoprotein synthesis: the exogenous pathway and the endogenous pathway. The exogenous pathway begins with dietary fat, namely, triglycerides, which are enzymatically degraded by pancreatic lipase and bile acids into fatty acids and monoglycerides. Following intestinal absorption, the triglycerides are reformed and packaged into chylomicrons with its specific apoproteins and outer shell components. Eventually, the chylomicrons enter systemic circulation and release free fatty acids into peripheral tissues. The hydrolysis of the triglyceride core is mediated through the action of lipoprotein lipase (LPL), a proteolytic enzyme bound to capillary endothelium. This process continues until only a chylomicron "remnant" exists. The new chylomicron "remnant" is now predominately composed of cholesterol ester acquired from circulating HDL molecules and is subsequently taken up by the liver for hepatic storage [2, 3].

The endogenous pathway of lipoprotein synthesis begins in the liver with the formation of VLDL molecules. The central core of the VLDL, like the chylomicron, is composed of triglycerides, which are derived from hepatic stores as well as circulating free fatty acids. As with chylomicrons, VLDLs are also cleaved by LPL until most of the triglycerides are removed and only a similar "remnant" remains. The VLDL remnant is called an intermediate density lipoprotein (IDL) and is ready to be taken up by the liver and degraded. The IDLs that escape hepatic uptake are stripped of their remaining triglyceride core and enter systemic circulation as LDLs.

LDLs deliver cholesterol esters to peripheral tissues where they can be converted into free cholesterol. Cholesterol is an essential component of many body tissues, including the selectively permeable cell membrane bilayer and myelin nerve sheaths. It also serves important roles in adrenal and gonadal steroidogenesis as well as the production of bile acids. Any excess cholesterol is re-esterified for hepatic storage [2, 3].

HDL also plays a very important and "protective" role in cholesterol metabolism. Its most important function is to "scavenge" free cholesterol from peripheral tissues so it can be esterified and transferred to other lipoproteins such as LDLs or remnants of chylomicrons and VLDLs for reverse transport or transport back to the liver. The esterification of free cholesterol is mediated by the enzyme lecithin cholesterol acyl transferase (LCAT).

Cholesterol homeostasis involves a complex interweaving of mechanisms. As such, disorders in lipid metabolism can occur in numerous ways. Inherited disorders resulting from genetic mutations (primary hyperlipoproteinemia) can yield absent or defective enzymes, receptors, or receptor ligands, with resultant overproduction or decreased clearance of lipoproteins. Several mutations are known to exist and are associated with a unique lipid profile. Additionally, secondary hyperlipoproteinemias due to an underlying disease that may disrupt lipid metabolism including diabetes mellitus, hypothyroidism, and nephrotic syndrome are not uncommon. Medications, such as oral retinoids, oral contraceptive pills, antiretroviral drugs to name a few can also lead to a hyperlipemic state [2, 3].

48.3 Clinical Presentation

Cutaneous xanthomas associated with hyperlipidemia are typically divided into five main groups depending on morphology and/or location: tuberous, tendinous, eruptive, planar, and palmar. Xanthelasma palpebrarum is the most common type of xanthoma presenting around the eyes. It is considered a subtype of planar xanthoma, although it is not necessarily associated with aberrant lipid metabolism (Fig. 48.1). Xanthoma disseminatum and verruciform xanthoma are not usually associated with any lipid abnormalities.

Tuberous xanthomas present as firm, painless, pink-to-yellow papules or nodules most commonly on extensor surfaces, especially the elbows and knees, as well as on pressure-prone areas such as the buttocks (Fig. 48.2). Tuberous xanthomas are particularly associated with hypercholesterolemic states such as *familial*

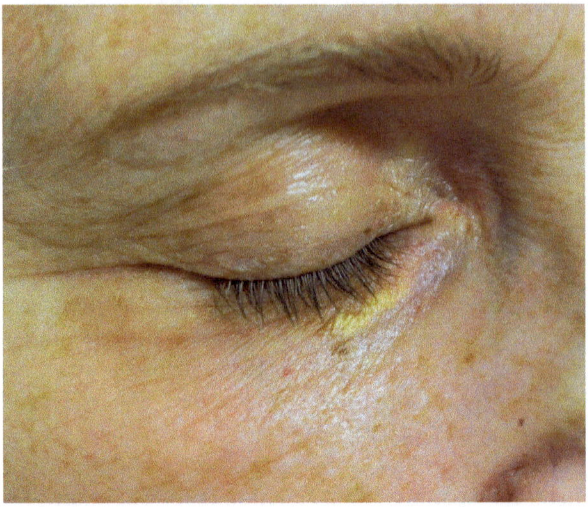

Fig. 48.1 Xanthelasma: yellow papules that commonly present around the upper and lower eyelids (Photo credit: Joshua A. Zeichner, M.D.)

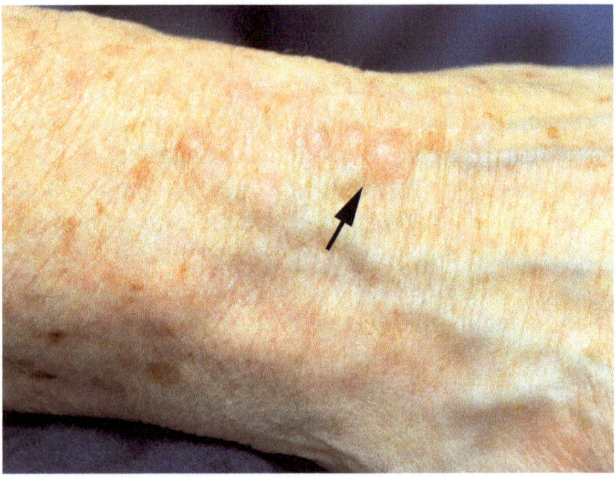

Fig. 48.2 Tuberous xanthomas: flesh-colored to erythematous papules that usually present around extensor surfaces of the elbows and knees. This patient had a family history of high cholesterol and developed lesions on the wrists (Photo credit: Joshua A. Zeichner, M.D.)

hypercholesterolemia (Type II) and *dysbetalipoproteinemia* (Type III). They may also be associated with secondary hyperlipidemias, including nephrotic syndrome and hypothyroidism. With treatment of the underlying disease, the lesions will usually resolve slowly over time.

Tendinous xanthomas are slowly progressing, firm, subcutaneous, nodular deposits of lipid that are associated with tendon sheaths. The Achilles tendon and extensor tendons of the hands and feet are most often affected. The overlying skin does not show any changes. Tendinous xanthomas are generally associated with significant serum lipid elevation, namely, elevated LDL. *Familial hypercholesterolemia* (Type IIa), *dysbetalipoproteinemia* (Type III), and hepatic cholestasis are all associated with this type of xanthoma [4].

Eruptive xanthomas appear suddenly as crops of red-to-yellow papules 1–4 mm in diameter on an erythematous base, sometimes imparting an inflammatory appearance to the lesions. They have a predilection for extensor surfaces of the extremities, buttocks, and hands. Patients often report pain and pruritus with the lesions, and koebnerization has been reported as a feature. Eruptive xanthomas are associated with primary (Types I, IV, V; elevated chylomicrons, VLDL, chylomicrons/VLDL, respectively) or secondary hypertriglyceridemia (diabetes mellitus). Triglyceride levels often exceed 3,000–4,000 mg/dl and can lead to acute pancreatitis or life-threatening atherosclerosis if not managed effectively. Unlike tuberous xanthomas, these lesions often resolve promptly upon treatment of the hypertriglyceridemia [5].

Planar xanthomas occur as yellow-to-orange macules, papules, patches, or plaques. They can occur anywhere, and often can give a clue to the underlying diagnosis depending on their location. For example, palmar crease lesions (*xanthoma striatum palmare*) are pathognomonic for *dysbetalipoproteinemia* (Type III), especially when tuberous xanthomas are also present. Antecubital fossae or finger web space lesions are nearly pathognomonic for *homozygous familial hypercholesterolemia* (Type II). Generalized lesions may cover the face, neck, and chest.

Xanthelasma, *xanthelasma palpebrarum*, is the most common type of xanthoma. Only about half are associated with an underlying lipid disorder, but a workup is generally still warranted, especially if the patient is younger and has a strong family history of dyslipidemia [3, 6].

Planar xanthomas may also be associated with cholestasis as a complication of biliary disease as well as in normolipemic patients. In the latter clinical scenario, a monoclonal gammopathy (IgG type), secondary to multiple myeloma, a lymphoproliferative disorder such as B-cell lymphoma or chronic myelomonocytic leukemia (CML), or Castleman's disease should be ruled out [3].

48.4 Workup

Xanthomas may be idiopathic or indicate more serious systemic disease. Key to the workup is diagnosing and treating any underlying hyperlipidemia in order to minimize the progression atherosclerotic disease. Any potential secondary causes of disease need to be excluded as well.

Primary, or inherited forms, of hyperlipidemia are generally a diagnosis of exclusion. Laboratory studies used to either primary or secondary hyperlipidemia should start with a serum lipid panel, including fasting plasma levels of triglycerides, cholesterol, and HDL cholesterol. LDL and VLDL concentrations can be calculated using the above information. Chylomicrons can be separated via ultracentrifugation and electrophoresis, then quantified using immunologic methods.

Certain xanthomas are highly suggestive of specific familial hyperlipoproteinemias and can guide the workup and diagnosis: xanthoma striatum palmare are seen in familial dysbetalipoproteinemia and intertriginous xanthomas in homozygous familial hypercholesterolemia. Rarely, plane xanthomas may be associated with an underlying monoclonal gammopathy, and urine or serum protein electrophoresis can be used as an initial test in this clinical setting. Xanthelasma palpebrarum, which is only loosely associated with underlying hypercholesterolemia, is characteristically found on the upper and lower eyelids. Imaging studies can aid in determining the extent of xanthomatous lesions as well as atherosclerotic disease [2–4].

The characteristic histologic finding in xanthomas is the foamy macrophage. The lipid droplets that fill the macrophage are often dissolved and removed during normal tissue processing, leaving behind artifactual clefting. Polarized microscopy can be used to detect cholesterol esters, which are doubly refractile, within the dermis. All xanthomas contain lipid within the dermal infiltrate, but they may vary in terms of the content, inflammatory infiltrate, amount and location of the infiltrate within the dermis, and the presence of extracellular lipid.

48.5 Treatment

Xanthomas are not always associated with hyperlipidemia, but when they are, a multidisciplinary approach to lowering the lipid levels is essential. First-line therapies include dietary modifications and lipid-lowering agents such as HMG-CoA reductase inhibitors ("statins"), bile acid-binding resins, fibric acid derivatives, and/or nicotinic acid. Cutaneous xanthomas generally resolve with correction of the underlying lipid disorder. Slower growing xanthomas such as tendinous or tuberous xanthomas may persist for years or never fully resolve in contrast to eruptive xanthomas, for example, which often disappear quickly with aggressive lipid-lowering therapy [1–3].

The cutaneous lesions, particularly xanthelasmas, can be treated by surgical excision or through locally destructive methods if they are a cosmetic or functional concern. Laser therapy (CO_2; pulsed-dye or erbium:YAG lasers; argon; Q-switched Nd:YAG; KTP), di- or trichloroacetic acid, electrodesiccation, cryotherapy, intralesional bleomycin, and intralesional corticosteroid injections have all been reported to be helpful [6]. Unfortunately, the xanthomas often recur despite initial success, and scarring, pigmentary changes, and koebnerization are potential adverse effects.

48.6 Conclusion

Several different forms of xanthomas exist. Patients often confuse xanthelasma on the face with acne vulgaris. The clinical appearance of xanthelasma differs from acne, and it is treated in different ways. The appearance of xanthomas on the skin may be a marker for systemic disease, including hyperlipidemia or monoclonal gammopathy, so a full workup should be performed.

References

1. Ford ES, Li C, Pearson WS, Zhao G, Mokdad AH. Trends in hypercholesterolemia, treatment and control among United States adults. Int J Cardiol. 2010 ;140(2):226–35.
2. Parker F. Xanthomas and hyperlipidemias. J Am Acad Dermatol. 1985;13(1):1–30.
3. Bolognia J, Jorizzo J, Rapini R. Dermatology. 2nd ed. New York: Elselvier Limited; 2008. Print.
4. Tsouli SG, Kiortsis DN, Argyropoulou MI, Mikhailidis DP, Elisaf MS. Pathogenesis, detection and treatment of Achilles tendon xanthomas. Eur J Clin Invest. 2005;35(4):236–44.
5. Streit E, Helmbold P. 65-year-old man with yellow-orange papules on both forearms. Eruptive xanthomas. Hautarzt. 2009;60(10):834–7.
6. Rohrich RJ, Janis JE, Pownell PH. Xanthelasma palpebrarum: a review and current management principles. Plast Reconstr Surg. 2002;110(5):1310–4.

Part VI
Pediatric Dermatoses Mimicking Acne

Chapter 49
Periorificial Granulomatous Dermatitis

Jacquelyn Levin, James Del Rosso, and Richard Miller

49.1 Introduction

Periorificial granulomatous dermatitis (PGD) was first reported in 1970 in the French literature by Gianotti et al. [1]. Gianotti et al. [1] described five Italian children ranging in age from 2.5 to 7 years with a distinctive eruption of monomorphous papules around the mouth with a granulomatous pattern noted histologically. In 1974, Marten et al. [2] reported 22 Black children with a similar eruption limited to the face. In 1989, Frieden et al. [3] termed this disease granulomatous perioral dermatitis in children. In 1990, Williams et al. [4] reported 5 very similar patients and coined the term facial Afro-Caribbean childhood eruption (FACE) to reflect that all their cases occurred in Afro-Caribbean children. In 1996, Knautz et al. [5] suggested the term childhood granulomatous periorificial dermatitis for this eruption to point out the frequent perinasal or periocular involvement and to avoid the term FACE which limits the diagnosis to Afro-Caribbeans.

Today, there is still no consensus about the nomenclature of the disease. This characteristic eruption has been reported in the literature as Gianotti-type perioral dermatitis [6], facial Afro-Caribbean childhood eruption (FACE) [4, 6–9], sarcoid-like granulomatous dermatitis [10], childhood granulomatous perioral dermatitis [3], and childhood granulomatous periorificial dermatitis [4, 5, 11]. In our opinion periorificial granulomatous dermatitis (PGD) best describes the clinical and

J. Levin, D.O. (✉)
Department of Dermatology, Largo Medical Center, 201 14th St SW, Largo, FL 33774, USA
e-mail: jlevin@hotmail.com

J. Del Rosso, D.O.
Touro University College of Osteopathic Medicine,
Henderson, NV, USA

R. Miller, D.O.
Nova Southeastern University College of Osteopathic Medicine,
Tampa, FL, USA

J.A. Zeichner (ed.), *Acneiform Eruptions in Dermatology: A Differential Diagnosis*,
DOI 10.1007/978-1-4614-8344-1_49,

histopathologic characteristics of this skin disease because PGD may not be limited to a perioral distribution and is histopathologically characterized by the presence of a granulomatous inflammatory reaction [12].

49.2 Background

The etiology of PGD is unknown, although several theories exist. Many believe that PGD is the less common granulomatous variant of perioral/periorificial dermatitis (PD) and that PD and PGD share the same etiologic factors [5, 13–17].

The main etiologic factors in PD are thought to be a decreased stratum corneum (SC) permeability barrier function [14] from intrinsic factors or deficiencies yet to be identified or from extrinsic causes such as topical products [15, 16]. The topical products implicated in PD include contact irritants or allergens in cosmetics and topical corticosteroids (TCs) [4, 11, 14, 17–20]. While there are no reports in the literature demonstrating SC permeability barrier dysfunction in PGD, there are conflicting reports regarding the pathogenic relationship of PGD to topical products. Some authors report a pathogenic relationship between PGD and TC use, or to topical allergens and irritants such as formaldehyde and antiseptic solutions [3, 6, 13, 21], while others specifically state that no etiologic relationship is present between TC and other products in PGD [22].

Whether the inciting factors are intrinsic or extrinsic, the initiating event for PD as well as PGD is believed to be the same; damage to the hair follicle which results in damage to the follicular wall, release of its contents into the surrounding dermis, and subsequent inflammation [14, 22]. The antigenic component of the ruptured follicle is unknown; however, it is thought in PGD to provoke a granulomatous response [22]. There are limited data available to support this theory of pathogenesis.

PGD is a rare skin disease that occurs mostly in children with skin of color [21, 23]. PGD has been seen healthy children ranging in age from 6 months to 18 years [17, 24, 25]. Afro-Caribbean, African American, and Asian children dominate the reports, but Caucasian patients are also susceptible [21, 23]. There have been reports of PGD being more common in boys versus girls [26, 27]; however, the majority of reports state that both sexes are affected equally [21].

49.3 Clinical Presentation

The primary lesions in PGD are discrete 1–3 mm asymptomatic monomorphous dome-shaped papules that can range in color from pink red to flesh colored to yellow brown (Fig. 49.1) [12, 13, 15, 22]. In some instances there is background erythema and overlying scale present; however, these features are not consistently present in published cases. The face is always involved in PGD, and lesions are typically concentrated around the mouth, nose, and/or eyes. PGD characteristically

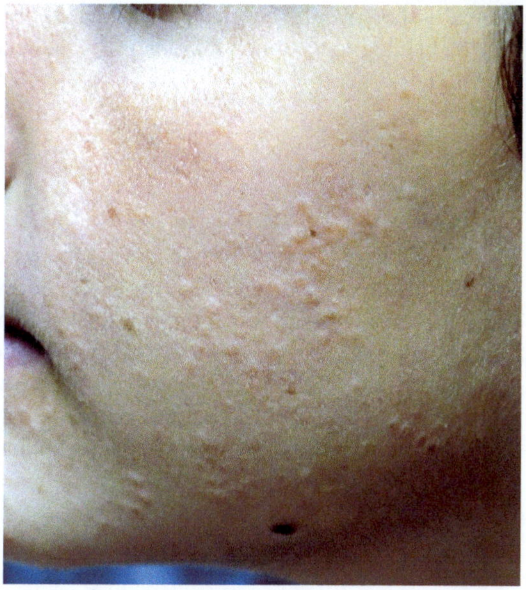

Fig. 49.1 Discreet, monomorphic, dome-shaped papules on the cheek of a teenage girl

involves the vermillion border of the lip which helps distinguishes this eruption from other diseases such as PD [23]. While the majority of cases reported in the literature are confined to the face, eight reported cases of PGD also had generalized skin lesions [21]. The patients with extrafacial involvement had lesions on the neck, upper trunk, extensor wrists, and vaginal area [28, 29]. Importantly, extensive skin involvement in PGD does not appear to change the duration of the eruption, the response to treatment, or have any association with any specific underlying internal diseases [15].

Scarring is variable in PGD. The initial cases described by Gianotti et al. [1] and several subsequent authors [6, 28, 30] reported the occurrence of small pitted scars after resolution of the papules. However, the majority of cases since then have reported no scarring or other sequelae after the resolution of PGD [4, 13, 23].

In the majority of cases where skin biopsies were performed, a dermal granulomatous infiltrate was seen concentrated around the upper half of the hair follicles [12, 13, 15]. In some biopsy specimens, the granulomatous infiltrate was more diffuse, and in some rare cases no granulomas were detected on histologic examination [2, 4]. Focal epidermal spongiosis is occasionally described; however, there is never caseation necrosis, and the results of special stains and cultures for acid-fast bacilli and fungi are always negative [15].

This granulomatous histologic appearance of PGD is not diagnostic. The differential diagnosis of small papules with granulomatous histologic features in children includes sarcoidosis, fungal or mycobacterial infection, familial juvenile systemic granulomatosis (Blau syndrome), and granulomatous rosacea in addition to PGD [15]. In typical cases of PGD, these entities can be differentiated clinically; however, in cases with extrafacial involvement, a more thorough workup may be needed to establish the diagnosis and exclude other entities in the differential diagnosis.

49.4 Workup

There is some disagreement concerning the recommended workup when the diagnosis of PGD is suspected. Because PGD occurs in healthy children and spontaneously resolves within a few months to years without scarring or sequelae, it is often difficult to justify a biopsy or a thorough systemic evaluation [4]. However, it can be difficult at times to differentiate PGD from other more serious conditions with extracutaneous manifestations and potential long-term detrimental sequelae [23]. For this reason, when clinical presentation is not sufficient to diagnose PGD [4, 31], histopathologic evaluation is recommended, with additional workup directed by the clinician based on the needs of the individual case. Examples of tests that may be included in the workup are chest radiograph, ophthalmologic examination, tuberculin skin test, serum calcium, serum angiotensin-converting enzyme level, and the use of special stains and tissue cultures for fungal or mycobacterial organisms on histologic sections (Table 49.1) [15, 22, 31, 32].

In the literature, PGD has been likened to many dermatologic disorders with both cutaneous involvement and cutaneous plus systemic involvement. The main differential diagnoses of PGD include acne vulgaris, periorificial dermatitis (PD), granulomatous rosacea, sarcoidosis, lupus miliaris disseminatus faciei (LMDF), and seborrheic dermatitis. Many of the facial dermatoses listed the differential of PGD are discussed in detail elsewhere in the book as they are also difficult at times to differentiate from acne vulgaris and other facial dermatoses. Table 49.2 summarizes the defining characteristics of PGD while Table 49.3 lists the characteristics that help differentiate the skin diseases listed above from PGD [4, 12, 18].

Table 49.1 Summary of possible workup for selected cases of periorificial granulomatous dermatitis[a,b]

- Skin biopsy
  - Confirm consistency with diagnosis and evaluate for other potential diagnoses such as sarcoidosis, infectious etiologies, others (see text)
  - Specimen must contain adequate depth to fully evaluate follicular structures
  - Special stains and cultures to detect fungal or mycobacterial organism if present
- Chest radiograph
- Ophthalmologic examination
- Tuberculin skin test
- Serum calcium
- Serum angiotensin-converting enzyme level

[a]Workup to be determined based on judgement of clinician in cases where clinical diagnosis alone is questionable

[b]References [15, 22, 31, 32]

Table 49.2 Summary of defining characteristics of periorificial granulomatous dermatitis

• Epidemiology
Rare
Common in darker skin types
• Onset
6 months to 18 years
• Clinical presentation
Healthy children
Recent history of steroid use
1–3 mm asymptomatic, monomorphous, multiple dome-shaped papules
Color variable: pink, red, yellow brown, flesh colored
Individual and/or with confluence
Lesions around the mouth, nose, and/or eyes
Can involve vermillion border
Can involve extrafacial skin
Face always involved
No systemic symptoms or internal organ involvement
Spontaneous resolution in months to years
Usually no scarring
• Histology
Mixed granulomatous infiltrate around hair follicles

References [4, 11–13, 15, 17, 21–24]

Less commonly reported skin diseases which should be included in the differential diagnosis of PGD include allergic/irritant contact dermatitis, impetigo, acrodermatitis enteropathica, tinea faciei, lip-lickers dermatitis, atopic dermatitis, benign cephalic histiocytosis, granulosis rubra nasi, glucagonoma syndrome, Blau syndrome, Haber syndrome, and facial demodicosis.

49.5 Treatment

Patients and parents should be reassured that PGD is a benign, self-limited condition. Since the disease is benign and self-limited, treatment may be unnecessary. However, the average reported time for spontaneous resolution is between 1 and 3 years [1, 6, 10, 30, 33–36], and the resolution may be hastened with the use of appropriate therapy [15]. The time to resolution with treatment varies greatly in the literature ranging from 1 week to 6 months [17, 20, 37].

There are no available randomized controlled trials providing guidance for the best treatment in PGD because of the rare nature of this skin disease. Some reviews dictate the first step in management to be discontinuation of all TCs or any other

Table 49.3 Differentiation of periorificial granulomatous dermatitis from other simulant dermatoses

• *Acne vulgaris*
Comedones, pustules, nodule, and cysts present
High incidence in puberty
• *Perioral dermatitis*
Most common in young women in third to fourth decade
Pustules present
Spares the vermillion border
No extrafacial eruptions
• *Granulomatous rosacea*
Most common in young women in third to fourth decade
Centrofacial distribution
Background erythema, flushing, telangiectasias, pustules may be present
No spontaneous resolution
• *Sarcoidosis*
Rarely presents in children
Multiorgan involvement
Systemic symptoms present
Granulomas on histology do not have surrounding infiltrate and are not centered around a follicle
• *Seborrheic dermatitis*
Ears, nasolabial folds, eyebrows, and scalp commonly involved
Scale or hyperkeratosis often present
• *Lupus miliaris disseminatus faciei*
Scarring is present
Most common in Japanese adults
Caseation necrosis on histology

References [4, 12, 18]

possible inciting chemicals or products [12, 13, 24, 34]. Because there may be an associated rebound or exacerbation of the skin disease after stopping TC use, many physicians recommend the use of a mild topical corticosteroids daily for a few weeks to effectively wean patients off more potent TCs; however, there is no scientific evidence that this approach is beneficial [25, 37, 38]. The authors suggest discontinuation of TCs without a weaning approach [39].

In the literature there are several case reports demonstrating the effectiveness of treatment with topical metronidazole, sulfacetamide-sulfur, topical erythromycin, oral tetracyclines, or oral erythromycin for PGD [4, 15, 21]. Nguyen and Eichenfeld [17] recommend a 1–2-month trial of topical metronidazole with the addition of oral erythromycin. Urbatsch states that the administration of oral macrolides or tetracyclines, alone or in combination with topical erythromycin, metronidazole, or sulfur-based lotions, hastens resolution in most patients [15, 21]. Although oral tetracyclines can be effective in treating PGD, they should not be used in PGD patients less than 8 years old as tetracyclines have been known to cause dental enamel discoloration [24, 39]. The availability of subantimicrobial dosing of doxycycline offers an option that may be effective without exposing the patient to antibiotic selection pressure [39].

49.6 Conclusion

PGD is a chronic and potentially disfiguring dermatosis, often affecting the face. It may commonly be mistaken for acne vulgaris, but clinically appears as monomorphic papules rather than the comedones, papules, and pustules observed in patients with acne vulgaris. Treatment can be challenging and requires often long-term combination therapy with both topical and oral medications.

References

1. Gianotti F, Ermacora E, Bennelli MG, Caputo R. Particuliere dermatite peri-orale infantile. Observations sur 5 cas. Bull Soc Fr Dermatol Syphiligr. 1970;77:341.
2. Marten RH, Presbury DG, Adamson JE, Cardell BS. An unusual papular and acneiform facial eruption in the negro child. Br J Dermatol. 1974;91:435–8.
3. Frieden IJ, Prose NS, Fletcher V, Turner ML. Granulomatous perioral dermatitis in children. Arch Dermatol. 1989;125:369–73.
4. Williams HC, Ashworth J, Pembroke AC, Breathnach SM. FACE-facial Afro-Caribbean childhood eruption. Clin Exp Dermatol. 1990;15:163–6.
5. Knautz MA, Lesher Jr JL. Childhood granulomatous periorificial dermatitis. Pediatr Dermatol. 1996;13:131–4.
6. Georgouras K, Kocsard E. Micropapular sarcoidal facial eruption in a child: Gianotti-type perioral dermatitis. Acta Derm Venereol. 1978;58:433–6.
7. Williams HC. Childhood granulomatous periorificial dermatitis. Pediatr Dermatol. 1996;13(6):515.
8. Laude TA, Salvemini JN. Perioral dermatitis in children. Semin Cutan Med Surg. 1999;18(3): 206–9.
9. Smitt JH, Das PK, Van Ginkel JW. Granulomatous perioral dermatitis (facial Afro-Caribbean childhood eruption [FACE]). Br J Dermatol. 1991;125:399.
10. Falk E. Sarcoid-like granulomatous periocular dermatitis treated with tetracycline. Acta Derm Venereol. 1985;65:270–2.
11. Tarm K, Creel NB, Krivda SJ, Turiansky GW. Granulomatous periorificial dermatitis. Cutis. 2004;73(6):399–402.
12. Zalaudek I, Di Stefani A, Ferrara G, Argenziano G. Childhood granulomatous periorificial dermatitis: a controversial disease. J Dtsch Dermatol Ges. 2005;3(4):252–5.
13. Kim YJ, Shin JW, Lee JS, Park YL, Whang KU, Lee SY. Childhood granulomatous periorificial dermatitis. Ann Dermatol. 2011;23(3):386–8.
14. Dirschka T, Tronnier H, Folster-Holst R. Epithelial barrier function and atopic diathesis in rosacea and perioral dermatitis. Br J Dermatol. 2004;150:1136–41.
15. Urbatsch AJ, Frieden I, Williams ML, Elewski BE, Mancini AJ, Paller AS. Extrafacial and generalized granulomatous periorificial dermatitis. Arch Dermatol. 2002;138(10):1354–8.
16. Dirschka T, Weber K, Tronnier H. Topical cosmetics and perioral dermatitis. J Dtsch Dermatol Ges. 2004;2:194–9.
17. Nguyen V, Eichenfield LF. Periorificial dermatitis in children and adolescents. J Am Acad Dermatol. 2006;55:781–5.
18. Ahmed I. Clinicopathologic challenge. Childhood granulomatous peri-orificial dermatitis with extra-facial lesions. Int J Dermatol. 2007;46(2):143–5.
19. Cochran RE, Thomson J. Perioral dermatitis: a reappraisal. Clin Exp Dermatol. 1979;4(1): 75–80.
20. Wilkinson DS, Kirton V, Wilkinson JD. Perioral dermatitis: a 12-year review. Br J Dermatol. 1979;101:245–57.

21. James W, Berger T, Elston D. Andrews' diseases of the skin: clinical dermatology. 11th ed. USA: Elsevier Health; 2011.
22. Makkar R, Ramesh V. On the diagnosis of facial granulomatous dermatoses of obscure origin. Int J Dermatol. 2005;44(7):606–9.
23. Choi YL, Lee KJ, Cho HJ, Kim WS, Lee JH, Yang JM, et al. Case of childhood granulomatous periorificial dermatitis in a Korean boy treated by oral erythromycin. J Dermatol. 2006;33(11):806–8.
24. Kuflik JH, Janniger CK, Piela Z. Perioral dermatitis: an acneiform eruption. Cutis. 2001;67: 21–2.
25. Coskey RJ. Perioral dermatitis. Cutis. 1984;34:8.
26. Kim MS, Kim BS, Koh WS, Cho JJ, Chun DK. A case of childhood granulomatous perioral dermatitis. Korean J Dermatol. 2000;38:526–9.
27. Lee WJ, Yang JH, Lee MW, Choi JH, Moon KC, Koh JK. A case of childhood granulomatous periorificial dermatitis. Korean J Dermatol. 2008;46:1570–2.
28. Andry P, Bodemer C, Teillac-Hamel D, Fraitag S, DeProst Y. Granulomatous perioral dermatitis in childhood: eight cases [abstract]. Pediatr Dermatol. 1995;12:76.
29. Hansen KK, McTigue K, Esterly NB. Multiple facial, neck, and upper trunk papules in a black child: childhood granulomatous perioral dermatitis with involvement of the neck and upper trunk. Arch Dermatol. 1992;128:1396–7.
30. Husz S, Korom I. Periocular dermatitis: a micropapular sarcoid-like granulomatous dermatitis in a woman. Dermatologica. 1981;162:424–8.
31. Frieden IJ, Prose NS, Fletcher V, Turner ML. Granulomatous perioral dermatitis or sarcoid? Arch Dermatol. 1990;126(9):1237–8.
32. Gupta AK, Goldfarb MT, Rasmussen JE. Papular midfacial eruption in a child. Cutaneous Sarcoidosis. Arch Dermatol. 1989;125(12):1704–5. 1707–8.
33. Gianotti F. Cutaneous benign histiocytosis of childhood. Mod Probl Paediatr. 1975;17: 193–203.
34. El-Saad E-RM. Perioral dermatitis with epithelioid cell granulomas in a woman: a possible new etiology. Acta Derm Venereol. 1979;60:359–60.
35. Hansen KK, McTigue K, Esterly NB. Multiple facial, neck, and upper trunk papules in a black child: childhood granulomatous perioral dermatitis with involvement of the neck and upper trunk. Arch Dermatol. 1992;128:1396–7.
36. Antony FC, Buckley DA, Russell-Jones R. Childhood granulomatous periorificial dermatitis in an Asian girl—a variant of sarcoid? Clin Exp Dermatol. 2002;27(4):275–6.
37. Manders SM, Lucky AW. Perioral dermatitis in childhood. J Am Acad Dermatol. 1992;27:688–92.
38. Wilkinson DS, Kirton V, Wilkinson JD. Perioral dermatitis: a 12-year review. Br J Dermatol. 1979;101:245–57.
39. Del Rosso JQ. Management of papulopustular rosacea and perioral dermatitis with emphasis on iatrogenic causation or exacerbation of inflammatory facial dermatoses: use of doxycycline modified-release 40 mg capsule once daily in combination with properly selected skin care as an effective therapeutic approach. J Clin Aesthet Dermatol. 2011;4:20–30.

Chapter 50
Keratosis Pilaris Atrophicans

Omar Pacha and Adelaide Hebert

50.1 Introduction

Keratosis pilaris atrophicans faciei (KPAF), also commonly known as ulerythema ophryogenes, is a rare disorder characterized by erythematous small keratotic papules that resolve with atrophy and resultant focal alopecia. This uncommon condition always involves the face, especially the eyebrows. Similarities exist, both genetically and clinically, to other scarring alopecias with follicular hyperkeratosis including atrophoderma vermiculatum and keratosis follicularis spinulosa decalvans. Some have characterized these clinical entities under a single term known as keratosis pilaris atrophicans [1]. Currently treatment options produce generally unimpressive clinical outcomes.

50.2 Background

Keratosis pilaris atrophicans faciei is an autosomal dominantly inherited disorder with incomplete penetrance. Originally described by Englishman Erasmus Wilson in 1878, the clinical findings were named folliculitis rubra [2]. In 1889, German Paul Taenzer coined the term ulerythema ophryogenes, meaning scarring of the eyebrows [3]. Efforts to determine the precise genetic cause are ongoing, but partial monosomy of chromosome 18 is the most frequently cited causation [4–6]. The association of chromosome 18 aneuploidy and KPAF indicates the absence of a gene, possibly for laminin $\alpha 1$, in the 18p area that regulates follicular keratinization and formation of sebaceous gland structures [6].

O. Pacha, M.D. (✉) • A. Hebert, M.D.
Department of Dermatology, University of Texas Health Science Center,
6655 Travis Street, Suite 600, Houston, TX 77030, USA
e-mail: omar.pacha@uth.tmc.edu

J.A. Zeichner (ed.), *Acneiform Eruptions in Dermatology: A Differential Diagnosis*,
DOI 10.1007/978-1-4614-8344-1_50, © Springer Science+Business Media New York 2014

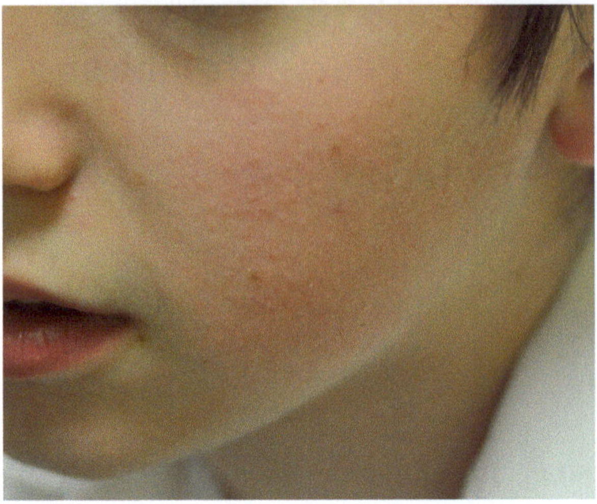

Fig. 50.1 Follicular papules on the cheek of an adolescent boy

Onset of the disease is noted a few months after birth, with the usual phenotype being Fitzpatrick skin type II, blond-haired boys, with the inherited findings occurring as an autosomal dominant disease with variable penetrance [7]. Pathogenesis is felt to occur as the result of a plug that forms in the follicular ostium that causes keratotic follicular papules and hair shaft deformation. Histologically, evidence of hyperkeratosis and hypergranulosis of the isthmus and infundibulum of the follicle lead to surrounding inflammation in the dermis. Subsequently, mononuclear cells appear around the superior follicle with surrounding mucin and destructive changes to connective tissue. After the disintegration of the follicle, reactive changes surrounding a naked hair shaft result in further inflammation and finally scarring in the final chronic phase [1].

50.3 Clinical Presentation

KPAF begins shortly after birth and is generally clinically evident before 5 years of age with erythema and small horny follicular papules emerging laterally from the eyebrows, often extending to the cheeks and forehead (Fig. 50.1). This condition is often associated with atopic dermatitis, asthma, and seasonal allergies. On exam many patients also often have keratosis pilaris on extremity extensor surfaces [8]. Eventually the affected areas become atrophic with residual scarring alopecia. The cycle continues through adolescence but generally halts with the beginning of puberty.

50.4 Workup

Diagnosis is based on clinical findings and may be made soon after birth. Since KPAF is believed to be inherited and is considered a marker of certain genetic syndromes such as Noonan syndrome [9–11], Rubinstein-Taybi syndrome [12],

Cornelia de Lange syndrome [13], and cardiofaciocutaneous syndrome [14, 15], workup and appropriate treatment for coexisting disease may be initiated.

Histology depends on disease stage. All follicular keratoses form keratotic plugs at the follicular orifice of the infundibulum which makes pathologic diagnosis difficult without relevant clinical history. Therefore, the initial stage of disease is impossible to distinguish between the various forms based on histology alone. The superficial dermis contains a predominantly lymphocytic infiltrate surrounding the follicle with a few neutrophilic granulocytes that progresses to perifollicular fibrosis with fewer lymphocytes over the course of disease. Further, the atrophic stage is characterized by dermal sclerosis, atrophy of hair follicles, and formation of horn cysts. Less commonly, dilated lymph vessels and blood vessels can also be seen. In the final atrophic phase, the disease has the appearance of a cicatricial alopecia.

50.5 Treatment

There is no apparent universally effective treatment for KPAF. Initial attempts at treatment were tried with antibiotics including sulfa-based medications, macrolides, tetracyclines, and penicillin; all have been shown to be ineffective. Oral isotretinoin has been described as effective by some authors at doses of 1–1.5 mg/kg [16] but marginal to ineffective by others [1, 17]. Topical keratolytics and topical corticosteroids may reduce keratin plugging, obtain mild improvement in the erythema, and slow progression of the alopecia [1, 18]. Immunomodulators such as cyclosporine and methotrexate have been reported in other cicatricial alopecias [19–21] but not KPAF and may represent a viable option. Surgical hair transplantation is a viable option for many patients and appears to produce durable hair growth, at least in the eyebrows, that is not susceptible to the lost native facial hair [22, 23].

50.6 Conclusion

KPAF is a progressive scarring condition affecting the face and the eyebrows. While treatment is challenging, aggressive therapy early after diagnosis may halt progression of the disease and minimize the onset of permanent scarring and alopecia later in life.

References

1. Baden HP, Byers HR. Clinical findings, cutaneous pathology, and response to therapy in 21 patients with keratosis pilaris atrophicans. Arch Dermatol. 1994;130:469–75.
2. Wilson, Erasmus (1878) Lectures on Dermatology. London. p 217
3. Paul Taenzer (1889) "Ueber das Ulerythema ophryogenes," Monats. f. prakt. Derwnat. Hamburg. pp 197–208.viii
4. Nazarenko SA, Ostroverkhova NV, Vasiljeva EO, et al. Keratosis pilaris and ulerythema ophryogenes associated with an 18 p deletion caused by a Y/18 translocation. Am J Med Genet. 1999;85:179–82.

5. Fiorentini C, Bardazzi F, Bianchi T, Patrizi A. Keratosis pilaris in a girl with monosomy 18p. J Eur Acad Dermatol Venereol. 1999;12 suppl 2:S221.
6. Stratakis, Zouboulis, Gollnick HPM, Orfanos. Keratosis pilaris/ulerythema ophryogenes and 18p deletion: is it possible that theLAMA1 gene is involved? J Med Genet. 2001;38:127.
7. Oranje AP. Others. Keratosis pilaris atrophicans: one heterogeneous disease or a symptom in different clinical entities? Arch Dermatol. 1994;130:500.
8. Davenport DD. Ulerythema ophryogenes. Arch Dermatol. 1964;89:134–40.
9. Pierini DO, Pierini AM. Keratosis pilaris atrophicans faciei (Ulerythema ophryogenes): a cutaneous marker in the Noonan syndrome. Br J Dermatol. 1979;100:409–16.
10. Snell JA, Mallory SB. Ulerythema ophryogenes in Noonan syndrome. Pediatr Dermatol. 1990;7:77–8.
11. Turner AM. Noonan syndrome. J Paediatr Child Health. 2011. doi:10.1111/j.1440-1754.2010.01970.x.
12. Centeno PG, Roson E, Peteiro C, Pereiro M, Toribio J. Rubinstein-Taybi syndrome and Ulerythema ophryogenes in a 9-year-old boy. Pediatr Dermatol. 1999;16:134–6.
13. Florez A, Fernandez-Redondo V, Toribio J. Ulerythema ophryogenes in Cornelia de Lange syndrome. Pediatr Dermatol. 2002;19:42–5.
14. Manci EA, Martinez JE, Horenstein MG, Gardner TM, Ahmed A, Mancao MC, et al. Cardiofaciocutaneous syndrome (CFC) with congenital peripheral neuropathy and nonorganic malnutrition: An autopsy study. Am J Med Genet A. 2005;137A:1–8. doi:10.1002/ajmg.a.30834.
15. Borradori L, Blanchet-Bardon C. Skin manifestations of cardio-facio-cutaneous syndrome. J Am Acad Dermatol. 1993;28:815–9.
16. Layton AM, Cunliffe WJ. A case of ulerythema ophryogenes responding to isotretinoin. Br J Dermatol. 1993;129:645–6.
17. Burnett JW, Schwartz MF, Berberian BJ. Ulerythema ophryogenes with multiple congenital anomalies. J Am Acad Dermatol. 1988;18:437–40.
18. Callaway SR, Lesher JL. Keratosis pilaris atrophicans: case series and review. Pediatr Dermatol. 2004;21:14–7.
19. Ross EK, Tan E, Shapiro J. Update on primary cicatricial alopecias. J Am Acad Dermatol. 2005;53(1):1–37. doi:10.1016/j.jaad.2004.06.015. ISSN 0190–9622.
20. Di Lernia V, Bisighini G. Discoid lupus erythematosus during treatment with cyclosporine. Acta Derm Venereol. 1996;76:87–8.
21. Mirmirani P, Willey A, Price VH. Short course of oral cyclosporine in lichen planopilaris. J Am Acad Dermatol. 2003;49:667–71.
22. GoldmanGD.EyebrowTransplantation.DermatolSurg.2001;27:352–4.doi:10.1046/j.1524-4725.2001.00209.x.
23. Barankin B, Taher M, Wasel N. Successful hair transplant of eyebrow alopecia areata. J Cutan Med Surg. 2005;9:162–4.

Chapter 51
Neonatal and Infantile Acne

Hilary Baldwin

51.1 Introduction

Acne vulgaris is a disease that typically affects teenagers but may continue into adulthood in some cases. However, acneiform eruptions can occur in the pediatric population from birth onward. Neonatal acne refers to lesions that develop in the neonatal period, from birth through 4 weeks old. Some consider neonatal acne to be synonymous with neonatal cephalic pustulosis. Infantile acne refers to the acneiform eruption that typically presents in children between 1 month and 1 year old [1]. Making the correct diagnosis can be a challenge, and in some cases the diagnosis of infantile acne is given whenever comedones are clinically present even if the patient is a neonate.

51.2 Background

It is estimated that up to 20 % of newborns develop an acneiform eruption. Neonatal acne occurs much more frequently in boys than girls. Two main theories exist regarding the condition's pathophysiology. First, maternal androgens are thought to stimulate sebaceous glands in neonates [2, 3]. Second, it is postulated that an increase in neonatal dehydroepiandrosterone (DHEA) stimulates the adrenal glands. There is a questionable association between neonatal acne and the development of acne later in adolescence [3].

Neonatal cephalic pustulosis (NCP) is another name given to acneiform eruptions seen in neonates. Some experts consider this a separate entity from true neonatal acne and attribute it to the presence of *Malassezia* yeast on the skin [4].

H. Baldwin, M.D. (✉)
Department of Dermatology, SUNY Downstate School of Medicine, Brooklyn, NY, USA

J.A. Zeichner (ed.), *Acneiform Eruptions in Dermatology: A Differential Diagnosis*,
DOI 10.1007/978-1-4614-8344-1_51, © Springer Science+Business Media New York 2014

In one study, pustules of the necks of 8 of 13 neonates with acne revealed *M. furfur* [5]. However, not all patients with the eruption have positive cultures, suggesting hypersensitivity to yeast as the causative factor rather than level of colonization itself [6–8].

Little epidemiological data is available on infantile acne, as it so uncommon. Expert opinions suggest that it occurs more commonly in boys than girls. Infantile acne usually presents between 3 and 6 months of age, but it may develop as early as immediately after birth or as late as 1 year old. While pustular lesions may be present in both NCP and infantile acne, the presence of comedonal lesions distinguishes infantile acne from the pustular lesions of neonatal acne/ NCP [6].

51.3 Clinical Presentation

Neonatal acne typically presents with pustules and erythematous papules on the cheeks, chin, and forehead (see Fig. 51.1). Lesions less commonly affect the neck, chest, or scalp. Comedones may occasionally be present as well. Most cases are mild in severity and self-limited, resolving spontaneously within 3 months [2]. NCP patients may present predominantly with pustules and inflammatory papules, but characteristically lack comedones.

Infantile acne may begin in the neonatal period with the presence of comedones that persist as the child ages. Unlike in neonatal acne, patients with infantile acne tend to develop inflammatory lesions, including papules, pustules, and in some cases nodules or cysts [9]. While infantile acne typically resolves by the age of 1 year, it may rarely persist for several years [10]. Inflammatory disease can result in scarring if not appropriately treated. It also may be associated with the development of severe acne later in life during adolescence [6].

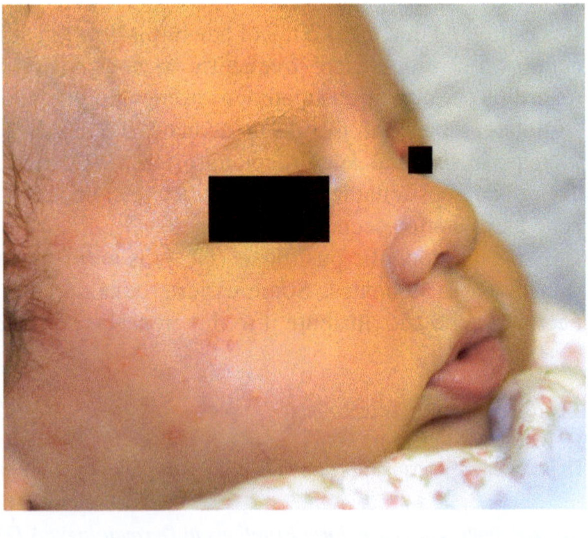

Fig. 51.1 Neonatal acne in a 1-month-old baby girl. Erythematous papules and pustules developed on the cheeks and chin (Photo credit: Joshua A. Zeichner, M.D.)

51.4 Workup

When evaluating a newborn with an acneiform eruption, all causes of a pustular eruption should be considered. Common conditions in the differential diagnosis seen in this population are erythema toxicum neonatorum, transient neonatal pustular melanosis, and miliaria. Less commonly, a bacterial, viral, or fungal infection may be present. Other dermatoses to be considered include keratosis pilaris, milia, molluscum contagiosum, sebaceous hyperplasia, or warts. Maternal medications such as lithium or corticosteroids might be causative. In most cases, laboratory evaluation is not necessary. Exceptions are cases in which the neonate demonstrates significant developmental abnormalities [6, 11].

In cases of suspected infantile acne, especially in those with inflammatory lesions, disorders associated with excess corticosteroids or androgens must be evaluated. These include congenital adrenal hyperplasia, a virilizing tumor, or another underlying endocrinopathy. High blood pressure, hand or foot growth, and development of secondary sex characteristics are all signs of an underlying disorder. In children with no signs of abnormalities other than acne, no further workup is needed [6, 11].

51.5 Treatment

Neonatal acne/NCP is a benign and self-limited condition that resolves within weeks without therapy. However, parents are often concerned and request treatment. In these cases, topical azole antifungals may be prescribed [12]. Some experts suggest ketoconazole 2 % cream twice daily for 1 week. If lesions persist past 1 month, the patient may in fact have early-onset infantile acne requiring treatment with topical retinoids, benzoyl peroxide, or topical antibiotics [6, 11].

First-line therapy for infantile acne is the use of topical medications. Combination therapy may be used as needed with topical retinoids and benzoyl peroxide, with or without topical antibiotics [6, 11]. In some moderate to severe cases, systemic medications may need to be added. Caution should be taken to avoid tetracycline class oral antibiotics in children under 8 years old, as they are associated with bone and tooth abnormalities [13]. Intralesional steroids may be administered and expert opinions report use oral isotretinoin in select severe patients [6, 11].

51.6 Conclusion

While most common in adolescence, acne can occur as early as the neonatal period. The lesions observed in newborns is most commonly associated with Malassezia yeast on the skin surface. However, true comedonal disease does occur. Therapy should be initiated based on clinical appearance and the parents' preferences.

References

1. Friedlander SF, Eichenfield LF, Fowler Jr JF, et al. Acne epidemiology and pathophysiology. Semin Cutan Med Surg. 2010;29:2–4.
2. Cantatore-Francis JL, Glick SA. Childhood acne: evaluation and management. Dermatol Ther. 2006;19:202–9.
3. Antoniou C, Dessinoti C, Stratigos A, Katsambas AD. Clinical and therapeutic approaches to childhood acne: an update. Pediatr Dermatol. 2009;26:373–80.
4. Bergman J, Eichenfield LF. Neonatal acne and cephalic pustulosis: is Malassezia the whole story? Arch Dermatol. 2002;138:255–7.
5. Rapelanoro R, Mortureux P, Couprie B, Malleville J, Taieb A. Neonatal *Malassezia furfur* pustulosis. Arch Dermatol. 1996;132:190–3.
6. Eichenfield LF, Baldwin HE, Friedlander SF, Mancini AJ, Yan AC. Pediatric acne management: optimizing outcomes. Semin Cutaneous Med Surg. 2011;30 Suppl 1:3S.
7. Bernier V, Weill FX, Hirigoyen V, et al. Skin colonization by Malassezia special in neonates: a prospective study and relationship with neonatal cephalic pustulosis. Arch Dermatol. 2002;138:215–8.
8. Ayhan M, Sancak B, Karaduman A, Arikan S, Sarhin S. Colonization of neonate skin by Malassezia species: relationship with neonatal cephalic pustulosis. J Am Acad Dermatol. 2007;57:1012–10128.
9. Tom WL, Friedlander SF. Acne through the ages: case-based observations through childhood and adolescence. Clin Pediatr (Phila). 2008;47:639–51.
10. Chew EW, Bingham A, Burrows D. Incidence of acne vulgaris in patients with infantile acne. Clin Exp Dermatol. 1990;15:376–7.
11. Krakowski AC, Eichenfield LF. Pediatric acne: clinical presentations, evaluation, and management. J Drugs of Dermatol. 2007;6(6):589–93.
12. Sancak B, Ayhan M, Karaduman A, Arikan S. In vitro activity of ketoconazole, itraconazole and terbinafine against Malassezia strains isolated from neonates. Microbiyol Bul. 2005;39: 301–8.
13. Gollnick H, Cunliffe W, Berson D, et al. Management of acne: a report from a Global Alliance to Improve Outcomes in Acne. J Am Acad Dermatol. 2003;49(1 Suppl):S1–37.

Chapter 52
Papular Granuloma Annulare

Rebecca Smith

52.1 Introduction

Granuloma annulare (GA) is a common benign dermatosis usually presenting as annular plaques composed of intradermal papules. Skin findings were first described by Fox in 1895 [1], and the designation "granuloma annulare" was introduced by Radcliff-Crocker in 1902 [2]. The eruption is generally asymptomatic and can spontaneously resolve. While the localized type is clinically most common, variants include disseminated, subcutaneous, and perforating lesions. Although clinically a ringed lesion is generally seen in the localized form of GA, the less common papular presentation of granuloma annular is not ringed and therefore could potentially mimic an acneiform eruption.

52.2 Background

The cause of GA is unknown although it has been reported to follow trauma [3], viral infections [4], tuberculin skin tests, malignancies [5], solar radiation, and insect bites [6]. It is hypothesized that a cell-mediated delayed-type hypersensitivity reaction to an unknown antigen is the inciting event. It has been postulated that the characteristic rings may form in response to a centralized insult that sets off an inflammatory chain reaction [7].

Granuloma annulare can occur at any age, but is most commonly diagnosed in children and young adults. Females are affected twice as commonly as males [8].

R. Smith, M.D. (✉)
Fort Mill Dermatology, LLC, 1700 First Baxter Crossing, Suite 101,
Fort Mill, SC 29708, USA

J.A. Zeichner (ed.), *Acneiform Eruptions in Dermatology: A Differential Diagnosis*,
DOI 10.1007/978-1-4614-8344-1_52,

The disseminated form is more common in adults [9]. The condition is usually seen in otherwise healthy patients but has occasionally been associated with diabetes or thyroid disease [10]. While the disease is usually sporadic, inherited cases have been described with an increased incidence of HLA-Bw35 in Israel [11], HLA-B8 in Denmark [12], and HLA-A29, B14, and B15 in Belfast [13]. The association with these particular phenotypes, however, may simply be population specific.

52.3 Clinical Presentation

GA presents with skin findings only. The most common form of GA is the localized type which presents as ringed, firm, and flesh-colored to slightly erythematous papules without scale or epidermal change (insert Fig. 52.1); the ringed papules can affect any skin surface, but is most commonly found on the extremities. The face and scalp are only rarely affected. The distribution of GA is approximately 60 % isolated to hands and arms, 20 % to legs and feet, and 7 % on both the upper and lower extremities. Fewer than 5 % of patients present with lesions on the trunk [14]. The rings vary in size and slowly expand reaching up to several centimeters in diameter with central clearing. Many patients have only a single ring, but multiple lesions are common. Over half of the patients with localized disease experience spontaneous resolution within 2 years. A papular umbilicated form of GA without perforation has been described in school age children on the dorsal hands and fingers [15].

Only rarely would papular GA be confused clinically with acne due to the difference in location and the lack of epidermal change. A localized papular eruption of GA on the chest or back could mimic an acneiform eruption, but the lack of comedones or pustules and the more monomorphous nature of GA would argue against acne. Papular GA would more often be in the differential diagnosis of arthropod assault reaction, secondary syphilis, xanthomas, or non-X-histiocytosis.

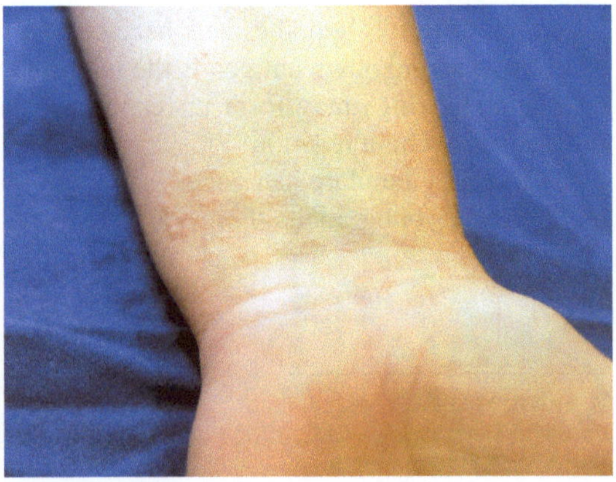

Fig. 52.1 Flesh-colored, occasionally pruritic papules without scale on the inner wrist (Photo credit: Joshua A. Zeichner, M.D.)

With papular GA, the diagnosis is often difficult due to the lack of the more typical annular plaques.

The differential diagnosis for classic GA includes annular lichen planus and tinea corporis. Often children have been unsuccessfully treated for tinea before presenting to a dermatologist for definitive diagnosis. A potassium hydroxide preparation, the lack of scale, and/or a confirmatory biopsy can differentiate these entities.

Generalized or disseminated GA consists of hundreds to thousands of individual, small papules that may form small annular plaques, are usually symmetrical, and can coalesce into reticulated, circinate, or linear patterns [10]. Unlike other forms of GA, the trunk is usually involved with a propensity for the neck, forearms, legs, and extensor elbows. This form may exhibit a slightly more violaceous color. It is unusual to see involvement of the face, palms, soles, or mucous membranes [9].

Subcutaneous GA is a variant generally seen in young children with large, asymptomatic, skin colored, rapidly enlarging deep dermal or subcutaneous nodules [16]. They may be solitary or multiple and have a predilection for pretibial skin, palms, soles, buttocks, fingers, toes, and periorbital areas. The skin overlying the lesions can ulcerate and often these nodules spontaneously regress. Deep GA can clinically resemble rheumatoid nodules, deep granulomatous infections, and subcutaneous sarcoid.

Perforating GA is a more rare form consisting of asymptomatic, superficial small-grouped papules with central umbilicated ulcerations and scale crust. These occur most frequently on the dorsal hands and fingers [17]. Differential diagnosis of perforating GA includes perforating collagenosis, Kyrle disease, and elastosis perforans serpiginosa.

52.4 Workup

Patients with GA are generally healthy and laboratory tests are usually normal and not recommended. The disseminated form may be seen more commonly in immunocompromised patients such as those with human immunodeficiency virus and lymphomas. Such patients may also have GA in atypical locations.

Often, the diagnosis can be made clinically, but a confirmatory punch biopsy can be helpful especially with the less common variants. Histologically, GA is a granulomatous dermatitis exhibiting focal degeneration of collagen and elastin fibers, mucin deposition, and a perivascular and interstitial lymphohistiocytic infiltrate in the upper and mid-dermis [18]. It is the increased mucin that is the hallmark of GA [19]. If not readily apparent on routine stains, using colloidal iron or Alcian blue to highlight mucin can be helpful. Palisaded granuloma with central connective tissue degeneration surrounded by histiocytes and lymphocytes is a common pattern seen microscopically. Often, the pattern is more infiltrative or interstitial with scattered histiocytes infiltrating between collagen fibers. In perforating GA there is transepidermal elimination of the degenerating collagen bundles.

52.5 Treatment

GA is rarely symptomatic, and due to the benign and often self-limited nature, clinical observation and reassurance are often the treatment of choice. While lesions can have a chronic relapsing course, they usually persist for only 1–4 years, and 73 % of all lesions disappear within 2 years. Cosmetic disfigurement can prompt the need for intervention and many modalities have been utilized. First-line therapies include topical steroids with or without occlusion or intralesional injections of triamcinolone. Complete involution of the entire lesion has been reported to follow biopsy. Other treatment modalities include cryosurgery [20], topical calcineurin inhibitors, PUVA [21], and CO_2 laser [22].

In general, systemic agents are reserved for more severe generalized cases. GA has been treated with short-term oral corticosteroids, chlorpropamide, pentoxifylline [23], nicotinamide, niacinamide [24], isotretinoin [25], etretinate [26], salicylates, potassium iodide, vitamin E, fumaric acid esters, antimalarials [27], dapsone [28], cyclosporine [29], and infliximab. Spontaneous resolution of the disease makes evaluation of the efficacy of such treatments more difficult. No large, randomized placebo-controlled double-blind studies have been performed.

52.6 Conclusion

The papular form of GA may mimic acne vulgaris in some cases. The lack of comedones and pustules and the monomorphic papular appearance of this rash clinically distinguish it from acne. While self-limited in most cases, lesions can persist for months to years, so therapies are targeted towards symptomatic relief and the unsightly appearance.

References

1. Colcott Fox T. Ringed eruption of the fingers. Br J Dermatol. 1895;7:91.
2. Radcliffe-Crocker H. Granuloma annulare. Br J Dermatol. 1902;14:1–9.
3. Mills A, Chetty R. Auricular granuloma annulare. A consequence of trauma? Am J Dermatopathol. 1992;14:431–3.
4. Spencer SA, Fenske NA, Espinoza CG, Hamill JR, Cohen LE, Espinoza LR. Granuloma annulare-like eruption due to chronic Epstein-Barr virus infection. Arch Dermatol. 1988;124:250–5.
5. Barksdale SK, Perniciaro C, Halling KC, et al. Granuloma annulare in patients with malignant lymphoma: clinicopathologic study of 13 new cases. J Am Acad Dermatol. 1994;31:42–8.
6. Moyer DG. Papular granuloma annulare. Arch Dermatol. 1964;89:41–5.
7. Dahl MV. Is actinic granuloma really granuloma annulare? Arch Dermatol. 1986;122:39–40.
8. Wells RS, Smith MA. The natural history of granuloma annulare. Br J Dermatol. 1963; 75:199–205.
9. Muhlbauer JE. Granuloma annulare. J Am Acad Dermatol. 1980;3:217–30.

10. Dabski K, Winkelmann RK. Generalized granuloma annulare: clinical and laboratory findings in 100 patients. J Am Acad Dermatol. 1989;20:39–47.
11. Friedman-Birnbaum R, Gideoni O, Bergman R, Pollack S. A study of HLA antigen association in localized and generalized granuloma annulare. Br J Dermatol. 1986;115:329–33.
12. Andersen BL, Verdich J. Granuloma annulare and diabetes mellitus. Clin Exp Dermatol. 1979;4:31–7.
13. Middleton D, Allen GE. HLA antigen frequency in granuloma annulare. Br J Dermatol. 1984;110:57–9.
14. Cronquist SD, Stashower ME, Benson PM. Deep dermal granuloma annulare presenting as an eyelid tumor in a child, with review of pediatric eyelid lesions. Pediatr Dermatol. 1999;16:377–80.
15. Lucky AW, Prose NS, Bove K, White WL, Jorizzo JL. Papular umbilicated granuloma annulare. Arch Dermatol. 1992;128:1375–8.
16. Felner EI, Steinberg JB, Weinberg AG. Subcutaneous granuloma annulare: a review of 47 cases. Pediatrics. 1997;100:965–7.
17. Shimizu H, Harada T, Baba E, Kuramochi M. Perforating granuloma annulare. Int J Dermatol. 1985;24:581–3.
18. Elder D, Elenitsas R, Jaworsky C, Johnson B. Lever's Histopathology of the skin. 8th ed. Philadelphia, PA: Lippincott-Raven Publishers; 1997.
19. Dabski K, Winkelmann RK. Generalized granuloma annulare: histopathology and immunopathology. Systematic review of 100 cases and comparison with localized granuloma annulare. J Am Acad Dermatol. 1989;20:28–39.
20. Blume-Peytavi U, Zouboulis CC, Jacobi H, Scholz A, Bisson S, Orfanos CE. Successful outcome of cryosurgery in patients with granuloma annulare. Br J Dermatol. 1994;130: 494–7.
21. Hindson TC, Spiro JG, Cochrane H. PUVA therapy of diffuse granuloma annulare. Clin Exp Dermatol. 1988;13:26–7.
22. Rouilleault PH. CO_2 laser and granuloma annulare. J Dermatol Surg Oncol. 1988;14:120.
23. Rubel DM, Wood G, Rosen R, Jopp-McKay A. Generalised granuloma annulare successfully treated with pentoxifylline. Australas J Dermatol. 1993;34:103–8.
24. Ma A, Medenica M. Response of generalized granuloma annulare to high-dose niacinamide. Arch Dermatol. 1983;119:836–9.
25. Ratnavel RC, Norris PG. Perforating granuloma annulare: response to treatment with isotretinoin. J Am Acad Dermatol. 1995;32:126–7.
26. Botella-Estrada R, Guillen C, Sanmartin O, Aliaga A. Disseminated granuloma annulare: resolution with etretinate therapy. J Am Acad Dermatol. 1992;26:777–8.
27. Simon Jr M, von den Driesch P. Antimalarials for control of disseminated granuloma annulare in children. J Am Acad Dermatol. 1994;31:1064–5.
28. Steiner A, Pehamberger H, Wolff K. Sulfone treatment of granuloma annulare. J Am Acad Dermatol. 1985;13:1004–8.
29. Fiallo P. Cyclosporin for the treatment of granuloma annulare. Br J Dermatol. 1998;138: 369–70.

Chapter 53
Precocious Puberty and Acne

Maria Miyar and Moise L. Levy

53.1 Introduction

Precocious puberty is defined as the onset of breast or pubic hair development before age 8 in girls and the onset of testicular development of more than 3 ml before age 9 in boys. The age limit is based on the data from a 1969 study done by Marshall and Tanner [1]. There is evidence to show that normal puberty in the USA and Europe is occurring earlier in children [2, 3]. A 2012 study suggested that puberty in boys might be occurring 6 months to 2 years earlier than documented in the previous Marshall and Tanner study [4]. In 1999 the Pediatric Endocrine Society proposed lowering the age limit for precocious puberty to be less than 7 years old in white girls and less than 6 years old in African-American girls [5]. Some argue that if the age limit of normal puberty is lowered, children between the ages of 6 and 8 with precocious puberty will be missed, resulting in a loss of height potential [6]. This chapter will describe precocious puberty as it relates to acne and address when an evaluation and treatment for precocious puberty should be undertaken when a young child presents with acne.

M. Miyar, M.D.
Department of Dermatology, UT Southwestern, Austin, TX, USA

M.L. Levy, M.D. (✉)
Department of Pediatric Dermatology, Dell Children's Medical Center, 4900 Mueller Blvd., Austin, TX 78723, USA
e-mail: mlevy@sfcasustin.com

J.A. Zeichner (ed.), *Acneiform Eruptions in Dermatology: A Differential Diagnosis*, DOI 10.1007/978-1-4614-8344-1_53, © Springer Science+Business Media New York 2014

53.2 Background

Precocious puberty is centrally mediated in approximately 90 % of cases through activation of the hypothalamic-pituitary-gonadal (HPG) axis [7]. It occurs more often in girls and it is usually attributed to a sporadic cause. In males, however, it is attributed to a central nervous system abnormality in 75 % of cases. Peripheral or precocious pseudopuberty, a much less common form of precocious puberty, occurs when hormones that initiate puberty are produced from a gonadotropin-independent source or a peripheral source. There is no activation of the HPG axis in peripheral precocious puberty but some secondary sex characteristics appear. Examples of peripheral precocious puberty in females include ovarian tumors, autonomously functioning ovarian cysts, feminizing adrenal tumors, McCune-Albright syndrome, and exogenous sources of estrogens. Examples in males include congenital adrenal hyperplasia (CAH), adrenal tumors, Leydig cell tumors, chorionic gonadotropin-producing tumors, and familial male precocious puberty. Sometimes peripheral precocious puberty can activate the HPG axis, and this is known as a mixed type of precocious puberty and occurs in McCune-Albright syndrome, CAH, and familial male-limited precocious puberty. A person with precocious puberty normally exhibits the sequences of normal puberty with sexual development beginning at an earlier age than normal [8].

Acne may be the presenting sign of the onset of puberty in children associated with the onset of adrenarche. In girls this may precede breast or pubic hair development [9]. The increase of androgenetic steroids such as dehydroepiandrosterone sulfate (DHEA-S) stimulates sebum production [10, 11] and plays a role in contributing to the retention hyperkeratosis central to the pathogenesis of acne [12]. The prevalence and severity of acne often increases as pubertal maturation occurs [13].

There is normally little androgen production in children between the ages of 1–7 years old [14]. So children presenting to the office with acne at younger ages should be evaluated for hyperandrogenism [15]. Potential causes include premature adrenarche, mild forms of congenital adrenal hyperplasia, gonadal or adrenal tumors, Cushing's syndrome, and true precocious puberty as described above [12]. Premature adrenarche is an incomplete form of precocious puberty, with evidence of early development of pubic and or axillary hair without breast development in girls or testicular development in boys [8].

53.3 Clinical Presentation

The presence of acne in a child between 1 and 7 years old is unusual and raises a concern for precocious puberty or hyperandrogenemia [16, 17]. Severe or recalcitrant acne are especially suspicious [17, 18]. These patients usually present with comedones on the central face, including the mid-forehead, nose, and chin (Fig. 53.1). Comedones in the concha of the ear are also suspicious (Fig. 53.2).

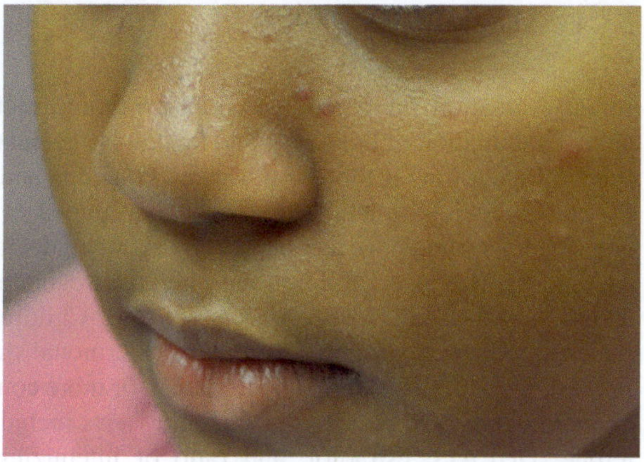

Fig. 53.1 Comedones on the nose of a 6-year-old girl. In addition, she had scattered inflammatory papules on the cheeks (Photo credit: Joshua A. Zeichner, M.D.)

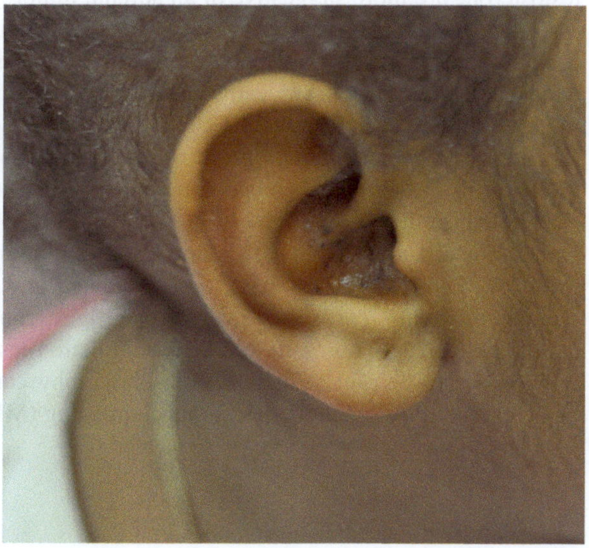

Fig. 53.2 Open comedones on the conchal bowl of the ear (Photo credit: Joshua A. Zeichner, M.D.)

Inflammatory lesions may be present as well [9]. The child should be examined for signs of advanced pubertal development, such as axillary or pubic hair development and breast development in girls or testicular development in boys. Other signs of precocious puberty include advanced osseous maturation and a high height and weight for age [8]. The increased rate of bone maturation can result in premature epiphyseal closure translating to a shorter adult stature. Approximately 30 % of girls and an even higher percentage of boys with precocious puberty grow to less than the 5th percentile of height as adults [2, 8]. While cognitive development is normal, these children may have emotional and behavioral issues [8].

53.4 Workup

Initial evaluation for precocious puberty should include a review of the growth chart, examination of bone age, and laboratory evaluations. Bone age measurement can help determine if there is advanced bone age and is considered by some to be the best screening evaluation for precocious puberty [16–19]. Children with precocious puberty often have a bone age 2–3 standard deviations above their chronological age [8]. Moreover, children with high androgen levels have accelerated growth across standardized growth percentiles [19]. Children with suspected precocious puberty or hyperandrogenism require a hormonal evaluation, which can be performed by the dermatologist, pediatrician, or more commonly, referral to a pediatric endocrinologist [20, 21]. Initial screening tests include serum free and total testosterone, DHEA-S, estradiol, and ratio of luteinizing hormone (LH) to follicle-stimulating hormone (FSH) [19]. Moderate elevation of DHEA-S is suggestive of an adrenal pathology (e.g., CAH), while extremely high levels of DHEA-S and/or testosterone are more suggestive of an adrenal tumor [22].

Concentrations of sex hormones may be used to help stage puberty. In both early normal puberty and the early phase of sexual precocity, serum estradiol is low or undetectable in girls. Serum testosterone levels are detectable or slightly elevated at the time of diagnosis in boys. LH levels are also elevated in children with central sexual precocity. The gonadotropin-releasing hormone (GnRH) stimulation test is also helpful in diagnosing precocious puberty. The test shows whether there is a predominance of LH over FSH [23]. Females with poor LH response in the GnRH stimulation test may also have a leuprolide stimulation test to evaluate for estradiol levels [8]. Other laboratory tests to be evaluated in working up hyperandrogenism include prolactin, cortisol, 17α-hydroxyprogesterone, androstenedione, and an adrenocorticotropic hormone (ACTH) stimulation test [16–18, 22]. Imaging technology is also helpful as pelvic ultrasonography can detect ovarian and uterine enlargement in girls. Magnetic resonance imaging (MRI) of the brain is indicated if true central precocious puberty is suspected [2].

53.5 Treatment

Acne treatment in a child with precocious puberty depends on severity of the acne. In general, mild cases of comedonal acne can be treated with topical retinoids like tretinoin or adapalene. Combination therapy is usually most successful using comedolytic agent like a retinoid along with topical benzoyl peroxide or salicylic acid [17]. Mild inflammatory lesions can be treated with topical benzoyl peroxide and/or topical antibiotics like clindamycin or erythromycin [19]. Fixed-dose combination products containing more than one active ingredient in one product are good options for children, as only one product needs to be used. For more severe or recalcitrant disease, oral antibiotics or oral retinoids may be needed. However, tetracyclines should not be used in children younger than 8 years old due to the potential damage to the developing bones and teeth [24]. If antibiotics are to be used in children less than 8 years old, erythromycin and trimethoprim/sulfamethoxazole are treatment options [18].

If a patient is suspected of precocious puberty, early involvement of a pediatric endocrinologist is advised. While acne may be managed by dermatologists, current hormonal therapies that may be prescribed by endocrinologists include GnRH agonists and growth hormone (GH). Treatment with GnRH agonists such as leuprolide helps prevent early fusion of the epiphyseal plates to avoid unnecessary short stature [25].

References

1. Marshall WA, Tanner JM. Variations in pattern of pubertal changes in girls. Arch Dis Child. 1969;44(235):291–303.
2. Sørensen K, Mouritsen A, Aksglaede L, Hagen CP, Mogensen SS, Juul A. Recent secular trends in pubertal timing: implications for evaluation and diagnosis of precocious puberty. Horm Res Paediatr. 2012;77(3):137–45.
3. Biro FM, Galvez MP, Greenspan LC, Succop PA, Vangeepuram N, Pinney SM, et al. Pubertal assessment method and baseline characteristics in a mixed longitudinal study of girls. Pediatrics. 2010;126(3):e583–90.
4. Herman-Giddens ME, Steffes J, Harris D, Slora E, Hussey M, Dowshen SA, et al. Secondary sexual characteristics in boys: data from the Pediatric Research in Office Settings Network. Pediatrics. 2012;130(5):e1058–68.
5. Kaplowitz PB, Oberfield SE. Reexamination of the age limit for defining when puberty is precocious in girls in the United States: implications for evaluation and treatment. Drug and Therapeutics and Executive Committees of the Lawson Wilkins Pediatric Endocrine Society. Pediatrics. 1999;104(4 Pt 1):936–41.
6. Midyett LK, Moore WV, Jacobson JD. Are pubertal changes in girls before age 8 benign? Pediatrics. 2003;111(1):47–51.
7. Cisternino M, Arrigo T, Pasquino AM, Tinelli C, Antoniazzi F, Beduschi L, et al. Etiology and age incidence of precocious puberty in girls: a multicentric study. J Pediatr Endocrinol Metab. 2000;13 Suppl 1:695–701.
8. Kliegman RM. Nelson textbook of pediatrics. 19th ed. Philadelphia, PA: Elsevier/Saunders; 2011.
9. Lucky AW, Biro FM, Huster GA, Leach AD, Morrison JA, Ratterman J. Acne vulgaris in premenarchal girls. An early sign of puberty associated with rising levels of dehydroepiandrosterone. Arch Dermatol. 1994;130(3):308–14.
10. Pochi PE, Strauss JS, Downing DT. Skin surface lipid composition, acne, pubertal development, and urinary excretion of testosterone and 17-ketosteroids in children. J Invest Dermatol. 1977;69(5):485–9.
11. Lucky AW, Biro FM, Simbartl LA, Morrison JA, Sorg NW. Predictors of severity of acne vulgaris in young adolescent girls: results of a five-year longitudinal study. J Pediatr. 1997;130(1):30–9.
12. Mancini AJ, Baldwin HE, Eichenfield LF, Friedlander SF, Yan AC. Acne life cycle: the spectrum of pediatric disease. Semin Cutan Med Surg. 2011;30(3 Suppl):S2–5.
13. Lucky AW, Biro FM, Huster GA, Morrison JA, Elder N. Acne vulgaris in early adolescent boys. Correlations with pubertal maturation and age. Arch Dermatol. 1991;127(2):210–6.

14. Reiter EO, Fuldauer VG, Root AW. Secretion of the adrenal androgen, dehydroepiandrosterone sulfate, during normal infancy, childhood, and adolescence, in sick infants, and in children with endocrinologic abnormalities. J Pediatr. 1977;90(5):766–70.
15. Goldberg JL, Dabade TS, Davis SA, Feldman SR, Krowchuk DP, Fleischer AB. Changing age of acne vulgaris visits: another sign of earlier puberty? Pediatr Dermatol. 2011;28(6):645–8.
16. Paller AS, Mancini AJ. Hurwitz clinical pediatric dermatology. 4th ed. Edinburgh, NY: Elsevier Saunders; 2011.
17. Cantatore-Francis JL, Glick SA. Childhood acne: evaluation and management. Dermatol Ther. 2006;19(4):202–9.
18. Antoniou C, Dessinioti C, Stratigos AJ, Katsambas AD. Clinical and therapeutic approach to childhood acne: an update. Pediatr Dermatol. 2009;26(4):373–80.
19. Lucky AW. A review of infantile and pediatric acne. Dermatology (Basel). 1998; 196(1):95–7.
20. De Raeve L, De Schepper J, Smitz J. Prepubertal acne: a cutaneous marker of androgen excess? J Am Acad Dermatol. 1995;32(2 Pt 1):181–4.
21. Eichenfield LF, Fowler Jr JF, Friedlander SF, Levy ML, Webster GF. Diagnosis and evaluation of acne. Semin Cutan Med Surg. 2010;29(2 Suppl 1):5–8.
22. Lucky AW. Hormonal correlates of acne and hirsutism. Am J Med. 1995;98(1A):89S–94S.
23. Iughetti L, Predieri B, Ferrari M, Gallo C, Livio L, Milioli S, et al. Diagnosis of central precocious puberty: endocrine assessment. J Pediatr Endocrinol Metab. 2000;13 Suppl 1:709–15.
24. Ray WA, Federspiel CF, Schaffner W. Prescribing of tetracycline to children less than 8 years old. A two-year epidemiologic study among ambulatory Tennessee medicaid recipients. JAMA. 1977;237(19):2069–74.
25. Appelbaum H, Malhotra S. A comprehensive approach to the spectrum of abnormal pubertal development. Adolesc Med State Art Rev. 2012;23(1):1–14.

Part VII
Drug-Induced Acneiform Eruptions

Chapter 54
Drug-Induced Acneiform Eruptions

Ha K. Do, Navid Ezra, and Stephen E. Wolverton

54.1 Introduction

Acne vulgaris is a polymorphic inflammatory skin disease, clinically characterized by mixture of comedones, superficial and deep inflamed papules, pustules, and nodules. It is a chronic inflammation of the pilosebaceous unit. Acneiform drug eruptions are a monomorphic inflammatory skin disease lacking comedones with lesions typically in the same stage. This type of drug eruption has an abrupt onset and is often associated with various medications (Table 54.1). The pathogenesis of acneiform drug eruptions is poorly understood; documented evidence when available will be presented under the specific drug categories in this chapter.

54.2 Drugs Associated with Acneiform Eruption

54.2.1 Hormones

54.2.1.1 Corticosteroids

Systemic corticosteroids causing acneiform eruption were first reported in 1950s [1]. Exposure to high levels of systemic (oral [2] or intravenous [3]), topical [4, 5], and inhaled [6–8] corticosteroids can induce or exacerbate acne. Perioral (periorificial)

H.K. Do, M.D. • N. Ezra, M.D. • S.E. Wolverton, M.D. (✉)
Department of Dermatology, Indiana University School of Medicine,
New York, NY, USA
e-mail: hado@iupui.edu; nezra@iupui.edu; swolvert@iu.edu

J.A. Zeichner (ed.), *Acneiform Eruptions in Dermatology: A Differential Diagnosis*,
DOI 10.1007/978-1-4614-8344-1_54,

Table 54.1 Drugs involved with acneiform eruption

Hormones
Oral, inhaled, and topical corticosteroids
Anabolic steroids and androgens
Danazol
Hormonal contraceptives (levonorgestrel)
Neuropsychotropic agents
Tricyclic antidepressants
Amineptine
Maprotiline
Imipramine
Lithium
Antiepileptics
Hydantoin (phenytoin)
Lamotrigine
Valproate
Antipsychotics
Aripiprazole
Targeted therapies
Epidermal growth factor receptor inhibitors (EGFR inhibitors)
Erlotinib
Gefitinib
Imatinib
Epidermal growth factor receptor monoclonal antibodies
Cetuximab
Panitumumab
TNF-α inhibitors
Infliximab
Lenalidomide
G-CSF
Vemurafenib
Retinoids
Etretinate
Cardiac medication
Propranolol
Quinidine
Immunosuppressive agents
Sirolimus
Tacrolimus
Cyclosporine
Azathioprine
Antituberculosis drugs
Isoniazid
Rifampicin
Thiacetazone
Other medications
Gold

(continued)

Table 54.1 (continued)

Dactinomycin
Dapsone
Halogens
Bromides
Dioxin
Iodides
Vitamins
Vitamin B6 and B12
White petrolatum
Cow udder ointment
Tetraethylthiuram disulfide
Dantrolene
PUVA

dermatitis is an example of a corticosteroid-induced eruption around the mouth [9] that is often associated with high-potency (class I and II) corticosteroid usage. These lesions might lack the erythema due to the anti-inflammatory effect of the topical corticosteroid [10]. However, when the topical agent is discontinued, an exuberant flare can occur. The acneiform eruptions have a variable onset after a new drug introduction, usually 2–4 weeks, but can take up to several months [11, 12]. Most lesions clinically present as small, similar-appearing skin colored to pink and red dome-shaped inflamed papules and pustules, lacking comedones, distributed on seborrheic areas on face and trunk, and potentially involve the shoulders. A full discussion of perioral dermatitis is found in a separate chapter of this book.

Some studies have shown topical corticosteroids lead to increased free fatty acids in skin surface lipids with resultant increased numbers of bacteria within the pilosebaceous unit [13, 14]. The breakdown of free fatty acid by *P. acnes*, consequently, leads to the development of inflammatory papules. Toll-like receptor (TLR), particularly TLR-2 subtype, has been linked to the pathogenesis of acne vulgaris. Activated TLR-2, which is stimulated by *P. acnes,* contributes to the inflammation seen acne vulgaris. It has been shown that cultured human keratinocytes will increase TLR-2 gene expression [15] when corticosteroids are added, which is further stimulated by *P. acnes,* tumor necrosis factor-α (TNF-α), and interleukin 1-α. These findings suggest that corticosteroids have the potential to exacerbate acne vulgaris and to cause drug-induced acneiform eruptions.

54.2.1.2 Androgens and Anabolic Steroids

In adolescent acne, androgens are known to increase sebum production by acting on sebocytes to proliferate and differentiate. Likewise, anabolic steroids or other synthetic hormones with androgenic activity will have similar effects on sebaceous glands [16, 17]. In a Norwegian prospective study, pubertal boys who were treated with injectable testosterone for premature closure of epiphyseal growth zones had an increased acne incidence [18]. There is also an increase in acne incidence in young athletes who take anabolic-androgenic steroid to increase muscle mass ("body builder acne" or "doping acne") [19–21].

54.2.1.3 Danazol

Danazol is a derivative of 2,3-isoxazole-17b-ethinyltestosterone. It has an antigonadotropic property by decreasing the production of follicle-stimulating hormone (FSH) and luteinizing hormone (LH). Consequently, danazol is often used to treat endometriosis, sexual precocity, and hereditary angioedema. An acute eruption of nodulocystic acne was reported in a female patient who was on danazol for treatment of endometriosis [22].

54.2.1.4 Hormonal Contraceptives

Hormonal contraceptives containing progestogens with androgenic activity or low-dose estrogens can cause or exacerbate acne. New onset of acne after placement of levonorgestrel-releasing intrauterine device can also occur [23, 24]. These patients developed inflammatory papules along the jaws 1–3 months after device insertion.

54.2.2 Neuropsychotropic Agents

54.2.2.1 Tricyclic Antidepressants

Amineptine is a non-halogenated tricyclic antidepressant that was widely used in France before its withdrawal from the market in 1999 [25–27]. This drug may induce florid acneiform eruption consisting of monomorphic noninflammatory papules and micro- and macrocysts. These lesions were located mainly on the face, auricles, neck, chest, back, and genitalia. It is rare, but other tricyclic antidepressants, such as maprotiline [28] and imipramine, can occasionally have been known to trigger acneiform eruption.

54.2.2.2 Lithium

The first few cases linking lithium to causing acneiform eruption appeared in the early 1970s [29–31]. Lithium triggers neutrophilic cutaneous conditions such as neutrophilic folliculitis, acneiform, and psoriasiform eruptions [32–34]. Acne induced by lithium occurs more frequently in males and patients with an allergic (atopic) history. Inflammatory papules and pustules are distributed on face, axillae, groin, arms, and buttocks. There is no direct correlation between lithium dose and acne appearance or severity. However, high level of lithium can be detected in the affected areas.

54.2.2.3 Antiepileptics

Various antiepileptic agents have been linked to drug-induced acneiform eruption [35]. Hydantoin [36] (i.e., phenytoin) and phenobarbital are the two most common culprits followed by lamotrigine [37] and valproate [38]. In 1980, a case of severe facial neonatal acne in an infant who had "fetal hydantoin syndrome" was reported [39]. Phenytoin can cross the placenta and is known to cause several skin manifestation ranging from acneiform eruption to hypertrichosis on extensor surface of extremities and gingival hyperplasia [40]. The acne improves when the treatment was stopped.

54.2.2.4 Antipsychotic Agents

Aripiprazole is an atypical quinolinone antipsychotic agent with antidepressant properties. It is a partial agonist at the dopamine$_2$ and 5-HT$_{1A}$ receptors but an antagonist at the 5-HT$_{2A}$ receptors. Common adverse effects include insomnia, internal restlessness (akathisia), nausea, and vomiting. Acneiform eruptions have been reported to occur 10 days after initiating the medication and improve within 10 days after discontinuing it [41].

54.2.3 Targeted Therapies

Acneiform eruptions are becoming a hallmark side effect for several therapies that target a specific key molecule involved in the pathophysiology of the disease. This therapeutic group of targeted therapies includes epidermal growth factor receptor (EGFR) inhibitors (gefitinib [42], erlotinib [43, 44], and imatinib [45]), EGFR monoclonal antibodies (i.e., cetuximab [46, 47] and panitumumab [48]), TNF receptor inhibitors [49] (i.e., infliximab and lenalidomide), and BRAF-V600E inhibitors.

54.2.3.1 EGFR Inhibitors

EGFRs belong to the tyrosine kinase family and are thought to play a crucial role in the development and progression of cancer. Several solid tumors of the head and neck, breast, lungs, ovary, prostate, and colon overexpress EGFRs. Consequently, EGFR inhibitors are used to treat these cancers.

Acneiform eruptions have quickly become the hallmark cutaneous adverse effects in patients receiving targeted EGFR inhibitor chemotherapy [50, 51]. Acneiform eruptions occur in 66 % of patients receiving gefitinib, in 75 % of patients receiving erlotinib, and in 86 % of patients receiving cetuximab during clinical trials. Patients with past history of adolescent acne or folliculitis are more prone to have acneiform development. Lesions can occur after the first cycle of treatment but more often occur between the third and fourth week. Worsening of acneiform lesions can be observed immediately after each cycle of treatment. The typical EGFR-induced acneiform eruption consists of inflamed papules and pustules distributed in seborrheic areas on the scalp, face, retroauricular skin, upper trunk, and shoulders. Comedones are lacking. Pruritus can accompany the rash.

Crusted or hemorrhagic lesions, along with Sweet syndrome-like lesions, have been reported in more severe forms [52]. A few studies have reported that acneiform lesion development is a prognostic factor for a good response to the treatment with longer survival time compared to no acneiform development [53, 54]. A severe cutaneous adverse effect, however, can require cessation of EGFR inhibitor therapy. Incidence and severity of acneiform eruption appear to be dose dependent. Tetracyclines (such as doxycycline or minocycline) can be used to control severe lesions but do not decrease the incidence of acneiform eruption.

Histologically, EGFR inhibitor-induced acneiform lesions display neutrophilic folliculitis and perifolliculitis. *P. acnes* has not been found in the affected hair follicles. The exact pathogenesis of EFGR inhibitor-induced acne still needs further elucidation. EGFRs are expressed in epidermal keratinocytes, sebocytes, and the hair follicle outer root sheath. In addition, EGFRs are involved in normal cell growth and differentiation. p27 is a cell cycle inhibitor that normally prevents progression from G1 to S phase in the cell cycle. EGFR inhibitors appear to unregulate the inhibitory effect of p27 and allow hyper-proliferation of the stratum corneum in follicular infundibulum and abnormal desquamation and, consequently, lead to the follicular plugging [55]. It is also possible for monoclonal antibodies to activate the inflammatory cascades by activating neutrophils and complements through the binding of their Fc domains.

54.2.3.2 TNF Inhibitors

Tumor necrosis factor (TNF) inhibitors are used to treat a wide range of autoimmune diseases such as inflammatory bowel disease, rheumatoid arthritis, psoriasis and psoriatic arthritis, and ankylosing spondylitis. Of the TNF inhibitors, infliximab is the most reported agent associated with an acneiform eruption [56]. Likewise, lenalidomide, a second generation of thalidomide, has major TNF inhibitory activity. Lenalidomide-induced acute acneiform eruption in a multiple myeloma patient has been reported [57]. The acneiform eruption was cleared with oral doxycycline 100 mg daily after 3 months without stopping lenalidomide therapy.

54.2.3.3 G-CSF

Granulocyte colony-stimulating factor (G-CSF) is a potent stimulator for bone marrow to produce neutrophils. There is a case report of worsening of preexisting acne vulgaris in an adolescent male while receiving chemotherapy and G-CSF for treatment of mixed germ cell testicular tumor [58].

54.2.3.4 Vemurafenib

Vemurafenib, a BRAF (V600E) inhibitor, was FDA approved in January 2012 for the treatment of advanced metastatic melanoma. Among the most common cutaneous adverse effects associated with vemurafenib are verrucous papillomas and hand-foot syndrome, along with keratoacanthomas and squamous cell carcinomas. More recently, a case report of acneiform eruption associated with vemurafenib has been published [59].

54.2.4 Retinoids

In the late 1980s, several case reports appeared in the medical literature linking acneiform eruption with oral etretinate [60, 61]. These patients developed acute onset of severe cystic acne within the first few weeks after the initiation of oral etretinate for psoriasis treatment. The acneiform eruption gradually improved when etretinate was discontinued and with using topical erythromycin or oral tetracyclines. Etretinate is no longer available in the United States.

54.2.5 Cardiac Medications

An acneiform eruption has been reported in a young adult who started propranolol for migraine prophylaxis [62]. The lesions completely resolved after propranolol was discontinued. These lesions recurred within 3 weeks when the patient was started on nadolol for migraine prophylaxis. Facial acne resolved soon after nadolol was discontinued. In general, cutaneous adverse effects from beta-blockers class are rare. The exact pathogenesis linking acneiform eruptions with beta-blockers is still unclear.

In 1981, the case of a 57-year-old man who develop papulopustules on the chest and back soon after initiating quinidine for treatment of premature ventricular contractions was reported [63]. The acneiform eruption responded well to topical erythromycin lotion and topical benzoyl peroxide.

54.2.6 Immunosuppressive Agents

54.2.6.1 Sirolimus

Sirolimus, an immunosuppressive drug often used after organ transplantation, has been associated with acneiform eruptions in several instances [64–67]. The most commonly observed cutaneous adverse effects of sirolimus include alterations of the pilosebaceous apparatus, chronic edema, angioedema, and mucous membrane disorders [68, 69]. Lesions primarily involve the sebaceous regions; however, lesions often extend to the forearms, inner surface of the arms, cervical area, and scalp [70, 71]. Sirolimus is thought to have a direct toxic effect on follicles, chemically modify sebum, and alter EGF and testosterone synthesis [70]. Sirolimus inhibits EGF action by inhibiting the mTOR pathway [69]. Testosterone upregulates EGFR synthesis, and sirolimus downregulates testosterone synthesis. Sirolimus might induce acneiform lesions predominantly in men because of the downregulation of the EGFR by testosterone suppression [70].

54.2.6.2 Tacrolimus

Tacrolimus is a macrolide derivative which blocks the calcineurin-dependent signal transduction pathway resulting in T-cell-specific immunosuppressive activity. Topical tacrolimus is primarily used for treatment of atopic dermatitis but has also been used to treat other inflammatory and immunologic skin disorders, including vitiligo. A case of focal acne was reported during topical tacrolimus therapy for vitiligo [72]. Rosacea-like dermatitis has also been reported during treatment of facial inflammatory dermatoses with tacrolimus ointment [73]. A similar rosaceiform eruption has been reported with use of pimecrolimus [74].

54.2.6.3 Cyclosporine

Cyclosporine (CsA) is a potent immunosuppressive agent used after organ transplantation and in the treatment of psoriasis and atopic dermatitis. There have been reports of cyclosporine-associated acneiform eruptions presenting as severe nodulocystic acne and acne keloidalis nuchae [75, 76]. Highly lipophilic, one of the possible routes of elimination of CsA may be via the sebaceous gland, which is the major cutaneous site for the elimination of lipids through sebum. Potentially, CsA may modify the structure, function, and/or integrity of the pilosebaceous follicle, thereby inducing an acneiform eruption [77].

54.2.6.4 Azathioprine

Azathioprine is a thiopurine analogue that suppresses the immune system by a wide variety of mechanisms. It is changed in the liver to a related drug, 6-mercaptopurine, and then into 6-thioguanine metabolite nucleotides which inhibit cell growth.

Transplant recipients are at increased risk of developing acneiform eruptions from azathioprine [78]. One case of azathioprine-induced acneiform drug eruption during treatment of multiple sclerosis has been reported [79].

54.2.7 Other Medications

54.2.7.1 Gold

Gold has been reported to be associated with acne. In one case report, a patient with rheumatoid arthritis first developed an eruption consistent with lichen planus and subsequently developed acneiform lesions on the face and trunk after gold sodium thiomalate treatment [80]. Gold is retained in the body for a prolonged duration and is especially bound in the kidneys, liver, and skin [80].

54.2.7.2 Dactinomycin

Dactinomycin, used in the treatment of solid tumors, has been associated with occasional development of an acneiform eruption. A case was reported of a prepubertal girl who received dactinomycin in combination with other chemotherapeutic agents (vincristine and cyclophosphamide), none of which have been implicated in the development of acne lesions [81]. A rise and fall of serum androstenedione, dehydroepiandrosterone, and testosterone levels over a period of time, defined by two courses of therapy inclusive of dactinomycin, was documented. Gradual improvement of the acneiform eruption was also noted as hormone levels diminished, which supported a relationship between drug exposure, the presence of the eruption, and the tested hormone levels [82].

54.2.7.3 Isoniazid

Isoniazid (INH) is a first-line medication in prevention and treatment of tuberculosis. INH-associated acneiform eruptions were reported to occur in 16 % of 2,600 patients receiving a combination of INH and aminosalicylic acid, with 11 % of these acne patients reported to be slow metabolic inactivators of INH [83]. In another report, seven patients developed acneiform eruptions associated with INH therapy, with five of these patients presenting with extensive eruptions and slow INH metabolic inactivation status [83]. A German study suggested acneiform skin lesions caused by INH are within the concept of acne vulgaris [84]. Factors which should be taken into account when considering a diagnosis of INH-associated acne are occurrence in persons older than those typically affected by acne vulgaris, absence of recent or remote history of acne vulgaris, and a sudden emergence of acneiform lesions with widespread involvement [83].

54.2.7.4 Rifampin

Rifampin (also named rifampicin) is a bactericidal antibiotic drug of the rifamycin group. Papular acneiform lesions of the face, neck, and shoulders developed in 8 of 24 males with genitourinary tuberculosis treated with rifampin [85]. Discontinuation of the medication led to resolution of the acneiform lesions within 3 weeks [85].

54.2.7.5 Dapsone

Dapsone inhibits bacterial synthesis of dihydrofolic acid via competition with para-aminobenzoate for the active site of dihydropteroate synthetase [86]. A young female with preexisting mild facial acne vulgaris was treated with oral dapsone following poor response to oral tetracyclines [87]. She soon developed acne fulminans and hemolysis which resolved with prompt administration of high doses of vitamin C, oral prednisone, and intravenous methylene blue [87].

54.2.7.6 Halogens

Acneiform eruptions may originate from skin exposure to various industrial chemicals, such as fumes generated in the manufacture of chlorine and its byproducts. These chlorinated hydrocarbons may cause chloracne, consisting of cysts, pustules, folliculitis, and comedones. The most potent acneiform-inducing agents are the polyhalogenated hydrocarbons, notably dioxin (2,3,7,8 tetrachlorodibenzodioxin) [88]. Notoriously difficult to treat, chloracne can persist for extended time periods without known additional exposure to chloracnegens [89]. The most acne-prone locations to “chloracnegens” are the malar crescent (inferior and lateral to the eye) and the postauricular region. The genitalia, both penis and scrotum, are also vulnerable anatomic regions. If sufficient exposure has occurred, lesions may involve the shoulders, chest, back, and, eventually, the buttocks and abdomen. The axillary regions have been commonly involved only in those patients who have ingested or inhaled the chloracnegens as the sole or major route of exposure. Cutting and lubricating oils, crude coal tar applied to the skin for medicinal purposes, heavy tar distillates, coal tar pitch, and asbestos are known to cause acneiform eruptions. Acne venenata is another term applied to this process [90].

Inflammatory acneiform flares have been reported in association with ingestion of iodides and bromides [91]. Common sources of halogens include some thyroid medications, expectorants containing potassium iodide, radiographic contrast media, iodized salt, vitamin and mineral preparations, and some sedatives of historical interest only. Stimulation of neutrophil function has been suggested, although the pathogenesis of this reaction is unknown. Initial lesions are often follicular pustules, and later, comedonal lesions can emerge, possibly related to a hyperkeratotic reaction to chronic inflammation [92].

54.2.7.7 Vitamins B6 and B12

Megadoses of vitamins B6 and B12 have been reported to induce a facial acneiform eruption [93]. The histology shows parakeratosis overlying a focally spongiotic epidermis with a mononuclear, perivascular inflammatory infiltrate in the papillary dermis. There was dramatic improvement in the acneiform lesions upon discontinue of the nutritional supplement [93].

Exacerbation or onset of inflammatory acne lesions correlated with vitamins B2 (riboflavin), B6 (pyridoxine), and B12 (cyanocobalamin) intake has been reported in the European literature [93]. This manifests as an exacerbation of preexisting acne vulgaris with onset of multiple papules and papulopustules or as an explosive facial pustular eruption. The pathogenesis is unknown, although it has been postulated that the origin of B6/B12-induced acne may be similar to that of INH-induced acne [93, 94].

54.2.7.8 White Petrolatum

Most uses for petroleum jelly exploit its lubricating, coating, and moisturizing potentials. White petrolatum-associated unilateral acne developed in a young woman attempting to relieve the effects of unilateral facial paralysis (Bell's palsy) by massaging the substance onto her face nightly [95]. While generally thought to be noncomedogenic and safe to use in acne-prone skin, its occlusive properties could induce a pustular reaction in selected individuals [95].

54.2.7.9 Cow Udder Ointment

Application of cow udder ointment used for treatment of atopic eczema and psoriasis was associated with development of widespread and atypical acneiform eruptions in two patients [96]. Cow udder ointment contains boric acid and starch in a wax and oil base.

54.2.7.10 Tetraethylthiuram Disulfide

Tetraethylthiuram disulfide (disulfiram) is commonly used to treat chronic alcoholism by producing an acute sensitivity to alcohol ingestion by blocking acetaldehyde dehydrogenase conversion of acetaldehyde leading to a higher concentration of the aldehyde in the blood producing symptoms of a severe hangover. A repeated nodulocystic acneiform eruption involving the face, anterior chest, and back, associated with concurrent ingestion of tetraethylthiuram disulfide, has been reported [97]. With each recurrent episode of acneiform lesions, withdrawal of the drug repeatedly resulted in resolution of the eruption [97].

54.2.7.11 Dantrolene

Dantrolene is a muscle relaxant that acts by abolishing excitation-contraction coupling in muscle cells. Two middle-aged females undergoing treatment with dantrolene for spasticity were reported to have a predominantly comedonal acneiform eruption [98]. Histologic examination demonstrated keratin-filled cysts in communication with the surface of the epidermis. In addition to facial involvement, acneiform lesions also favored sites of friction and chronic trauma, a distribution specific to dantrolene acneiform eruptions [98, 99].

54.2.7.12 Psoralen Plus UVA (PUVA)

Oral and topical methoxsalen (8-methoxypsoralen) used along with subsequent long-wave ultraviolet A (UVA) light exposure (PUVA) is commonly used to treat psoriasis. Several cases of acne believed to be induced by PUVA treatment have been reported [100–102]. The distributions reported include the chest and back, periorally, and localized on the forehead. Acne-like eruptions on the face, induced by light, were first described using the term "light-sensitive seborrheid" [101, 102]. The designation acne aestivalis (Mallorca acne) is used for papular eruption occurring after intense sun exposure in an anatomic distribution characteristic of acne vulgaris [101, 102]. Overall, acne vulgaris usually improves during the summer months with exposure to sunshine, although it may be aggravated in some patients. This exacerbation is thought to be secondary to eccrine sweating.

54.3 Conclusion

Acne vulgaris and acneiform drug eruptions can easily be overlooked in daily clinical practice. There are no specific diagnostic criteria to define drug-induced acne. However, several key clinical characteristics (Table 54.2) may help clinicians to

Table 54.2 Acne versus acneiform drug eruption

	Acne	Acneiform drug eruption
Age of onset	Adolescent or early adulthood years	Unusual age of onset (>30 years)
Lesion morphology	Polymorphic lesions (mixture of comedones, papules, pustules, and inflamed subcutaneous nodules)	Monomorphic lesions, lacking comedones and cysts
Lesion distribution	Face, upper chest, and upper back where there are high density of sebaceous glands	Unusual location that extends beyond seborrheic area such as arms, lower back, and genitalia
Temporal relationship	No temporal relationship with medication	Lesions started shortly after new drug introduction Improvement after drug withdrawal Recurrence after drug introduction

recognize and diagnose acneiform drug eruptions. Two useful clinical keys to help diagnose acneiform drug eruptions are the temporal relationship (acne-like eruption after introduction of a new medication) and the monomorphic lesions (all lesions are in the same stage and lacking comedones).

References

1. Brunner MJ, Riddell Jr JM, Best WR. Cutaneous side effects of ACTH cortisone and pregnenolone therapy. J invest Dermatol. 1951;16:205–10.
2. Clementson B, Smidt AC. Periorificial dermatitis due to systemic corticosteroids in children: report of two cases. Pediatric Dermatol. 2012;29:331–2.
3. Fung MA, Berger TG. A prospective study of acute-onset steroid acne associated with administration of intravenous corticosteroids. Dermatology. 2000;200:43–4.
4. Plewig G, Kligman AM. Induction of acne by topical steroids. Arch Dermatol Forsch. 1973;247:29–52.
5. Hengge UR, Ruzicka T, Schwartz RA, Cork MJ. Adverse effects of topical glucocorticosteroids. J Am Acad Dermatol. 2006;54:1–15. quiz 6–8.
6. Monk B, Cunliffe WJ, Layton AM, Rhodes DJ. Acne induced by inhaled corticosteroids. Clin Exp Dermatol. 1993;18:148–50.
7. Hughes JR, Higgins EM, du Vivier AW. Acne associated with inhaled glucocorticosteroids. BMJ. 1992;305:1000.
8. Guillot B. Adverse skin reactions to inhaled corticosteroids. Exp Opin Drug Saf. 2002; 1:325–9.
9. Cohen HJ. Perioral dermatitis. J Am Acad Dermatol. 1981;4:739–40.
10. Wells K, Brodell RT. Topical corticosteroid "addiction". A cause of perioral dermatitis. Postgrad Med. 1993;93:225–30.
11. Hurwitz RM. Steroid acne. J Am Acad Dermatol. 1989;21:1179–81.
12. Bedane C, Souyri N. Induced acne. Ann Dermatol Venereol. 1990;117:53–8.
13. Gloor M, Funder H, Franke M. Effect of topical application of dexamethasone on Propionibacteria in the pilosebaceous duct. Eur J Clin Pharmacol. 1978;14:53–6.
14. Gloor M, Mildenberger KH. On the influence of an external therapy with dexamethasone-21-sodium-m-sulfobenzoate on the amount of free fatty acids in the skin surface lipids. Arch Dermatol Res. 1978;261:33–8.
15. Shibata M, Katsuyama M, Onodera T, Ehama R, Hosoi J, Tagami H. Glucocorticoids enhance Toll-like receptor 2 expression in human keratinocytes stimulated with Propionibacterium acnes or proinflammatory cytokines. J Invest Dermatol. 2009;129:375–82.
16. Scott III MJ, Scott AM. Effects of anabolic-androgenic steroids on the pilosebaceous unit. Cutis. 1992;50:113–6.
17. Scott Jr MJ, Scott 3rd MJ. Dermatologists and anabolic-androgenic drug abuse. Cutis. 1989; 44:30–5.
18. Fyrand O, Fiskaadal HJ, Trygstad O. Acne in pubertal boys undergoing treatment with androgens. Acta Derm Venereol. 1992;72:148–9.
19. Heydenreich G. Testosterone and anabolic steroids and acne fulminans. Arch Dermatol. 1989;125:571–2.
20. Melnik B, Jansen T, Grabbe S. Abuse of anabolic-androgenic steroids and bodybuilding acne: an underestimated health problem. J Dtsch Dermatol Ges. 2007;5:110–7.
21. Gerber PA, Kukova G, Meller S, Neumann NJ, Homey B. The dire consequences of doping. Lancet. 2008;372:656.
22. Greenberg RD. Acne vulgaris associated with antigonadotropic (Danazol) therapy. Cutis. 1979;24:431–3.

23. Ilse JR, Greenberg HL, Bennett DD. Levonorgestrel-releasing intrauterine system and new-onset acne. Cutis. 2008;82:158.
24. Olsson SE, Odlind V, Johansson E. Androgen levels in women using Norplant implants. Contraception. 1986;34:157–67.
25. Grupper C. New iatrogenic acne: acne caused by amineptin (Survector). Ann Dermatol Venereol. 1988;115:1174–6.
26. Thioly-Bensoussan D, Charpentier A, Triller R, et al. Iatrogenic acne caused by amineptin (Survector). Apropos of 8 cases. Ann Dermatol Venereol. 1988;115:1177–80.
27. Vexiau P, Gourmel B, Husson C, et al. Severe lesions of acne type induced by chronic amineptin poisoning: apropos of 6 cases. Ann Dermatol Venereol. 1988;115:1180–2.
28. Ponte CD. Maprotiline-induced acne. Am J Psychiatry. 1982;139:141.
29. Kusumi Y. A cutaneous side effect of lithium: report of two cases. Dis Nerv Syst. 1971;32:853–4.
30. Ruiz-Maldonado R, Perez de Francisco C, Tamayo L. Lithium dermatitis. JAMA. 1973;224: 1534.
31. Yoder FW. Letter: acneiform eruption due to lithium carbonate. Arch Dermatol. 1975;111: 396–7.
32. Rifkin A, Kurtin SB, Quitkin F, Klein DF. Lithium-induced folliculitis. Am J Psychiatry. 1973;130:1018–9.
33. Heng MC. Lithium carbonate toxicity. Acneiform eruption and other manifestation. Arch Dermatol. 1982;118:246–8.
34. Heng MC. Cutaneous manifestations of lithium toxicity. Br J Dermatol. 1982;106:107–9.
35. Hesse S, Berbis P, Lafforgue P, Acquaviva PC, Pastor MJ, Privat Y. Acne and enthesiopathy during anti-epileptic treatment. Ann Dermatol Venereol. 1992;119:655–8.
36. Jenkins RB, Ratner AC. Diphenylhydantoin and acne. New Engl J Med. 1972;287:148.
37. Nielsen JN, Licht RW, Fogh K. Two cases of acneiform eruption associated with lamotrigine. J Clin Psychiatry. 2004;65:1720–2.
38. Joffe H, Cohen LS, Suppes T, et al. Valproate is associated with new-onset oligoamenorrhea with hyperandrogenism in women with bipolar disorder. Biol Psychiatry. 2006;59:1078–86.
39. Stankler L, Campbell AG. Neonatal acne vulgaris: a possible feature of the fetal hydantoin syndrome. Br J Dermatol. 1980;103:453–5.
40. Norris JF, Cunliffe WJ. Phenytoin-induced gum hypertrophy improved by isotretinoin. Int J Dermatol. 1987;26:602–3.
41. Mishra B, Praharaj SK, Prakash R, Sinha VK. Aripiprazole-induced acneiform eruption. Gen Hosp Psychiatry. 2008;30:479–81.
42. Warthan MM, Jumper CA, Smith JL. Acneiform eruption induced by Iressa (gefitinib) tablets used to treat non-small cell lung cancer. J Drugs Dermatol. 2004;3:569–70.
43. Schalock PC, Zug KA. Acneiform reaction to erlotinib. Dermatitis. 2007;18:230–1.
44. Kardaun SH, van Duinen KF. Erlotinib-induced florid acneiform rash complicated by extensive impetiginization. Clin Exp Dermatol. 2008;33:46–9.
45. Martin JM, Jorda E, Monteagudo C, Alonso V, Garcia L, Villalon G. Follicular acneiform eruption induced by imatinib. J Eur Acad Dermatol Venereol. 2006;20:1368–70.
46. Lee JE, Lee SJ, Lee HJ, Lee JH, Lee KH. Severe acneiform eruption induced by cetuximab (Erbitux). Yonsei Med J. 2008;49:851–2.
47. Molinari E, De Quatrebarbes J, Andre T, Aractingi S. Cetuximab-induced acne. Dermatology. 2005;211:330–3.
48. Rowinsky EK, Schwartz GH, Gollob JA, et al. Safety, pharmacokinetics, and activity of ABX-EGF, a fully human anti-epidermal growth factor receptor monoclonal antibody in patients with metastatic renal cell cancer. J Clin Oncol. 2004;22:3003–15.
49. Sun G, Wasko CA, Hsu S. Acneiform eruption following anti-TNF-alpha treatment: a report of three cases. J Drugs Dermatol. 2008;7:69–71.
50. Jacot W, Bessis D, Jorda E, et al. Acneiform eruption induced by epidermal growth factor receptor inhibitors in patients with solid tumours. Br J Dermatol. 2004;151:238–41.

51. DeWitt CA, Siroy AE, Stone SP. Acneiform eruptions associated with epidermal growth factor receptor-targeted chemotherapy. J Am Acad Dermatol. 2007;56:500–5.
52. Eames T, Landthaler M, Karrer S. Severe acneiform skin reaction during therapy with erlotinib (Tarceva), an epidermal growth factor receptor (EGFR) inhibitor. Eur J Dermatol. 2007;17:552–3.
53. Journagan S, Obadiah J. An acneiform eruption due to erlotinib: prognostic implications and management. J Am Acad Dermatol. 2006;54:358–60.
54. Perez-Soler R, Saltz L. Cutaneous adverse effects with HER1/EGFR-targeted agents: is there a silver lining? J Clin Oncol. 2005;23:5235–46.
55. Segaert S, Van Cutsem E. Clinical signs, pathophysiology and management of skin toxicity during therapy with epidermal growth factor receptor inhibitors. Ann Oncol. 2005;16: 1425–33.
56. Sladden MJ, Clarke PJ, Mitchell B. Infliximab-induced acne: report of a third case. Br J Dermatol. 2008;158:172.
57. Michot C, Guillot B, Dereure O. Lenalidomide-induced acute acneiform folliculitis of the head and neck: not only the anti-EGF receptor agents. Dermatology. 2010;220:49–50.
58. Lee PK, Dover JS. Recurrent exacerbation of acne by granulocyte colony-stimulating factor administration. J Am Acad Dermatol. 1996;34:855–6.
59. Petukhova TA, Novoa RA, Honda K, Koon HB, Gerstenblith MR. Acneiform eruptions associated with vemurafenib. J Am Acad Dermatol. 2013;68:e97–9.
60. Lowe L, Herbert AA. Cystic and comedonal acne: a side effect of etretinate therapy. Int J Dermatol. 1989;28:482.
61. Menter A, Boyd A. Cystic acne in psoriatic patients undergoing etretinate therapy. J Am Acad Dermatol. 1988;18:751–2.
62. Bajwa ZH, Sami N, Flory C. Severe acne as a side effect of propranolol and nadolol in a migraineur. Headache. 1999;39:758–60.
63. Burkhart CG. Quinidine-induced acne. Arch Dermatol. 1981;117:603–4.
64. Fidan K, Kandur Y, Sozen H, Gonul II, Dalgic A, Soylemezoglu O. How often do we face side effects of sirolimus in pediatric renal transplantation? Transplant Proc. 2013;45:185–9.
65. Kunzle N, Venetz JP, Pascual M, Panizzon RG, Laffitte E. Sirolimus-induced acneiform eruption. Dermatology. 2005;211:366–9.
66. Lubbe J, Sorg O, Male PJ, Saurat JH, Masouye I. Sirolimus-induced inflammatory papules with acquired reactive perforating collagenosis. Dermatology. 2008;216:239–42.
67. Momin SB, Peterson A, Del Rosso JQ. A status report on drug-associated acne and acneiform eruptions. J Drugs Dermatol. 2010;9:627–36.
68. Mahe E, Morelon E, Lechaton S, et al. Acne in recipients of renal transplantation treated with sirolimus: clinical, microbiologic, histologic, therapeutic, and pathogenic aspects. J Am Acad Dermatol. 2006;55:139–42.
69. Mahe E, Morelon E, Lechaton S, et al. Cutaneous adverse events in renal transplant recipients receiving sirolimus-based therapy. Transplantation. 2005;79:476–82.
70. Bakos L, Bakos RM. Focal acne during topical tacrolimus therapy for vitiligo. Arch Dermatol. 2007;143:1223–4.
71. Antille C, Saurat JH, Lubbe J. Induction of rosaceiform dermatitis during treatment of facial inflammatory dermatoses with tacrolimus ointment. Arch Dermatol. 2004;140:457–60.
72. El Sayed F, Ammoury A, Dhaybi R, Bazex J. Rosaceiform eruption to pimecrolimus. J Am Acad Dermatol. 2006;54:548–50.
73. el-Shahawy MA, Gadallah MF, Massry SG. Acne: a potential side effect of cyclosporine A therapy. Nephron. 1996;72:679–82.
74. Azurdia RM, Graham RM, Weismann K, Guerin DM, Parslew R. Acne keloidalis in caucasian patients on cyclosporin following organ transplantation. Br J Dermatol. 2000;143: 465–7.
75. Bencini PL, Crosti C, Sala F, et al. Gingival hyperplasia by nifedipine. Report of a case. Acta Derm Venereol. 1985;65:362–5.

76. Formicone F, Fargnoli MC, Pisani F, Rascente M, Famulari A, Peris K. Cutaneous manifestations in Italian kidney transplant recipients. Transplant Proc. 2005;37:2527–8.
77. Schmoeckel C, von Liebe V. Acneiform exanthema caused by azathioprine. Hautarzt. 1983; 34:413–5.
78. Hjortshoj A. Lichen planus and acne provoked by gold. Acta Derm Venereol. 1977;57: 165–7.
79. Blatt J, Lee PA. Severe acne and hyperandrogenemia following dactinomycin. Med Pediatr Oncol. 1993;21:373–4.
80. Bereston ES. Reactions to antituberculous drugs. J Invest Dermatol. 1959;33:427–39.
81. Cohen LK, George W, Smith R. Isoniazid-induced acne and pellagra. Occurrence in slow inactivators of isoniazid. Arch Dermatol. 1974;109:377–81.
82. Amann W. Can acneiform skin lesions caused by Inh-medication Be considered as being within the concept of acne vulgaris? Dermatol Wochenschr. 1964;150:647–51.
83. Holdiness M. Adverse cutaneous reactions to antituberculosis drugs. Int J Dermatol. 1985;24:280–5.
84. De D, Dogra S, Kaur I. Dapsone induced acute photosensitivity dermatitis; a case report and review of literature. Lepr Rev. 2007;78:401–4.
85. Ismail R. Acne fulminans with dapsone induced haemolysis: a case report. Med J Malaysia. 1987;42:124–6.
86. Pelclova D, Urban P, Preiss J, et al. Adverse health effects in humans exposed to 2,3,7,8-tetrachlorodibenzo-p-dioxin (TCDD). Rev Environ Health. 2006;21:119–38.
87. Tindall JP. Chloracne and chloracnegens. J Am Acad Dermatol. 1985;13:539–58.
88. Plewig G, Jansen T. Acneiform dermatoses. Dermatology. 1998;196:102–7.
89. Webster GF. Pustular drug reactions. Clin Dermatol. 1993;11:541–3.
90. Fisher AA. Drug eruptions in geriatric patients. Cutis. 1976;18:402–9.
91. Sherertz EF. Acneiform eruption due to "megadose" vitamins B6 and B12. Cutis. 1991;48: 119–20.
92. Braun-Falco O, Lincke H. The problem of vitamin B6/B12 acne. A contribution on acne medicamentosa (author's transl). MMW Munch Med Wochenschr. 1976;118:155–60.
93. Frankel EB. Acne secondary to white petrolatum use. Arch Dermatol. 1985;121:589–90.
94. O'Brien TJ. Acneiform eruption associated with the use of a cow udder ointment. Australas J Dermatol. 1990;31:119.
95. Barefoot S. Acneiform eruption produced by use of tetraethylthiuramdisulfide. JAMA. 1951;147:1653.
96. Pembroke AC, Saxena SR, Kataria M, Zilkha KD. Acne induced by dantrolene. Br J Dermatol. 1981;104:465–8.
97. Joynt RL. Dantrolene sodium: long-term effects in patients with muscle spasticity. Arch Phys Med Rehabil. 1976;57:212–7.
98. Jones C, Bleehen SS. Acne induced by PUVA treatment. Br Med J. 1977;2:866.
99. Nielsen EB, Thormann J. Acne-like eruptions induced by PUVA-treatment. Acta Derm Venereol. 1978;58:374–5.
100. Humbert P. Induced acne. Rev Prat. 2002;52:838–40.
101. Frumess GM, Lewis HM. Light-sensitive seborrheid. AMA Arch Derm. 1957;75:245–8.
102. Hjorth N, Sjolin KE, Sylvest B, Thomsen K. Acne aestivalis–Mallorca acne. Acta Derm Venereol. 1972;52:61–3.

Index

J.A. Zeichner (ed.), *Acneiform Eruptions in Dermatology: A Differential Diagnosis*,
DOI 10.1007/978-1-4614-8344-1, © Springer Science+Business Media New York 2014

T

MIX
Papier aus verantwortungsvollen Quellen
Paper from responsible sources
FSC® C105338

If you have any concerns about our products,
you can contact us on
ProductSafety@springernature.com

In case Publisher is established outside the EU,
the EU authorized representative is:
Springer Nature Customer Service Center GmbH
Europaplatz 3, 69115 Heidelberg, Germany

Printed by Libri Plureos GmbH
in Hamburg, Germany